Extraordinary
HEALING

Extraordinary
HEALING

The Amazing Power of
Your Body's Secret Healing System

Arthur H. Brownstein,
M.D., M.P.H.

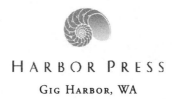

HARBOR PRESS
GIG HARBOR, WA

Library of Congress Cataloging-in-Publication Data

Brownstein, Arthur H., 1950–
   Extraordinary healing: the amazing power of your body's secret healing
   system / Arthur H. Brownstein
      p. cm.
   Includes bibliographical references.
   ISBN 0-936197-49-8 (alk. paper)
Healing. 2. Health. 3. Mind and body. I. Title.

RZ401.B825 2 005
615.5—dc22

2 004040615

EXTRAORDINARY HEALING
The Amazing Power of Your Body's Secret Healing System

Printed in the United States of America.

10 9 8 7 6 5 4 3

Harbor Press, Inc.
P.O. Box 1656
Gig Harbor, WA 98335

HARBOR PRESS and the nautilus shell design are registered trademarks of
Harbor Press, Inc.

This book is dedicated to Norman Cousins (1915–1990) and to his surviving family members. A rare and most unusual human being, Cousins was an international emissary of peace; a political advisor to statesmen, politicians, popes, and presidents; a prolific, best-selling author; a musician; a humorist; and an extraordinary healer. Considered "healer of the medical profession" and "founding father of mind-body medicine," he was also a pioneering researcher and outspoken proponent of psychoneuroimmunology, a new branch of medical science that studies the interactions among the mind, the nervous system, and the immune system to help us better understand how our beliefs, thoughts, feelings, and attitudes can affect our physical health.

Even though he was in the middle of intense fundraising and research in psychoneuroimmunology when we met in his office at the UCLA School of Medicine, Norman Cousins took time out of his busy schedule to tell me about the healing system. He spoke at length about why he considered it the most important system in the body, and how research needed to be conducted in this vital area of human health. Although, over the past 15 years, I have since heard and read about the healing system many times, and have gone on to conduct my own clinical studies and observations about it, Norman Cousins was the first one to make me aware of it and its profound importance to humanity's ongoing battle against disease. I credit him for making me a better doctor, and for the inspiration to write this book.

CONTENTS

FOREWORD

Modern medicine rarely succeeds in teaching doctors how to get their patients to actively participate in their own healing. This is one of the major problems with medicine today and with doctors trained to focus on external solutions to their patients' health problems. The modern-day approach of quick-fix solutions and an emphasis on "wonder" drugs often disregards the remarkable potential we all have to awaken our own extraordinary healing powers when we're sick, and to use these healing powers to prevent disease from ever occurring. But in order to use these healing powers that we all have, we must tap into a system of the body that has been virtually ignored until now—the healing system. True and lasting healing can only occur when you work with this strong and seemingly mysterious power within you.

Through the years, I have seen patients with diseases and conditions of all kinds work with their healing systems in a variety of ways to combat sickness and restore their bodies and minds to a healthy state. I have even seen unconscious patients in intensive care units of hospitals heal themselves with a strong will to live that stimulates the healing system to go into high gear. Pay attention to the stories Dr. Brownstein shares in this book. They are all dramatic examples of the incredible power we all have to heal ourselves and the critical importance of looking within for permanent solutions to health problems.

If you are sick or weak, or even if you're just not feeling as good as you'd like to feel, your healing system may be slumbering, but it is just waiting to be called into action—and it is as necessary to your good health as your respiratory system and your digestive system. Try waking it up with the strategies and techniques you'll find in this book, and you'll experience the full range of your potential to achieve maximum health. Begin with a simple first step: "Program" yourself to think and feel in a positive way about yourself and others, and, before long, you'll see extraordinary changes in the way you feel physically. Use the power of your mind to affect your body, and your healing system will respond in a myriad of ways to your thoughts and attitudes, and it will begin healing and strengthening all of the other systems in your body. Just as patients who are in extreme circumstances, such as in intensive care units of hospitals, can rally and recover, so can you if you learn to acknowledge and work with your own healing powers.

You are about to begin quite an unusual and remarkable book, one that deserves to be read carefully and then kept close at hand for future reference in times of need. Let Dr. Brownstein show you how to strengthen and fortify the extraordinary healing system within you, and you'll see remarkable changes in the health of your mind, body, and spirit.

Claes Frostell, M.D.
Karolinska University Hospital Huddinge
Stockholm, Sweden

ACKNOWLEDGMENTS

Many people are due my thanks for the publication of this book. Many more simply could not be listed here. To them I offer my sincere apologies.

I would like to acknowledge the following people for their contribution to this work:

Norman Cousins was the original inspiration that led to the writing of this book.

Gary David Saldana, M.D., of Kauai, Hawaii, regularly encouraged me for five years and additionally contributed by seeing my patients each week so I would have the time to write.

Dr. Dean Ornish, the first person in the world to prove that heart disease could be reversed, provided a strong, scientific foundation for the ideas presented here. During the 10 years that I was fortunate enough to work with him, I was able to witness, firsthand, the miraculous workings of the healing system in patients with severe, advanced heart disease. I shall be forever grateful to Dr. Ornish for his wisdom and generosity.

Dr. Lee Lipsenthal, medical director of the Ornish Program and originator of the Physician Heal Thyself program, has been a continuous source of encouragement for this project.

Other staff and participants of the Ornish Program I would like to personally thank include Melanie Elliot, R.N.; Ruth Marlin, M.D.; Rob Saper, M.D.; Jim Billings, Ph.D.; Dr. Conrad Knudsen; Dennis Malone; Glenn Perelson; Werner and Eva Hebenstreit; Hank and Phyllis Ginsberg; and the entire Ornish staff.

Erminia M. Guarneri, M.D., cardiologist and current head of the Scripps Clinic Center for Integrative Medicine; Bruno Cortis, M.D., cardiologist; and Andy Meyer, M.D., cardiologist, provided lessons in cardiology and how important the heart is to the healing system.

Bernie Siegel, M.D., has been a mentor and friend. His work with Exceptional Cancer Patients therapy, described in his best-selling classic book, *Love, Medicine and Miracles*, and his many other books have been a source of great inspiration in the writing of this book.

Andrew Weil, M.D., colleague and friend, is one of the world's most authoritative experts in the practical and responsible use of complementary and alternative medicines, and one of the first doctors to write about the healing system. I thank him for his courage and wisdom in helping me advance the scientific and practical ideas presented.

Larry Dossey, M.D., colleague and medical expert on spirituality and prayer, has contributed greatly to the ideas included here.

Edgar Mitchell, Ph.D., was an Apollo 14 astronaut who made history by walking on the moon. He went on to found the Institute of Noetic Sciences, which helps fund scientific research on the cutting edge of healing and consciousness. He has been a major source of inspiration over the years in my investigation into the workings of the healing system.

David Simon, M.D., a colleague and conventionally trained neurologist who has studied and written about Ayurveda and yoga, has contributed greatly to this work through his insights and deep understanding of the healing system.

Joan Borysenko, Ph.D., best-selling author and scientist, has been a mentor and source of great inspiration in my personal and professional life. Over the years she has provided me with many case histories and other important clinical evidence shared in these pages.

Herbert Benson, M.D., is a Harvard cardiologist, an expert in the treatment of stress-related illnesses, and the first person in the world to prove that meditation can lower blood pressure. His work has been invaluable to my ongoing investigations into the field of relaxation and how it can benefit our healing systems.

James Banta, M.D., M.P.H., was the medical director of the Peace Corps during the Kennedy administration, former dean of the School of Public Health and Tropical Medicine at Tulane University in New Orleans, and currently is professor of epidemiology at George Washington University School of Medicine, and professor emeritus at many medical schools around the world. I thank him for sending me to India, where I had the opportunity to study yoga and traditional Indian medicine. Because of him, I was able to observe ancient, natural, effective methods for treating diseases that worked with the healing system.

Larry Payne, Ph.D., founder of the International Association of Yoga Therapists, internationally acclaimed yoga teacher and best-selling author, has been a huge support in my work with the body's healing system and in the writing of this book.

Steve Schwartz, M.D., colleague and classmate in medical school, and his wife, Alma Schwartz, M.D., both long-time advocates of the body's natural ability to heal itself, have made a significant contribution to my career and the birth of this project.

Roberto Masferrer, M.D., military medicine colleague, and world-class neurosurgeon, Dr. Tom Higginbotham, D.O., an osteopathic physician with incredibly gifted healing hands, and Dr. Bud Hockley, dermatologist, have been sources of great support and inspiration in my career and as I put together this material.

David Elpern, M.D., has been a wise colleague and major support for my career over the years. He was kind enough to contribute case histories from his patient archives that I have included within.

Bernard Towers, M.D. (deceased), was my advisor in the department of psychoneuroimmunology for the research I was proposing to do with Norman Cousins at UCLA. He, along with the entire team of researchers in the Norman Cousins Program in psychoneuroimmunology at UCLA, which included George Solomon, M.D., Fawzy Fawzy, M.D., Carmen Clemente, M.D., Herbert Weiner, M.D., and others, contributed to the book's ideas. I thank them all for their pioneering work and early conceptualization of these ideas.

Tuck Craven, M.D.; Betty Craven, M.D.; Professor Len Eisenman, Ph.D., from Jefferson Medical College in Philadelphia; and Dr. Frank Marstellar were all instrumental in my medical education and contributed to many of the ideas expressed here.

Marty Rossman, M.D., and David Bressler, Ph.D., founders of the Academy for Guided Imagery, were my instructors in the two-year clinical training program I completed in guided imagery and healing, and they taught me what a powerful tool imagery can be in the activation of the healing system.

S. Kuvalayananda, pioneering researcher in yoga and founder of the Kaivalyadhama Yoga Institute in India, where I have studied during the past 20 years, and his wise and devoted students, Swami Digambarji; Sri O. P. Tiwari; V. Pratap, Ph. D.; and Dr. Sri Krishna, M. B.B.S., Ph.D., all served as my teachers and caretakers in India and taught me about the invaluable therapeutic benefits of yoga and how it can strengthen and fortify the healing system.

Claes Frostell, M.D., Ph.D., chairman of the department of anesthesiology at the Karolinska Institute in Stockholm, Sweden; Rosario Porrovecchio, M.D., of Italy; and Pedro de Vicente, M.D., of Spain, have all encouraged and inspired me in my work of integrating body, mind, and spirit in support of the healing system.

Virender Sodhi, a brilliant yet down-to-earth Ayurvedic physician and naturopathic doctor, has continued to inspire, encourage, and support my career and the writing of this book.

Rob Ivker, D.O., author of numerous books and past president of the American Holistic Medical Association, as well as Len Wisneski, M.D., a holistic endocrinologist and healer, have supported and encouraged me in this project.

Hawaii-based physicians Ira Zunin, M.D., M.P.H., M.B.A, president of the Hawaii State Consortium of Integrative Medicine; and Terry Shintani, M.D., M.P.H., J.D., founder of the Hawaiian Diet Program, have both, through their work, contributed significantly to the ideas presented in this book.

Tim Crane, M.D.; Donald Traller, P.A.; Robert Teichman, M.D.; Ph.D.; Nicholas Zina, M.D.; Jeff Goodman, M.D.; Ron Burkhart, M.D.; Stephen DeNigris, M.D.; Roger Netzer, M.D.; Bill Evslin, M.D.; Neal Sutherland, M.D.; all my colleagues at the Wilcox Hospital in Kauai; and my colleagues at the University of Hawaii supported and encouraged me in the completion of this project.

The staff, my colleagues and coworkers, and my many patients at the Princeville Medical Clinic; Kilauea North Shore Clinic; Kapaa Clinic; and Family Practice Walk-In Clinic at Wilcox Hospital in Lihue, Kauai, have, over the years, had an open mind to give me feedback on the many unconventional methods I have recommended here.

Debby Young is the best editor in the whole world. Over a four-year period, she was instrumental in helping me to organize, clarify, and strip down the huge volume of material I had gathered for this book into a cohesive, clear, readable manuscript. Because of her, the ideas flow smoothly and are easy to grasp. Since I have begun working with her, I have become a much better writer. She has also served as my spiritual cheerleader by encouraging me to keep going when I was overwhelmed with both clinical duties and writing. Thank you, Debby.

Bert Holtje and Gene Brissie are my agents and I thank them for representing me in this literary work.

Harry Lynn, president of Harbor Press, published my first book, *Healing Back Pain Naturally*. I thank him for believing in me enough to publish this work, as well. I also want to thank his staff and associates and the rest of the folks at Harbor Press for being so helpful and cooperative.

Nutan, my wife, and Shantanu, my son, allowed me to be away from them for so many hours, which added up considerably over four years, while I wrote. Being married to a physician is hard enough, but to a physician who is also a writer—this is a most cruel and unusual punishment!

My father, S.R. Brownstein, M.D., encouraged me to do my best in all my endeavors while he practiced medicine in a career that spanned 50 years, including a professorship at the UCLA School of Medicine and a private practice in Beverly Hills, California. My mother, Fernlee Brownstein, relentlessly encouraged me to follow in my father's footsteps as a physician over the course of my childhood and early education.

"Natural forces within us are the true healers of disease."

—HIPPOCRATES (460–400 B.C.)

"The inner intelligence of the body is the ultimate and supreme genius in nature."

—THE VEDAS

"The physician is only nature's assistant."

—GALEN (129–199 A.D.)

"The physician knows that his little black bag can carry him only so far and that the body's own healing system is the main resource."

"The physician's ability to reassure the patient is a major factor in activating the body's own healing system."

"The more serious the illness, the more important it is for you to fight back, mobilizing all your resources—spiritually, emotionally, intellectually, and physically."

"We are becoming a nation of sissies and hypochondriacs, a self-medicating society easily intimidated by pain and prone to panic. We understand almost nothing about the essential robustness of the human body or its ability to meet the challenge of illness."

—NORMAN COUSINS

"There is a wide body of evidence suggesting that extraordinary healing, including regression of normally fatal tumors, takes place, with no known scientific explanation."

"We believe if there is one pressing argument for a thoroughgoing, urgent, and even passionate investigation of remarkable recovery, it is this: to discover and utilize the properties of another unmapped metasystem of the body and mind—the healing system."

—Drs. Brendan O'Regan and Caryle Hirshberg

"Your body can heal itself. It can do so because it has a healing system. If you are in good health, you will want to know about this system, because it is what keeps you in good health and because you can enhance that condition. If you or people you love are sick, you will want to know about this system, because it is the best hope for recovery."

—Andrew Weil, M.D.

"Medical students are not really taught about the healing system. They are taught about disease—how to diagnose and how to treat, but they are not taught how the body goes about treating itself. They will point to the immune system and let it go at that. But healing involves not just killing off disease germs or viruses but the process of reconstruction and repair."

—Dr. Omar Fareed

"We are at a turning point in medical history, when, having recognized the outer limits of technological medicine, doctors and lay people are together discovering the vast powers for creating health that we each inherit at birth."

"Far from being a passive victim to disease, the human body rallies its healing forces and removes the offender or repairs damaged tissue with as much vigor as the world's best-trained medical team."

—Hal Zina Bennet

"The land of healing lies within, radiant with happiness that is blindly sought in a thousand outer directions."

—S.S. Yukteswar

"When you are sick of your sickness you will cease to be sick."

—Lao Tzu

"There is no such thing as an incurable disease, only incurable people."

—Bernie Siegel, M.D.

"There are no incurable diseases, only those for which man has not yet found the cure."

—Rachelle Breslow

"Whenever a new discovery is reported to the scientific world, they say first, 'It is probably not true.' Thereafter, when the truth of the new proposition has been demonstrated beyond question, they say, 'Yes, it may be true, but it is not important.' Finally, when sufficient time has elapsed to fully evidence its importance, they say, 'Yes, surely it is important, but it is no longer new.'"

—Michel de Montaigne (1533–1592)

INTRODUCTION

Your body is an incredible creation. No other machine is like it in the world. For the most part, it is designed to last for about 100 years, and it can repair and heal itself from a whole host of injuries, traumas, illnesses, and diseases. It can do this because, in addition to the other systems of the body, it has a *healing system*, a system so powerful and efficient, so subtle and dynamic, and yet so obvious that it has been largely taken for granted and overlooked by most of modern science. Even if this system were more actively searched for, our most modern diagnostic technologies are currently inadequate to accurately map out the full extent of its realm. As a result, despite its supreme importance, your healing system remains the least studied, the least understood, and the least well known of all of your body's systems.

Although the concept of a healing system may seem relatively new to Western medicine, in reality, the idea that such a system exists is very old. More than two thousand years ago, Hippocrates, considered "the father of Western medicine," declared that "natural forces within us are the true healers of disease." Even today, doctors in China, India, Japan, and other countries in the Far East and Middle East continue to teach their patients how to activate and cooperate with their bodies' natural ability to heal themselves in times of illness and injury. And within the lofty ranks of our own modern medicine, every surgeon who has ever wielded a scalpel has relied on the body's natural ability to heal itself following each and every operation performed.

Norman Cousins, the famous author, healer, and diplomat, first spoke to me about the healing system more than a decade ago. At this time, he was at UCLA, pioneering a new scientific program in psychoneuroimmunology, or PNI, for short, which focused on understanding how the mind and nervous system influence the functioning of the immune system. His research findings helped usher in an important new era in medicine. When we met, he implored me to investigate and write about the healing system, but it wasn't until I came across the following extraordinary case that I became aware of the significance of Cousins' supplications.

Peter was a patient of mine who had undergone a major operation 25 years earlier, during which a part of one of his lungs had to be removed. To access his lungs, the surgeon surgically removed a rib from his chest wall. As we spoke about the operation, Peter mentioned that even though the entire rib had been removed from his spine to his chest, it had somehow grown back. As a physician, I had never heard of ribs growing back, so I asked whether he had proof. He said he had a copy of his X-ray, which verified that what he said was true. If I hadn't seen the X-ray, I wouldn't have believed it possible. And although the rib was mottled in appearance and distinctly thinner than his other ribs, there it was. One solid rib bone had grown in and connected from his sternum in the very front of his chest to the vertebra in the back of his spinal column.

Although it took his body 25 years to regrow the rib, his X-ray was proof of a healing system that was never discussed in my medical school training and was more amazing than I had ever known. To form a new complete rib where only a blank space existed is akin to salamanders growing new tails or a person growing a new limb. I still have a copy of Peter's X-ray in my office to remind me of how truly amazing this healing system within our bodies really is. It also reminds me that if we would devote more time to its study, we could learn countless other wondrous miracles about this incredible natural healing system that each one of us possesses, including how to access it to achieve optimum health.

Your body's healing system works in ways that modern science hasn't even begun to look at or understand. In addition, it has the titanic responsibility of monitoring all the other systems in your body and making sure that everything in your body is functioning at its optimum. This is especially challenging when our modern way of life, which can be fast-paced and stressful, is inherently very hard on our bodies. For this reason, it is important to get to know your healing system, to learn how to cooperate with it, and to explore and discover ways to strengthen and fortify it in the process.

In this book, I share basic information about your healing system. I also provide simple yet effective, time-honored, scientifically valid, practical strategies, exercises, techniques, and methods to help you take advantage of your natural internal healing resources. These tools will enable you to prevent and overcome a vast array of illnesses while improving the overall quality of your health and life.

Part One describes your extraordinary healing system and how it works, as well as specific strategies and techniques for strengthening and fortifying this remarkable system.

Chapter 1 explains how your body's natural state is one of health, how illness and disease are exceptions rather than the rule, how your body operates on the same principles that work in nature, and how your healing system's primary function is to help you maintain your natural state of health.

Chapter 2 presents evidence that demonstrates the existence of your healing system, with case reports and examples that reveal how your body uses specific mechanisms of repair and restoration of health that are adapted to a wide variety of medical scenarios.

Chapter 3 briefly describes the other important systems in your body that function synergistically and cooperate with your healing system to help keep you healthy.

Chapter 4 presents simple yet powerful strategies and techniques that will teach you how to cooperate with and enhance your healing system, strengthening and fortifying it so it can most efficiently do its job of preventing and healing illness and disease, while creating better overall health.

Chapter 5 covers the important area of nutrition and its role in influencing the performance of your healing system.

Chapter 6 explores the important relationship between your mind and your body, how your thoughts, attitudes, beliefs, and emotions influence your physical health and the functioning of your healing system, and what practical steps you can take to maximize the benefits of this relationship.

Chapter 7 reinforces the power of a strong and vibrant healing system as it relates to the aging process. In this chapter you'll find numerous stories of people who have lived very long lives with optimum health because of their strong healing systems. These stories illustrate the critical point that growing older doesn't have to be synonymous with sickness and deterioration. This important chapter shows that the most effective path to a long life with good health is to keep your healing system fortified and strong.

Chapter 8 includes stories of extraordinary healing that I've either witnessed myself or have heard about. This is a small sampling of the thousands and thousands of people whose healing systems have enabled them to heal from a wide variety of health problems, from very serious illnesses, such as cancer, to less life-threatening conditions, such as eczema.

Part Two is the prescriptive section of the book. It begins with general strategies to enhance your healing system that take minutes a day, but that will have a powerful cumulative effect on your healing system. Then you'll find step-by-step strategies to help you overcome specific medical problems and heal from a wide variety of common ailments. I organized this section by the systems of the body to make it easier for you to use. Part Two ends with additional relaxation methods, breathing techniques, and guided-imagery techniques to strengthen your healing system.

The bottom line is that you have many more internal healing resources available to you than you are currently aware. If you knew what your healing system was capable of, and how you could bring out its best, you would be able to overcome almost any malady or affliction that life could throw your way. In so doing, you would discover that just as illness does not occur randomly or spontaneously, neither does health. Simple things that you can do to support your healing system can combine to make a huge difference in your health and quality of life.

We are not helpless victims of circumstance. We can do much to heal ourselves from illness, and to live vibrant, healthy, happy lives.

PART ONE

Your Extraordinary
Healing System

CHAPTER 1

Your Healing System
and Your Natural State of Health

Throughout the universe and all of nature, there exists an abundantly flowing, vibrant energy that creates and sustains all of life. On earth, this energy permeates all living forms and is the underlying sustaining principle that allows species to be born, to grow, to multiply, to flourish, and to continue their life cycles for thousands and even millions of years. This energy, or *life force,* as it is often referred to, expresses itself as vitality or "aliveness." Although there may be exceptions, this is the overwhelmingly dominant theme that governs the life of each living creature and species, including human beings. In human beings, this vitality or aliveness expresses itself as a natural state of health.

Health is your body's fundamental, natural state. Health is programmed into the DNA of every one of your cells, as it is programmed into the DNA of the cells of every human being. In fact, if you were to conduct a simple experiment by leaving your body to its own devices, supplying it with just a few basic necessities, you would discover that, for the most part, it can remain healthy all on its own, with very little interference or intervention.

Your body's natural state of health explains why the average current life span for human beings is well over 75 years, with many people living to the age of 100 or more. Without this intrinsic state of health, humans could not possibly live this long and continue to exist generation after generation. If good health were not our species' natural, fundamental condition, we would have long since perished from the face of the earth.

Your natural state of health serves as a fundamental principle around which your body organizes, balances, and keeps itself vital and strong over the years. Because of this internal organizing principle, your body knows how to adjust and adapt to external forces and changes in the environment while keeping its order and balance. It can right and repair itself from life's myriad challenges, threats, and disturbances. Your body possesses an uncanny resiliency to spring back to health even after it has been subjected to tremendous forces of deprivation, starvation, and torture, life-threatening illnesses, and high-impact accidents.

Your body also displays an inner intelligence or wisdom that supports your natural state of health as you move through the various stages of life. Consider, for example, that your body knows how to grow a complete set of new teeth after you lose your baby teeth. How does the body know how to increase its size as it grows, to create facial hair in men as they go through puberty, and to enlarge the breasts in women? How does it know how to grow a new toenail in the place of the one that has been lost because of a stubbed toe, and to create new skin where the old layer has been lost during an abrasion? How does your body know how to knit together a fractured bone so that it is stronger than before, and to grow new blood vessels in the heart if there is a blockage in the old ones?

How does your body maintain its natural state of health, even when injuries occur and various diseases regularly assault it? How can it mend and heal itself, and return to a state of normal functioning, following infections from viruses, bacteria, fungi, and parasites, or major traumatic injuries and life-threatening illnesses? Think about childhood alone, and all the injuries children sustain, and the tears they shed throughout the early stages of growing up, as they learn to crawl, stand, walk, climb up and down stairs, run, ride a bicycle, and swim. Add to this the multitude of rashes, fevers, and infections they must endure, and it is difficult to imagine that any child could ever make it into adulthood in one piece. And yet, most of us did.

How does your body move forward through the rough and tumble, turbulent times of life and always spring back, continuing, for the most part, past the age of 50, to 75, and even 100 years or more? It accomplishes all this because of its incredible healing system, and the crucial ways in which that system works with your body's other tissues, organs, and systems.

Health Is Natural and Normal; Disease Is Unnatural and Abnormal

Because health is your natural, normal state, illness represents an unnatural, abnormal state. What do I mean by this?

The word *health* is related to the word *healing*, which is a movement toward wholeness and a sense of well-being. When you are healthy, you feel whole and well, and you have a comfortable, vibrant, free-flowing, easy feeling in your body. Your body feels light; your everyday movements and activities feel effortless. This is your natural state of health, a condition associated with a feeling of ease in the body and in the mind.

When you become ill, you lose your health. You lose your feeling of ease, and you become afflicted with "dis-ease." Understood in these terms, *disease* represents nothing more than a temporary departure from your natural state of health.

Disease represents a movement away from your central, orderly, naturally balanced state, into a more chaotic state. This condition is accompanied by a feeling of discomfort or even pain. Each movement in your body becomes difficult and full of effort. You expend great energy performing simple tasks. Your breathing is usually labored. Your heart rate is increased. Your appetite is decreased. Your body feels weak and vulnerable. This is an unnatural and abnormal state for your body.

When you have lost your health, instead of a natural feeling of lightness or ease, your body feels sluggish and heavy. You feel ill at ease because you are out of balance, and your body has become disoriented. It has become a huge distraction for your mind. To think about anything uplifting or creative is difficult, because your mental energies are completely consumed by your disease and discomfort. Your body has become a painful, heavy burden that keeps you from enjoying your life. Disease is not your body's natural, normal state. On the contrary, it is entirely abnormal and unnatural.

In the science of biology, the word *homeostasis* describes your body as a flexible, fluid form, with an ever-changing internal environment that is naturally resilient, always striving for order and balance. This order and balance that maintain your natural state of health are achieved through homeostasis as your body processes and adjusts to external forces and stimuli to maintain its natural state of health.

When external forces become harmful or toxic, and these forces are large or persistent enough to create significant imbalance in your body, order turns to chaos, with dis-ease, or illness resulting. According to the biological principle of homeostasis, or balance, illness and disease are only temporary states. Any illness or disease, then, when dissected to its essential nature, reflects only this: a breakdown in the orderliness of your body, a state of temporary imbalance and disorder.

Illness and disease not only create temporary, unnatural imbalance in your body; they also are the result of temporary, unnatural imbalances that have been created in the world. For example, in many developing countries, where the scales of material abundance have been tipped toward poverty, scarcity, and a lack of basic human necessities such as food, water, shelter, clothing, sanitation, and education, "diseases of lack" predominate. Enough of the basic human necessities simply are not available. In this deficient environment, the body becomes weak and vulnerable and can fall prey to any of a number of diseases. Alternatively, in the developed Western world, "diseases of excess" prevail, diseases caused by too much: too much food, too much luxury, too much overindulgence, too much stress, and so on. Again, this situation represents imbalanced conditions.

Nobody gets sick by accident, or out of the blue. If you take a closer look at the factors that govern your health, you will discover that illness does not strike randomly. Disease and illness, with very few exceptions, occur at predictable times, and for discernable reasons. Just as sunrise and sunset are predictable and occur in conjunction with the earth's rotation on its axis, just as the tides of the ocean are predictable and occur in conjunction with the lunar phases, so it is with illness and disease.

Listening to Your Body

As I've already mentioned, illness and disease occur when your body's internal environment has become imbalanced and disordered. This is usually the result of nature's basic laws of health being knowingly or unknowingly violated. These laws are simple and systematic. More important, your body, which is connected to nature, is constantly trying to remind you of these laws through its intelligent communications network. In fact, you are probably intuitively aware of what your body requires to remain healthy and strong.

Your body continually provides you with clear, updated information relayed directly from a precise, highly intelligent, early warning system designed to inform you when you are in danger of losing your health. You fall into illness or disease usually when you have ignored your body's basic communications and early warning signs. This occurs in spite of your body's pleading with you to change your unhealthy ways. These physical messages usually start as gentle incantations in the form of bodily discomfort, and then progress to shouting and screaming in the form of debilitating pain.

For instance, Greg, a patient of mine with chronic back problems, was building a house. After bending over, sawing wood, pounding nails, and lifting heavy lumber all day long, in the evening he'd be extremely sore and stiff. The next morning, the pain was so bad he could barely get out of bed. Rather than rest and take it easy, however, he'd take pain killers so he could finish his work. This pattern went on for several weeks, and it seemed to work, until one day he went too far. While he was bending over to lift a heavy laminated beam, he ruptured a disc in his spine and ended up on an operating table, where he underwent emergency spine surgery. As is often the case with many of my other back-pain patients, Greg had had plenty of warning from his body before his rupture; he just chose not to listen. To him, finishing his house was a higher priority than listening to and taking care of his body. As with most illness or injuries that are entirely preventable, Greg could easily have solved his back problem without having to go through surgery if he had taken the time to heed the messages from his body.

Jim, another patient of mine, had chronic obstructive lung disease, a condition very much like asthma. He needed regular prescriptions for inhalers that contained strong medicines, which he used daily just to be able to breathe. As a complication of his condition, he often came down with serious respiratory infections that required potent antibiotics to stop. Often, he would end up in the emergency room because he couldn't breathe. At these times, he needed oxygen, ventilating assistance, and strong intravenous medications, or he could easily have died. Although his breathing problems would flare up when he smoked, he continued to do so, to the tune of one to two packs of cigarettes a day, his pattern for more than 20 years. His body was constantly hacking, coughing, and spitting up foul-smelling mucous and phlegm. He finally got the message one day after a near-death episode, after which he ended up in the intensive-care unit for two weeks.

It has now been three years since Jim stopped smoking. Funny, he no longer requires inhalers to breathe, he hasn't had a respiratory infection in more than a year, and his chronic obstructive pulmonary disease has vanished. Jim decided to pay attention to his body's messages and work with its natural ability to maintain his health and well-being.

Sally is another patient of mine who ignored her body's messages. Sally was in a lot of pain and had been vomiting yellow, bilious material for two days before she came to my office in obvious distress. Her pain, which had lasted for almost one week, was located in the right upper aspect of her abdomen. She was significantly overweight, of fair complexion, and approximately 40 years of age. Her signs and symptoms pointed to an acute gall-bladder attack, which tests later confirmed to be the problem. In most cases, this condition, brought on largely by a high-fat diet, is completely preventable.

Almost every day for the week preceding her problem, Sally had eaten sausage and fried eggs for breakfast, burgers and fries with a milkshake for lunch, and pizza and ice cream for dinner. Even when her pain increased and the vomiting began, she continued to eat toast with butter, cheese sandwiches, and chocolate candy bars, all high-fat foods. She couldn't understand why she didn't feel better.

After I spoke with Sally at length, she mentioned to me that this wasn't the first incident of this nature. Over the past several years, after having eaten certain rich foods, she had noticed significant abdominal discomfort, bloating, and belching, things that she attributed to mere "indigestion." Her body had obviously been trying to get her attention to change her diet for a long time.

I placed Sally on a clear, liquid diet for 48 hours and also sent her down to the hospital for laboratory tests and an X-ray to confirm my diagnostic suspicions. After the diagnosis was confirmed, I referred Sally to a surgeon to have her gall bladder removed. During the 48 hours after she had come to see me, during which she drank only water and liquids and ate nothing solid, her vomiting and pain completely stopped, and she told me she hadn't felt that good in a long, long time. However, by then, the wheels of the system were turning, and the surgeon's knife was impatiently waiting. After three days, Sally was wheeled into the operating room, where her gall bladder was removed in less than 2 hours. Sally could have maintained her natural state of health by heeding the messages her body had been giving her. Instead, she ignored them and interfered with her body's natural ability to keep her healthy and strong.

Sam's body was talking to him, too, and, like Sally, he wasn't listening. Sam was a local Hawaiian who drank a case of beer each day and didn't think much about it. He and his buddies had been on this steady regimen for many years. They met at the local beach park after work, drank, and told their stories until well after dark and it was time to go home. One day, after many years of these drinking activities, Sam came in to see me. His abdomen was tender, and his liver was painful and swollen. He was nauseous and dehydrated, and he hadn't been able to eat or drink for more than a week. He was suffering from acute (and chronic) alcoholism that was affecting his liver. His feet and ankles were also extremely swollen, a bad sign that meant he was having circulation problems, as well.

Sam had had plenty of warnings from his body before this episode. He had not only experienced a tender, swollen belly and liver, nausea, and dehydration on several prior occasions, but he had also suffered from DTs (delirium tremens) and shakes when he had tried to quit drinking. After brief periods, however, once the storms of suffering had passed, he had resumed his drinking habits with his buddies.

I was very busy with other patients, and after hearing Sam's story, I thought I wouldn't have much of an impact on helping him to change his ways. I resigned myself to believing he was just another casualty of alcohol, and I referred him to an internist who could admit him to the hospital. I did, however, give my perfunctory speech about the need to stop drinking, which I thought would only fall on deaf ears.

Two years later, a man showed up in my office for a chest cold. Other than that, he looked healthy and in good, athletic shape. Because of his new beard, I didn't recognize who it was—Sam. He was a totally changed person!

Sam told me that what I had said to him that day did make an impact. He hadn't had a drink in two years. And it showed! Instead, he had been drinking lots of water, exercising, and doing hard physical labor; he had quit smoking, as well. Sam had finally listened to his body, and he was back to his natural state of health.

Who Gets Sick, and Why?

Many people come into my office blaming another family member, or the person sitting next to them on the airplane, for the bronchitis or throat infection they contracted. This attitude is only natural. However, because of the ubiquity of bacteria, viruses, and other organisms in our immediate environment and in the air we breathe, these microorganisms, in and of themselves, are usually not the only cause of the illness. If they were, all of us would be sick all the time. Also, if germs were spread from person to person so easily, then doctors, who spend every day around these germs and around the people who spread these germs, should be the sickest people of all. But they are not. Under normal conditions, bacteria and viruses in our environment usually do not bother us in the least. What, then, has changed that allows us to become infected and affected by them? Is it them, or something in us? Recent research points strongly in favor of the latter. *Epidemiology* is the science that studies disease outbreaks in the world, known as epidemics. A classic model known as the epidemiological triangle exists in this field. The epidemiological triangle illustrates that the existence of disease depends on three factors: 1) the host, which is the person who is the potential target of the disease; 2) the agent, which is the organism or disease-causing factor that initiates or transmits the disease;

and 3) the environment, in which both the host and agent reside or come in contact. Medical science needs to weigh and measure all three factors to help discover the true origins of illness, while it works to solve and prevent future epidemics from occurring.

Whereas previous medical research attributed more importance to the virulence of such agents as bacteria and viruses that caused the diseases, newer medical research places much greater emphasis on host resistance factors, which are factors within us that keep us healthy and help us resist illness. We can think of host resistance factors as the body's internal healing resources. They determine a person's susceptibility to illness and disease and reflect one's natural resiliency. Studying host resistance factors helps us to understand why some people get sick and why others don't, even when they are exposed to the same disease-causing agents; why certain people get sick more often than others; and why certain diseases seem to have an affinity for certain people.

Studies on host resistance factors show that, for people living in the modern, developed world, the most important factors in determining our state of health and susceptibility to illness are based on how well we take care of ourselves, how well we nurture and honor our bodies, and how well we respect our natural state of health. These factors are dependent on the personal choices we make in our every day lives.

Studies on host resistance factors have also led to the realization that, in addition to the immune system, there is another extremely important system in the body that is responsible for its natural resiliency, and its ability to heal itself and keep itself healthy. This system is the body's healing system, the most recently discovered system, and its most important one. The body knows how to heal itself and maintain its natural state of health because of its healing system.

Your Healing System
The Guardian of Your Body's Health

Imagine yourself outside on a beautiful, warm summer day. You're skipping down the street, feeling carefree and light-hearted. All of a sudden, you trip on an oversized crack in the sidewalk. As you feel yourself going down, you instinctively put out your arm to brace your fall. As you hit the ground and slide along the pavement, you immediately feel pain in your arm. As you slowly rise to your feet, you notice an area where a patch of skin has been ripped off. It is red, raw, and bleeding. Although you're thankful that it's only a scrape, it still hurts like the dickens. In doctor's language, you have just sustained an *abrasion!*

Over the course of the next several days, without much fuss, you watch your body go through interesting yet predictable changes at the site of the abrasion. First, it begins to secrete a clear-looking fluid that eventually turns into a brown, crusty covering that thickens and forms into a scab. When your body sheds the scab after a week or two, just as a snake or lizard sheds its skin, you notice you have a brand-new layer of skin. Several months later, there's not even a scar to mark the sight of the injury. Pretty common, everyday stuff, and yet, at the same time, when you think about the fact that you have new skin, you have to ask yourself, "How did my body know how to do that?"

Your body knows how to heal itself because of its healing system. For the most part, without your even knowing it, your healing system keeps your body resilient by repairing and healing it from a myriad of problems encountered every single day of your life. These events include not only the rapid mending of superficial problems such as abrasions and cuts and bruises on the skin, but also the supervising, monitoring, and continual adjusting of critical physiological processes that occur deep within your body's internal environment. When external forces seek to create imbalance within your body, when order becomes less orderly and may even turn to chaos, when dis-ease, or illness manifests, your healing system works hard to restore order and balance to help you reclaim your natural state of health. Here are just a few ways your healing system works to safeguard your health:

- Your healing system can expand and contract blood vessels to increase blood flow to specific areas of your body that need healing.

- Your healing system can speed up your heart rate and increase the strength of its contractions to rapidly deliver more blood, oxygen, and nutrients to specific sites that need healing; this process includes cases of life-threatening emergencies.

- Your healing system stimulates your glands to produce key hormones to initiate growth and repair processes within the cells of damaged tissues.

- Your healing system can increase body temperature to cause a fever and induce sweating, to remove toxins when an infection is present.

- Your healing system can modify the function of your kidneys to reduce urine output and help conserve water if you're dehydrated.

- Your healing system supervises the amazing process of bone remodeling, of knitting your bones together as it heals fractures.

- Your healing system can increase your breathing rate and lung capacity to bring in more oxygen for your cells and tissues when an illness or injury has occurred.

Your healing system can do all of these things and many, many more. In fact, for as long as you are alive, your healing system remains viable and committed to its role as the guardian of your body's health.

Even if there have been times in the past when you were quite ill and had to struggle against life's most serious adversities and setbacks, your healing system was there for you, attempting to pull you out of your suffering. Even if you are battling an illness right now, underneath the symptoms of illness, you will find your healing system working hard to reestablish balance and order in your body. The fact that you are alive today is indicative of your healing system's functioning to fulfill your body's underlying drive to heal and become healthy once again. Even if your health is currently compromised and not what you would like it to be, you can work with your healing system to strengthen and fortify it and regain your natural state of health.

Eliminating Obstacles to Your Healing System

In many cases, you unknowingly place obstacles in the way of your healing system, creating an unfair burden that hinders its work and jeopardizes its effectiveness. By understanding what these obstacles are and removing them, in many instances, your healing system, now unshackled to complete its task of healing, can quickly restore normal functioning to your body, enabling it to express its natural state of health.

For example, consider the case of a chronic lung infection in a person who continues to smoke cigarettes. Constant breathing of cigarette smoke is not natural. If cigarette smoking were natural, we'd all have been born with a cigarette in our mouth. Your body was designed to breathe fresh and healthy, clean, natural air. Although it can survive and tolerate cigarette smoke for a certain period of time, after a while, the smoke particles, the carbon monoxide, the tars, and the other toxic substances in the cigarette smoke create a burden on your healing system that causes an imbalance and a breakdown in your health. In this case, removing the harmful obstacle of the cigarette smoke is all that is required for your body to regain its natural state of health. With the burden of the cigarette smoke removed, it is an easy, routine task for your healing system to restore your body to its natural state of health.

Another example is evident with heart disease, the number-one killer in the Western world. Heart disease is caused by excess cholesterol accumulation. High cholesterol levels resulting from a lack of exercise, too many rich and fatty foods, and stress can clog the arteries of the heart and cause a heart attack. Removing these obstacles by restricting fat intake, increasing exercise, and managing stress allows the healing system to restore the body to its natural state of health. It is well known that this simple strategy can reverse even severe, advanced heart disease.

The major diseases of our time, including lung diseases, heart diseases, joint diseases, metabolic diseases, autoimmune diseases, and even cancer, have at their roots major obstacles that have been placed as burdens upon the healing system. Remove these burdens, and healing occurs because now the healing system is free to restore the body to its natural state of health.

Why the Healing System Has Been Overlooked

Sometimes, what we are looking for is right under our noses. This is exactly the case with the body's healing system. Until recently, we missed something very fundamental and essential about how our bodies work as intelligent, functional, whole living systems. As a consequence, we failed to recognize the significance of the most important system in our entire bodies.

The body's healing system has been overlooked until now for a number of reasons. The primary reason is that conventional medical science focuses, for the most part, on the structure and form of the body, rather than on its function, or how the body works. This view has an impact on medicine in these significant ways:

- Conventional medicine focuses more on structure and form than on function (how the body works), and so diseases and illnesses are viewed as localized problems within specific anatomical areas of the body. Instead of one unit working as a whole, the body is viewed as many individual parts working separately and surgery is often seen as the ultimate treatment for these separate problems.

- Conventional medicine has neglected to acknowledge the central role that energy plays in the body's growth, development, sustenance, and healing. Not recognizing that energy is the real, active, life-promoting, fundamental principle in our bodies, doctors once again tend to focus more on structure and form than on function. But the healing system is not confined to one anatomical area. The body is a functional system based on the flow and movement of energies within it. The body directs healing energy to where it is needed, much like a fireman directs water from the end of his hose to help put out a fire.

- A large part of scientific research has been devoted to the study of external agents of disease, such as bacteria and viruses, and the development of specific drugs, such as antibiotics, to kill them. This research has directed awareness away from the body's inner resources. For the most part, this focus has left us ignorant about how our bodies work and how they heal themselves.

- A large amount of research is currently devoted to genetics, which seeks to link certain diseases to specific gene defects. Genetic defects are currently being blamed for most diseases not caused by external agents such as bacteria, viruses, or injuries. Although genetics certainly has its place in a person's health, international public health data show that bad genes do not cause most diseases in the world. Most common diseases, such as heart disease, high blood pressure, diabetes, stroke, arthritis, and cancer, are linked to poor diets and unhealthy lifestyles rather than bad genes. Seeking to cure all diseases with genetic engineering through the removal of defective genes, while important for certain rare diseases, completely bypasses the importance of discovering how the body's healing system can help overcome the majority of diseases.

The Growth of Specialties in Medicine

Another significant reason that the healing system has been overlooked is the tremendous amount of information coming from so many different specialty fields in medicine today. Specialists, like surgeons, tend to treat each system of the body as a separate entity, rather than as part of a unified whole.

For example, we now have *cardiology* to study and treat the heart; *dermatology* to study and treat the skin; *neurology* for the nerves; *endocrinology* for the glands; *nephrology* for the kidneys; *pulmonology* for the lungs; *rheumatology* for the joints; *orthopedics* for the bones and muscles; *podiatry* for the feet; *otolaryngology* for the ears, nose, and throat; *urology* for the bladder and related organs; and so on. Because the healing system is integrated within the structure and function of all the other systems of the body, overspecialization has caused us to see only fragments of its existence while we continue to remain unaware of its total presence and significance.

Each specialty focuses on the study of only one system within the human body, and communication among the various specialty fields is often lacking. As a result, we physicians have developed a type of tunnel vision that prevents us from seeing the big picture, and organizing and sorting all of this specialized information into one complete, whole system. At times, it appears the left hand doesn't know what the right hand is doing. This is a major flaw of modern medicine.

The Healing System Is Not a New Discovery

Although many people regard the body's healing system as a recent discovery, in fact, ancient cultures and healers from other parts of the world have long known about it. Within the healing communities of these societies, whose members lived in close proximity to nature and respected her wisdom, the existence of a healing system has never been challenged. It is only in our modern age of skepticism, in which we need new ideas to be scientifically proven before we can accept them as fact, that the role of the healing system has been questioned.

Even today, most practitioners of the healing arts living abroad operate from the premise that our bodies are linked to nature, and that the body's healing system works with the same intelligent organizational principles that can be found in nature. Further, they believe that by studying these natural principles, we can discover and utilize important, natural, gentle, and supportive modalities that work in harmony with this healing system to help restore and maintain our health. Healing can occur when we work *with*, not *against*, the forces of nature that exist within the human body.

When confronted with a sick patient, any physician who understands the true value of the healing system will try to understand how the body's natural forces of health became unbalanced in the first place. What caused the body to become less orderly and more chaotic, and to fall out of its natural balanced state of health and into a state of disease? Factors such as stress, poor sleeping habits, poor diet, lack of regular exercise, problems at work or working too much, turmoil at home, erratic social relationships, mental and emotional conflict, and so on, are all possibilities. Discovering and investigating these factors is critical for a successful treatment outcome. Once the harmful culprits have been identified, the road back to health becomes clearer. Removing these obstacles and harmful forces allows the healing system to do its job more effectively.

Powerful Evidence of Your Healing System

Western medical science's discovery of the body's healing system is still in its early stages, and so much of the evidence for its existence is indirect. This situation, however, is to be expected of any new field of scientific exploration. Let me explain.

In the field of astronomy, when a new star or planet is first discovered, the first sign of its existence is often glimpsed through observing its influence on the behavior and orbiting characteristics of its closest known neighbor. Here, motion abnormalities can often be detected with the help of a high-powered telescope. Precise mathematical data about the new entity, based on mass, density, gravitational fields, and orbital motions, result in careful calculations and a closer look through the telescope, until the new star or planet comes into clear focus and is actually seen. Many new stars and planets, and even galaxies, have been discovered in this manner. In the vastness of the universe, if we don't actively look for something, the chances of finding it are almost nil.

Within our bodies also exists an entire, vast universe of its own: the healing system. Because we have spent more efforts investigating external agents of disease and haven't been actively looking for this internal system, we haven't amassed a great deal of information about it. The healing system's tremendous effect on us and how our bodies function is clear, even though we don't have scientific evidence yet of its existence. Given the limitations of our current technologies and mindset, which focus more on anatomical structures and less on energy and function, the healing system would still be difficult to accurately evaluate in all its exquisite detail and sophistication, even if we had been more aggressively looking for it.

If we can shift the current focus of scientific exploration away from the various bacteria and viruses and the pharmaceutical weapons produced to neutralize them, away from quick-fix surgical solutions, away from toxic chemicals to poison our malignancies, and away from "bad genes" that we suspect cause the majority of our other problems, and instead focus more on understanding how our bodies know how to heal themselves, then we will be much further along in learning how to cooperate with our healing systems to prevent illness, heal diseases, and enjoy long and healthy lives beyond our current expectations.

Centenarians
Living Examples of Your Healing System

In nature, each living species has a programmed lifespan, a maximum potential age to which members of that species can live. For example, most insects, such as mosquitoes, gnats, and butterflies, live to a maximum of only one to two weeks. For dogs, the lifespan is roughly 10 to12 years. For great white sharks, it is 300 years. For certain reptiles, such as desert tortoises, it is 400 years. For certain trees, such as the Giant Sequoias of Northern California, the life-span ranges from 2,000 to 3,000 years. For humans, the maximum potential lifespan is about 100 years.

If a group of people ever demonstrated the human body's natural ability to stay healthy, and the existence of its healing system, that group is the *centenarians*, who, by definition, are people who have lived to and beyond 100 years of age. Surprisingly, according to recent demographic surveys, the fastest growing segment of the U.S. popu-lation is people over the age of 100. Twenty years ago in the U.S., there were 6,200 reported centenarians. Today, there are more than 64,000 centenarians in the U.S. alone. People today are more health-conscious than they were 20 years ago, so they are better at cooperat-ing with and strengthening their healing systems. This change has enabled more people to live longer. Without the body's incredible ability to heal itself and return to its natural state of health over and over again, how is it possible for so many people to live so long?

By and large, centenarians have learned how to cooperate with their healing systems to reap and enjoy their maximum allotment of time on this earth. And most did it while staying active and main-taining their health until the very end. Looking at their lifestyles, and not merely their genes, we can learn a lot about the many ways that we too can cooperate and work with our healing systems.

Most centenarians I have met, although they are all unique indi-viduals with their own personal stories, share a common bond in how they have lived their lives. Most have eaten moderately, kept active, enjoyed good sleep, rested when necessary, stayed involved with friends and family, and generally enjoyed life. Although their diets, lifestyles, and genes have differed, many have had to endure extreme hardships over the course of their long lives, including the loss of their closest loved ones and family members. Still, most of these people have exhibited what I would call a "lighthearted atti-tude." It's rare to meet a centenarian without a great sense of humor and a smile on his or her face. An example of this was the world's oldest living Western woman, a French woman who lived to 122 years of age. Although she had lost her eyesight and recently had come to rely on a wheelchair, she had just quit smoking at the age of

121! When interviewed about the secrets of her longevity, she replied that the only thing she knew was that "I only have one wrinkle on my entire body, and I'm sitting on it!" This kind of light-hearted attitude typifies those who have reached the age of 100 or beyond.

The well-known comedian George Burns lived to be more than 100 years old, and he continued to perform and act in movies until his passing. He never stopped smoking cigars; more importantly, he also never stopped smiling and telling jokes! His positive attitude helped to strengthen his healing system and bring his body back to its natural state of health after illness.

I once treated a delightful 95-year-old woman who was dressed in a hot-pink outfit, sunglasses, and a shell necklace, and who had a big smile on her face, despite the fact that she had a large gash on her leg, which prompted her visit to me. She was taking a cruise and had stepped off the ship for a day's shopping in Hawaii. When she removed her sunglasses, I saw a pair of youthful, sparkling, blue eyes that easily revealed her carefree, optimistic attitude toward life. After several minutes of chatting as I attended to her wound, she asked whether I could speed things up. "Why?" I asked.

"Because my older sister is in your waiting room, and I don't want to keep her waiting. We only have one day on your island, and I promised to go bodysurfing with her!"

When I stepped out into the waiting room, I saw her sister, three years her elder. She was also vibrant and smiling, and dressed in a matching red outfit with a straw hat!

Many people come into my office and tell me that they are "getting old and falling apart!" I have had people in their thirties and forties tell me this. Conversely, I have seen many other patients who are learning how to surf and water ski at the age of 70, others who are taking yoga in their eighties and are more supple and graceful than people less than half their age, and still others who are dancing and gardening daily well into their nineties. Youth and health appear to be more connected to our states of mind, and reflect our attitudes more than pure chronology. A positive attitude and a zest for life are critical for enhancing and fortifying your healing system.

Take a lesson from the centenarians, and discover the many ways that you too can enjoy a long, healthy, and rewarding life, free from disease and debility, way beyond your present expectations, by learning to cooperate with your healing system, and respecting and honoring your natural state of health.

Closing Thoughts on Your Healing System and Your Natural State of Health

Health is your normal and natural state. This condition is founded on universal biological principles that apply to all living species, not just humans. Health is programmed into the DNA of every cell in your body and is the reason why the human species has been able to flourish and survive from one generation to the next for thousands of years. Health is the reason you are alive today. The maximum average potential lifespan for a human being is 100 years or more. Because your natural state is health, any deviation from this natural state represents an unnatural condition. You are actually programmed for good health the day you are conceived.

Disease and illness not only are undesirable conditions, but they also are fundamentally unnatural and abnormal. Their existence represents a departure from the natural laws that govern normal biological processes on earth. When you become ill, it usually means that unnatural, harmful, unhealthy forces have been imposed upon your body that cause it to become temporarily imbalanced and disordered. Restoring order and balance returns your body to its natural state of health. This is the job of your extraordinary healing system, which can be thought of as the guardian of your body's health.

Even though challenges and difficulties may seem to be an almost daily occurrence, your body can rise to meet these challenges and difficulties because it has an extraordinary healing system that has been designed to sustain, repair, and correct imbalances and problems, naturally and automatically. At times, disease may appear overwhelming and all-encompassing, but your healing system can help your body bounce back to reclaim its natural state of health, even in the face of death, and at times when you have abandoned all hope. Through your healing system, your body possesses an uncanny natural resiliency, like a buoy floating in the sea, to right itself in the midst of life's most devastating tempests.

In the next chapter, you will get a closer look at your healing system in action, including the opportunity to examine the evidence for its existence, and to understand what this system does and how it works. You will also discover why learning to cooperate with your healing system, and strengthening and fortifying it, are essential for you to achieve and enjoy optimum health.

CHAPTER 2

Your Healing System in Action

When you think about the number of threats and insults your body sustains over the course of a lifetime, the fact that it can remain healthy at all is truly amazing. To accomplish this incredible task, you need a single system in your body that can supervise and direct all the other systems into a unified, efficient, orchestrated healing response for your protection and the preservation of your natural state of health. That single, supervisory system is your healing system.

Your healing system not only maintains your natural state of health, but whenever you are sick or injured, or whenever your health is threatened, it also is in charge of damage control. It monitors and supervises all processes of repair, growth, and restoration of health and normal functioning of your body's cells, tissues, and organs. In fact, you wouldn't be alive today if it weren't for your body's remarkable healing system.

Illness or injury can strike at any time, and so your body needs a system it can count on to safeguard its health, 24 hours a day, 7 days a week, 365 days a year. In this regard, your body's healing system is a tireless workhorse because it never sleeps or even snoozes. It cannot even afford the luxury of a catnap. It remains alert at all times, ready to spring into action at a moment's notice. Like a 911 emergency-response, paramedic rescue crew, your healing system is on call continuously—no time off for sick leave, vacations, or even good behavior. It also has tremendous endurance and stamina, and it can remain operational for up to 100 years, or even longer.

Your healing system permeates every organ and tissue in your body; it is not confined to any one structure or specific location. It cannot be surgically removed, or even visibly seen on an X-ray, CAT scan, or MRI, as is the case with most other structures in your body. When you are healthy, it is difficult to even know that such a system exists; however, during times of injury or illness, as your body mounts a healing response, evidence of its existence becomes quite apparent.

Although your healing system is arguably the most important system in your body, you probably have never heard about it before, or, if you have, the information was sparse. Although you may be familiar with the other systems in your body, such as the digestive, respiratory, circulatory, nervous, and immune systems, you probably are reading about the healing system for the very first time. In fact, you may be confusing your healing system with your immune system right now, as many people do.

Differences Between Your Healing System and Your Immune System

When people first hear of the healing system, they often confuse it with the immune system. Even though on one level the two systems may be difficult to tell apart because they work together in a cooperative effort, on another level they are two very different systems that serve entirely different purposes.

The fundamental difference between the two systems is that your immune system is concerned with defending your body against infections, while your healing system is responsible for repairing tissue damage from injuries or illnesses, and restoring your body to its natural state of health. Your immune system's focus is largely on attacking and protecting your body from foreign invaders. Your healing system focuses more on healing, growth, regeneration, restoration of function, and maintaining health.

For example, if you were to come down with bronchitis, which is an infection in the respiratory system, your immune system would be expected to attack and eliminate the offending organisms that are causing the infection. However, if you were injured in a car accident and broke your arm, your healing system would be called upon to heal your injuries. Your immune system would not become involved because typically there is no infection with a broken bone. The mending of the broken bone would be a specific function of your healing system.

Similarly, if you had a heart attack, your healing system would immediately become activated. A heart attack is not caused by an infection, and so healing from it does not involve your immune system, but rather your healing system. After a heart attack, your healing system repairs the damage to your heart muscle while it restores normal functioning to your heart.

When you understand that most diseases and injuries are not caused by infection, the distinction between your healing system and your immune system becomes clearer, and the unique role of your healing system becomes much more significant.

All of this having been said, be aware that there are times when the division of labor between your immune system and healing system is not so clear. Your healing system and immune system work together and cooperate with each other to keep you healthy. For example, if your body has sustained damage from an infection, your healing system and immune system will work side by side to repair the damage as they fight against, neutralize, and remove the infectious agents to prevent further damage to your body. Your immune system will attack the infection that caused the problem, and your healing system will actually repair the damage the infection caused to your body.

Listening to Your Healing System

Because your body's natural state is good health, your physical needs are actually quite simple. However, when these needs are not being met, your body is not shy about giving warning signs to prompt you into taking immediate corrective action. When situations of urgency arise, or when you are not healthy, your body, through its communications system, which works closely with your healing system, will let you know immediately. For your healing system to repair, restore, and sustain your body most effectively, you must learn how to listen to your healing system when it talks to you.

For instance, when your water reserves become low, and there is danger of dehydration, your thirst mechanism kicks in, urging you to drink. When your body is low on energy and you need more calories, your hunger drive is activated, prompting you to eat. When you need sleep or rest, you will begin to yawn, and your eyes will feel heavy, urging you to lie down. When you become chilled in cold weather, your body will begin to shiver, forcing you to put on a sweater or jacket, or to seek shelter. If you eat foods that are too rich or too spicy, or the wrong combination of foods, you'll feel nauseous and might possibly even regurgitate. All these sensations and responses are part of your body's intelligence and communications network, which your healing system monitors and supervises to help restore normal function and maintain your natural state of health.

Two Essential Roles of Your Healing System

Your healing system functions in two critical ways. In its first important role, much like a foreman at a large building site who supervises, organizes, and dispatches workers, equipment, and machinery while he overlooks a construction project, your healing system meticulously monitors, surveys, and observes each and every part of your body to ensure that all organs and tissues remain healthy and function smoothly. It facilitates communication between your body's various systems and their respective cells and tissues. It monitors your body's complex internal environment, where literally millions of powerful chemical reactions occur each day. Your healing system troubleshoots problems anywhere in your body. Just like a mother who cares for and looks after her children, your healing system in its protective and nurturing role safeguards the integrity of your entire body, helping maintain its natural state of health.

In its second vital role, your healing system functions like an emergency-response paramedic crew, jumping into action whenever there is a threat to your health. In this more active phase, your healing system is able to perform a wide range of diverse functions, such as dispatching nerve messages and impulses; mobilizing immune and inflammatory cells; coordinating the release of powerful chemicals that can raise body temperature, dilate or constrict blood vessels, increase or decrease blood flow to specific areas; and performing many other vital functions. Your healing system directs the activities of the other systems in your body to cooperate with each other in providing a unified, concerted, and effective healing response.

In its first role, you may not even be aware of your body's healing system as it goes about the business of its crucial surveillance work silently and without much fanfare. In the second role, however, the presence of your healing system is much more noticeable, with specific changes that occur in your body as a result of its actions. The dual supervisory and emergency-response roles that your healing system plays in the general functioning of all the systems and structures in your body makes it the most powerful and important system in your body.

How Your Healing System Works

Understanding how your healing system functions requires a different way of thinking about how your body works. Although doing so may seem difficult at first, if you think of your body in terms of energy and function, rather than in terms of matter, structure, and form, it will all make perfect sense. Thinking in terms of energy does not ignore or nullify the existence of certain structures within your body; rather, this view gives you a deeper look into the dynamic forces that govern your health. When these dynamic forces become unbalanced, you can easily see how problems that create illnesses and diseases in your body arise. Armed with this knowledge and insight, you will be able to more effectively remedy these problems by working with, rather than against, your healing system. Let's examine a case that illustrates this point.

Al cut his finger with a kitchen knife while he was slicing vegetables. At first, there was no blood at all, and he imagined that maybe it didn't really happen, and that he'd get off easy. Then, as the first signs of blood began to ooze out of the wound, he realized the puncture was deep. In no time, the bleeding became profuse. Pain, delayed for several seconds, soon began to pulsate and throb throughout his fingertip and entire hand. Al applied pressure to prevent his blood from spilling onto the floor. After half an hour, he noticed the bleeding had slowed. An hour later, it eventually stopped.

From the very beginning of this incident, and over the course of the next several days, Al's healing system was busy activating a healing response that includes

- The nervous system, which first responds with messages of pain that warn Al an injury has occurred.

- The complex mechanisms of blood clotting, which are a sophisticated interaction of hormones, enzymes, and numerous chemicals and cells within the circulatory system. These components are naturally sticky and join together to seal off the wound to protect the body from further blood loss.

- The layers of the skin, deeper tissues, and various cells, which weave themselves together to form a transitional, intermediate layer of skin and fill in the gap created by the wound.

- The formation of a scab, which protects the deeper, more sensitive layers of new skin and tissues as the healing process continues.

When the scab sloughs off, Al's healing system miraculously manufactures new skin where the old skin had been completely severed. After several weeks, Al's finger looks the way it did before his injury, as if nothing had happened at all.

Even though Al's injury is a relatively simple one, if you look at the sequence of events, the various systems and components involved in the healing of his wound, and the synchronized flow of energy and movement during the entire healing process, you start to develop an appreciation for the degree of complexity and precision, and the incredible organization, speed, and efficiency your healing system requires to perform this specific task.

Keep in mind that your healing system supervises and coordinates all healing responses in your body, including illnesses and injuries that are far more complex and serious than Al's injury. And even though your healing system may appear to be hidden and difficult to pinpoint within any given part of your body, you can begin to understand the function and purpose of this amazing system by observing its powerful, swift, dynamic and efficient movements, and viewing the results of its actions. The subtle and dynamic aspect of your healing system is one of the reasons it has not been more widely recognized, acknowledged, and accepted until just recently.

The Immune System and the Healing System

The immune system and the healing system are both subtle and dynamic systems, and although they often work together, they serve different functions.

The healing system is even more subtle and more widespread in its distribution throughout the body than the immune system, permeating every organ, tissue, and cell in your body. It is also more powerful, more dynamic, and more diversified in its functions and tasks than your immune system.

Like the healing system, the immune system has many branches, is not limited to one particular area of the body, and operates on the microscopic level of cells and biochemicals. In fact, your immune system collaborates with your healing system and can be thought of as an aspect of the healing system that is concerned with preventing and eradicating infections from the body. The immune system also was poorly understood and not given much importance in the practice of modern medicine until the discovery of AIDS. Fortunately, with the shift of funds and resources, and research being directed from without to within the realm of our own bodies, we have learned more about our body's natural defense system than we ever imagined existed.

Your Healing System and the Other Systems in Your Body

Your healing system utilizes the special properties and functions of other systems in your body, integrating and supervising their activities into one organized, efficient healing response. To understand this more clearly, let's see what happens when you accidentally touch a hot electric iron and burn yourself.

Imagine an iron that is plugged into an electrical socket, sitting upright on the ironing board, and inadvertently left on for half a day. When you discover the iron and try to put it away, you accidentally touch the very hot bottom.

As soon as you touch the hot iron and hear the sizzling sound of your flesh burning, you instantaneously feel pain as you immediately jerk your hand back. In addition to the incredible burning pain, within a matter of minutes, you begin to notice blisters forming on your fingers and hands in the places that came in contact with the iron. From the vantage point of what is going on inside of your body, let's take a closer look at what is happening, step by step, as your healing system springs into action:

Step 1

Your healing system is immediately activated when you touch the hot iron, as the pain sensors in your fingers and hand send a signal to the brain through your nervous system. Your nervous system, working with your healing system, initiates a reflex response in the muscles of your arm to contract the arm, pulling it away to prevent further contact with the hot iron, which prevents further injury.

Step 2

Almost immediately, in collaboration with the skin, your healing system coordinates a response that first results in redness or inflammation as tiny blood vessels are directed to increase blood flow to the area of the scorched skin.

Step 3

Specialized cells known as *macrophages*, along with red blood cells, white blood cells, oxygen, and other essential nutrients, are pumped into the bloodstream and directed to the injury site to help nourish, fortify, and support the body's repair processes.

Step 4

Shortly thereafter, the skin secretes specific fluids to help form blisters at the burn sites. The blisters serve several protective and healing functions. First, the fluid-filled sacs act like shock absorbers to protect the raw, injured skin that lies underneath. They also act as sealed barriers against the possibility of infection. The fluid inside the blisters also contains nutrients to help nourish and feed the new layer of skin that will form underneath. Antibodies and immune cells also have been mobilized by the immune system in this fluid. These mechanisms also are under the direction of the healing system, to ward off any microorganisms that might cause infection. In addition, the body releases other important chemicals to cooperate in the healing response.

Step 5

With the healing response well under way, new cells, fluids, and chemicals are continuously pumped in and out of the burn site over the course of the next several days and weeks; the pain begins to subside and the new skin growth accelerates.

Step 6

Soon, the blisters gradually shrink as the fluid is reabsorbed back into the body, with new skin arising to take the place of the previously injured old skin.

Step 7

Continued healing mechanisms are activated on the microscopic level to finish the job, and, if all goes well, not even a scar will be present where the new skin has grown back.

Even with a simple injury such as a minor second-degree burn, you can see that a lot more is going on in your body beneath the surface of the skin than meets the eye. As with the more serious and complicated problems that occur within your body, again it is clear that the body needs a single system that can supervise and direct all the other key systems into one orchestrated and efficient healing response for the protection, self-preservation, and health of your body. This is the incredible job that your healing system does for you.

Healing System Responses vs. Symptoms of Disease
A New Way of Thinking About Your Health

When our healing system is initially activated, we might confuse the changes that occur in our body, which are normal healing responses, with symptoms of a particular disease. In fact, this is the common mistake most people make, including doctors and the medical profession in general. Again, until very recently, our culture has been disease-oriented in its approach to understanding health and healing, and so we have remained largely ignorant of the healing system and how our bodies continually strive to correct imbalances and keep us healthy.

When things begin to change in our bodies, we automatically assume we are sick, and that something is dreadfully wrong. If our bodies begin to reflect imbalance and function abnormally, if there is some discomfort or pain, our first assumption is most likely that we are becoming sick or that we have an allergy. This is because we are trying to account for our symptoms. This is a natural and normal interpretation of what is happening with our bodies.

Rather than jumping to the conclusion that something is wrong with your body, first try to understand how your healing system may be responding appropriately to correct an imbalance that has occurred. Let me explain what I mean.

Consider sneezing, for example. We usually think of sneezing as a symptom of the common cold, or the beginning of an allergy. In reality, sneezing is a normal healing-system response to expel foreign debris, flush out irritants, remove potential pathogens, rid the body of disease, and help the body maintain its integrity. Sneezing also is a protective mechanism that helps to prevent the further advance of unwanted foreign invaders into the deeper, more delicate structures of the respiratory system, such as our lungs and sinuses, and is another common way that our healing systems safeguard our health.

In addition to sneezing, most people, including doctors, confuse many other common healing responses with symptoms of a disease. These responses include the following:

- *Coughing.* Also considered a symptom of a respiratory illness or condition, coughing is a definitive response from your healing system to expel unwanted debris and invading microorganisms that have penetrated deeper into the respiratory system and are threatening to cause damage to your lungs. In medical circles, a good cough is known as a productive cough in that it successfully brings up phlegm, mucous, microorganisms, and infectious debris, which effectively clears the airways and makes for easier breathing. Coughing can be powerful; the speed at which foreign particles and debris exit the lungs with a cough has been clocked at approximately 660 mph, about the speed of an F4 Phantom fighter aircraft.

■ *Diarrhea.* Usually considered a symptom of an intestinal disease, diarrhea is a healing response that your body uses to eliminate toxins and contaminated material from your colon and large intestines. Diarrhea is fast and efficient, and it helps to flush out what is irritating or offending your intestinal tract. A number of potentially serious intestinal diseases or problems can be eliminated this way. Suppressing diarrhea through artificial medications can be dangerous, and doing so often backfires. When you clog up your body's natural eliminative processes through the suppression of diarrhea, harmful microorganisms have nowhere to go but further inside your body, where they can invade your liver or bloodstream and cause more serious illness. Of course, there are times when too much fluid and electrolyte loss from diarrhea may require medical intervention. However, by seeing diarrhea as a response of your healing system, and seeking out ways to cooperate with that system, you can often make simple, natural adjustments to restore balance and health to your body. These may include drinking more fluids, avoiding irritating foods and substances, and managing stress, which can be harmful to your intestines and digestive system. (We will look more closely at these factors in the chapters that follow.)

■ *Fainting.* Fainting occurs when a person temporarily loses consciousness and falls down. The causes of fainting can range from serious to benign, but the loss of consciousness is usually due to of a lack of blood flow to the head and brain. Falling down while fainting represents a compensatory response from your body's healing system. When the body has fallen and lies flat on the ground in a horizontal position, blood flow and oxygen to the brain increase, which can often restore consciousness. Most instances of fainting are totally benign, especially if no serious underlying diseases or conditions exist. However, there are occasions when serious underlying disease is present, and you will need to be brought to the hospital and treated. However, the correct treatment is to deal with the underlying causes that precipitated the fainting, not just with the fainting itself.

■ *Fever.* Commonly associated with an infection, fever is your healing system's way of heating your body up to kill offending organisms, most of which are extremely temperature sensitive and cannot tolerate excessive heat. Additionally, fever induces sweating, which helps the body eliminate toxins more rapidly. Learning to work with a fever through continuous rehydration (drinking plenty of water), rather than suppressing a fever with artificial medications, will support your healing system and result in a faster, more thorough healing response. Even at times when medical suppression of a fever may be necessary, fluid intake should be encouraged. With any fever, it is prudent to look for the underlying causes of the fever and to treat these, not just suppress the fever. Doing this works with your healing system to help restore health and balance to your body.

■ *Nausea.* Nausea occurs in the small intestines and stomach, and it is a specific response from your healing system that protects your body from more food entering into it. When you feel nauseous, you have lost your appetite for food. Your healing system does this when your body needs to limit solid food intake. Nausea occurs when you have a high fever and are in need of lots of fluids, or when you have a stomach virus or an ulcer, and solid foods would make these conditions worse. Nausea also helps to conserve energy and frees blood flow from the digestive tract so it can be rerouted to other areas of the body that have a greater immediate need for healing energy.

■ *Pus.* Your body's healing system, working with your immune system, produces pus, an unpleasant, smelly, yellowish substance, to help eliminate foreign material, both large and small. Pus commonly occurs with infection. In the case of a splinter or foreign body in the skin, your healing system will form a pus pocket to wall off the splinter, separating it from the rest of your body. Your healing system will attempt to digest and dissolve the splinter or foreign object; if this proves difficult, it will try to push the splinter out of the skin. In addition to fluids secreted to flush out microorganisms and foreign debris, pus contains white blood cells and digestive enzymes that break down and digest foreign material. In the case of a bacterial infection in any part of the body, the pus produced will attempt to kill off and digest the bacteria while it flushes out the infection.

- *Runny nose and nasal congestion.* Usually considered symptoms of the common cold or allergies, a runny nose and nasal congestion are actually specific responses from your body's healing system. The increased secretions, mucous, phlegm, and congestion are your healing system's way of attempting to flush out any offending organisms or foreign particles that may have invaded the entrance to your respiratory system. Although attempting to suppress these healing responses with nasal decongestants and other drugs gives temporary relief, doing so often backfires; it can prolong an illness and even make things worse. Because the pharmaceutical agents tend to dry up the secretions to eliminate symptoms, they work against the natural processes of your body's healing system to eliminate harmful substances.

- *Swelling and redness.* The first visible signs at the site of any injury, trauma, or infection in the body, swelling and redness, too, are specific responses of your healing system. Whether caused by a bruise, a contusion, a sprain, a fracture, or an infection, swelling is the result of increased fluids from the lymphatic system, leaky blood vessels, and other soft tissues. The fluid helps immobilize the site and serves as a shock absorber to prevent further injury to the area. Redness, known as inflammation, is often accompanied by pain and represents increased blood flow to the area. Inflammation is a complex response from your healing system, working with your immune system, to bring important cells and powerful chemicals to the injured area to help remove toxins, repair damaged tissues, and speed healing.

- *Tearing of the eyes.* Tearing is a specific healing response similar to what occurs in a runny nose. Tearing helps to flush foreign material or microorganisms out of the delicate and sensitive surfaces of the eyes. Sometimes, when infection or irritation is extreme, the eyes will remain glued shut because the tears and secretions have dried up. Keeping the eyelids glued shut is a further attempt of the healing system to protect the eyes from additional injury or damage.

■ *Vomiting.* Vomiting is a protective mechanism that your healing system uses to eliminate contaminated or noxious material that has somehow entered into your stomach and small intestines. Vomiting is a fast, efficient, and powerful way for your body to rid itself of toxins or other harmful substances. After you have eaten contaminated food, as in food poisoning, vomiting will occur to expel infectious organisms as well as unwanted food and toxins. People usually report feeling much better after they have vomited in these instances. If you have overeaten, eaten foods that are too rich, or drunk too much coffee or alcohol, which act as intestinal irritants and toxins when they're taken in excess, vomiting will occur to clean out and reduce the burden on the digestive system and body.

Although initially you may think these responses are associated only with the individual systems within the body, such as coughing and the respiratory system, or vomiting and the gastrointestinal system, remember that it is the healing system's presence within and its supervisory role over these systems that actually causes these responses. Keep in mind that the healing system is not a separate anatomical system. It is a functional, energetic, intelligent system that permeates every single system in your body.

As you read the rest of this book, think about your body, your bodily sensations, and any changes that are occurring in your body as well-measured responses produced by your body's healing system. Think of them as responses that are intended to correct imbalances and help you maintain your natural state of health, rather than symptoms of disease. Shift your awareness away from your symptoms, your discomfort, and your thoughts of an illness or allergy, even if these are real problems for you. Instead, trust that your healing system is making necessary physiological adjustments to correct imbalances and restore your body to its natural state of health.

I realize this perspective may be a radical departure from how you currently view your body and your health; however, learning to do this will make a significant difference in your health. If you can focus less on disease and more on health, less on what is wrong with your body, and more on what is functioning properly; if you can turn your attention away from the fear of external causes of disease and agents of disease that lie beyond your control, and instead look with confidence to the hidden treasure chest of healing resources that lies within your very own body, you will be able to reap the benefits of superior health. If you can learn to recognize the many ways your healing system responds to challenges, your dependence on drugs and doctors will be lessened, and the quality of your life will be vastly improved.

Benefits of Recognizing Your Healing System's Responses

You will gain a great deal by recognizing the responses of your healing system. Your healing system

- Empowers you to discover and make use of the vast supply of healing resources that lie within your own body.

- Directs your energies and efforts within your own body and away from blaming your discomfort or disease on external causes and forces beyond your control, which can be disempowering.

- Shifts your focus away from fear-based thinking that can be harmful to your health and well-being.

- Empowers you to take greater responsibility for your life, and helps you understand the connection between your own actions and thoughts, including your diet and lifestyle, and your health.

- Lessens your dependence on doctors, drugs, and external agents of treatment.

- Improves your confidence in your body's ability to remain healthy and heal itself.

- Helps in planning the treatment and healing of any health problem you might face.

You can see that the benefits of recognizing the power of your remarkable healing system and working with it will have a huge, positive impact on your health and your life.

Note: As you are learning this new way of thinking about your body, do not neglect to see your doctor if any physical discomfort or pain increases or does not go away on its own. Your doctor can be a valuable aid and support for your healing system.

Clinical Evidence of Your Healing System at Work

We've already looked at healing responses in general, and we've seen several different examples of the healing system at work to help heal superficial injuries. Now let's move deeper inside the body as we continue to examine the evidence that clearly demonstrates that your body has a healing system that keeps you alive and healthy. In each of the situations that follow, remember that the healing system is the essential element in the healing process and that, without it, healing would not occur.

Your Healing System and Fractures: Sam's Story

Sam was a 34-year-old senior staff sergeant with 15 years' experience as a veteran paratrooper and combat controller in the United States Air Force. During a routine training mission, he was required to jump from an altitude of 10,000 feet at nighttime over remote jungle terrain. Sam got caught up in a tree as he was landing and broke his ankle in several places. The bone pierced through the skin, making it a compound fracture. This type of injury has a high rate of infection and is notoriously difficult to treat. Infection that sets into the bones is known as *osteomyelitis*, a serious condition that is difficult to eradicate and that complicates the healing system's ability to knit the bones together to heal a fracture.

Sam was taken by airplane back to the Regional Medical Center in the Philippines, where I was required to follow his case to see whether he would ever be able to resume his career duties again. For all intents and purposes, it looked as if his military career was over.

Sam was hospitalized repeatedly, placed on numerous antibiotics, and operated on 11 times over a two-and-one-half-year period, in attempts to knit his bones together. During this period, he wore a cast almost continuously and was never able to walk on his own, relying instead solely on crutches. He underwent numerous painful scrapings and bone grafts in an attempt to clean the surfaces of the bones from infection while the doctors were trying to join the bones together. During these operations, numerous plates and screws were also attached to his bones.

At one point, when it looked as if the fracture might heal, Sam's cast was removed, and he was told he could participate in light sports. A week later, while he was fielding a grounder during a friendly squadron softball game, Sam's ankle snapped and broke in two pieces as his foot bent out at a 90-degree angle. After this, it was back to the operating room for him, with more scraping, more metal plates and screws, another cast, and more crutches.

After two and one-half years, Sam was not only in jeopardy of losing his job and being medically discharged from the Air Force, he was also being considered for a foot amputation. He consulted with the prosthetic specialist, who began fitting him for a prosthetic (artificial) foot in anticipation of the upcoming operation. This was a frightening proposition for such an active and previously healthy young man.

Back home in the U.S., a brilliant orthopedic surgeon named Robert Becker had invented an electrical bone stimulator to aid the healing system in cases of stubborn-healing fractures. Sam faced the prospect of either having his foot amputated, or having this tiny, electronic device, still in the experimental stages, temporarily implanted next to the fracture site in his ankle. He chose the new device, hoping against hope that it would work.

Several months later, Sam was back with a clean bill of health, jumping out of airplanes. His bones had mended together with the help of a device that worked with the healing system. Dr. Becker knew that, given half a chance, the body's healing system could take over and finish the job. As the famous physician of ancient times, Galen (129–199 AD), once said, "The physician is only nature's assistant."

A fractured bone is not a laughing matter, and it can be extremely painful and disabling. However, because of your healing system, even the largest bone in your body, your femur, under normal circumstances takes only six weeks to completely heal. Even if a fracture is displaced and the broken bones are not perfectly lined up, in most cases, your healing system can knit the bones together and realign them perfectly, so that when the healing has finished, there is little or no evidence that a fracture ever occurred. Even when fractures are complicated, and bones are totally displaced and out of alignment, and metal plates and screws are required to hold the bones together, your healing system can fuse them into one solid form. Without your healing system, fractures would be impossible to heal.

Whether or not a cast or splint is placed around the fracture site, if a fractured bone is allowed to rest and remain immobile, bone remodeling, initiated by your healing system, begins immediately after a fracture has occurred. Bone remodeling, when seen under the microscope, is one of life's true miracles. Tiny cells in the bone matrix, known as *osteoclasts*, digest the bone and release calcium into the bloodstream, while other cells, known as *osteoblasts*, act like civil engineers erecting a new suspension bridge and use the blood-calcium stores to deposit new bone at the fracture site. These deposits facilitate the process of knitting the bone back together again. No modern technological invention, surgical procedure, or synthetic drug can replace your healing system as it performs the important work of repairing a fracture. The natural healing of a fractured bone after it is healed is so effective that the fracture site is often stronger than the surrounding normal bone tissue.

Your Healing System and the Heart: Verne's Story

Verne's heart disease was discovered when he had his first heart attack in the emergency room at the age of 69. He had another attack about a year later. Over the course of the next several years, he was placed on numerous medications while he underwent several procedures, known as *angioplasties*, to unclog his arteries and slow the progression of his disease. But these methods were only temporarily successful. Over time, Verne's heart disease grew worse. He was plagued with constant chest pain, which increased when he walked up stairs or whenever he became angry or upset. It was quite scary.

When I met Verne, his heart disease had progressed to desperate proportions, and his doctors were recommending bypass surgery as the only way to keep him from dying. Even then, because of his advanced condition, they said his prognosis did not look good, and the bypass operation would only buy him a couple of extra years, at best. Verne was not too keen on having his chest cracked open, and by sheer persistence and determination, he was able to enroll in Dr. Dean Ornish's first experimental research study group to investigate whether or not heart disease could be reversed without drugs or surgery.

Dr. Ornish's program is based on the now-proven premise that if you can remove the obstacles to your body's natural healing processes, and work with your healing system, even severe heart disease can be healed. Dr. Ornish's program is simple and uncomplicated, and it consists of comprehensive lifestyle changes that include a healthy diet, exercise, stress management, and group support. Of course, at the time of his first study, these ideas and methods were considered radical by conventional medical standards. Even to this day, the thought of reversing heart disease is difficult to digest for those steeped in the "old school" ways of thinking about medicine and the treatment of disease.

Verne took to the program enthusiastically, and within several weeks his chest pain went away as his breathing became easier. He began to have more energy and at the same time felt more relaxed. His stress and anger diminished. Gradually, one by one, the 13 different heart medicines he was taking were reduced until he was down to one-half of a baby aspirin, every other day.

Today, at the age of 87, Verne is totally free of heart disease. All of his medical tests—*positron emission tomography* (PET) scans and *coronary angiograms*—have documented complete reversal of his condition. He hikes in alpine altitudes and travels the world extensively with his wife, teaching yoga and lecturing to senior citizens on the merits of the Ornish program and the body's natural ability to heal itself.

Although heart disease is still the number-one killer in the entire Western world, even this deadly condition can be reversed and healed when you learn to cooperate with your healing system, as Verne did, by correcting the unhealthy underlying factors that are causing blockages in the coronary arteries. As is possible for you, Verne discovered the tremendous healing resources within his own body, and, by adopting a healthier lifestyle, he became a partner in his own healing process. Thanks to the groundbreaking work of Dr. Ornish, we now know that by learning to listen to the body and working with its healing system, people can reverse even the most advanced cases of heart disease.

As a direct result of Dr. Ornish's work, we now know that the healing system can stimulate the growth of new blood vessels to the heart when its current blood supply is threatened. This process is known as *neovascularization* or *collaterization*. The new arteries can effectively bypass the old blockage, ensuring a continuous, uninterrupted flow of blood to the heart's muscles. The process can prevent heart attacks, and it is how you can literally grow your own coronary artery bypass, without having to go through an operation.

Even if you have suffered a heart attack, and the heart's muscle cells seem to have died, new evidence has demonstrated that through your miraculous healing system, and restoring blood flow to these heart muscle cells within a reasonable period of time, they can miraculously come back to life. The medical term for this new discovery, wherein heart tissue that is presumed dead can come back to life when circulation is re-established, is *hibernating myocardium*—like the sleeping bear who reappears when winter is over.

Your Healing System and High Blood Pressure: Mike's Story

Mike was a flight engineer in the Air Force, where he had served for 20 years. He had flown in Vietnam, was married with three children, and loved his job. However, because he had been recently diagnosed with high blood pressure, he was in danger of losing his job and possibly being kicked out of the Air Force. To prevent this from happening, he lost 25 pounds over six months by eating a low-fat diet and running every day for 30 minutes. However, his blood pressure still did not come down. To complicate things further, because of his flying status, he wasn't able to take medications of any kind. I was an Air Force flight surgeon at the time, and he came to me seeking help.

After I reviewed his records and his efforts to lower his blood pressure by losing weight through diet and exercise, I asked Mike whether he was under stress of any kind. He quickly responded with a confident and adamant "No!" This response let me know immediately that I might be in for a difficult case because I had yet to meet someone in the military who wasn't under a certain degree of stress. Additionally, I later found out that Mike was having some troubles with his marriage, which were causing even more stress. In spite of his finest efforts to lower his blood pressure through diet and exercise, stress was contributing to his continued high blood pressure.

After several meetings and long discussions, during which I explained the mechanisms of how prolonged stress can cause high blood pressure, Mike was finally able to own up to the stress in his life. He then consented to learning and practicing the simple, basic stress-management techniques (see Chapter 6) I recommended, which I thought would activate his healing system and lower his blood pressure.

After only six weeks, Mike's blood pressure returned to normal and remained there for the rest of his career. By removing the unhealthy factors that were responsible for creating the high blood pressure, particularly the extreme stress in his life, Mike's healing system could easily and effortlessly restore his body to its natural state of health. Of course, he still continues his healthy lifestyle, including a low-fat diet, and 30 minutes of exercise and 15 minutes of stress management each day.

As you can see, one of the most significant underlying factors in high blood pressure is stress, which can create significant imbalance in the body's internal environment. Dr. Herbert Benson, associate professor of medicine at Harvard Medical School and chief of the Division of Behavioral Medicine at the New England Deaconess Hospital, has conducted numerous studies on the benefits of stress management in lowering high blood pressure. By practicing simple yet powerful stress-management techniques similar to those taught by Dr. Benson (see Chapter 6), you can help your healing system restore your blood pressure to normal levels.

High blood pressure, or *hypertension*, is known as "the silent killer" because it can lead to more serious, and sometimes deadly, conditions such as heart disease and stroke. Although many medications are currently available for managing high blood pressure, they often have side effects, and, unfortunately, none of them can cure the problem. Once patients begin taking these medications, getting off them is difficult, and many people will be on two or three of them just to manage their high blood pressure.

Just as with heart disease, new evidence is proving that the healing system can reverse and heal high blood pressure once the underlying causes of the disease are addressed and such simple, natural methods as diet, exercise, and stress management are properly implemented. There is no mystery to this malady; the mechanisms for healing high blood pressure are not complex or difficult to understand. As with other diseases, removing the harmful causes of the disease allows the healing system to restore the body to its natural state of health.

Your Healing System and Stroke: Dean's Story

Dean was a young doctor with a heavy load on his heart. Not only was he physically overweight, but he was financially burdened by thousands of dollars of outstanding student loans and a family to support. Working more than 100 hours each week, sleep-deprived, eating high-fat junk food, getting no exercise, having no fun, and constantly fighting with his wife from the stress ended up costing Dean his health.

Dean was suffering from chronic high blood pressure, for which he was treating himself with the drug samples that the pharmaceutical representatives gave him. He was erratic in monitoring his blood pressure, and he didn't want his colleagues to know about his condition. At the young age of 32 years, Dean suffered a massive stroke that left him paralyzed in his right leg and arm. He was in the hospital for many weeks, and he underwent extensive physical therapy and rehabilitation to learn how to move his arm and walk again. He was extremely depressed during the therapy and felt as if he had nothing left to live for.

During this low period of Dean's life, he came across a man who also had had a stroke. But this man had completely recovered and gone on to enjoy greater health than ever before by completely revamping his diet and lifestyle, and learning how to manage his stress through simple yet effective stress-management methods. With his back up against the wall, on disability, and unable to practice his trade, Dean decided to give these methods a try.

He immediately shifted his diet to one that was low fat and consisted mostly of fruits, vegetables, grains, and other whole foods. He started exercising regularly, and he began practicing stress management along with gentle yoga. Even though he didn't consider himself a religious person, he also began to pray regularly to help relax and calm his mind.

His blood pressure slowly normalized, and he was gradually able to get off all his medications. As his health steadily improved over the next two years, he began to feel better than ever before. He eventually returned to active medical practice, and went on to write many best-selling books about his experiences. Because he learned to adopt a healthier lifestyle and incorporate methods that were in harmony with his body's healing system, Dean was able to completely reverse the effects of his stroke and live a far healthier, more active, and more fulfilling life than before.

Stroke is a serious condition usually caused by either a hemorrhage or a blood clot in the brain. It also can occur as a result of chronic high blood pressure or other circulatory disturbances. Stroke can be fatal. When it's less severe, it can cause paralysis of the extremities, most often on one side of the body, but it can also cause paralysis of the facial muscles, and affect speech, hearing, eyesight, and the ability to swallow.

Although stroke can be prevented by addressing its underlying causes, even after it occurs, the healing system can often miraculously restore the body to its natural state of health. Numerous studies have documented that when one side of the brain is damaged, if the individual receives proper training and makes a sincere effort, the body's healing system can facilitate the transfer of information from the damaged side to the healthy side of the brain to restore normal function to once-paralyzed limbs and muscles.

Your Healing System and Diabetes: Eric's Story

Eric was a 65-year-old, active man with advanced heart disease complicated by longstanding diabetes. For the past 20 years, he injected himself with insulin daily to control his high blood sugar. His usual daily dose of insulin was 45 units, not a small amount. If he didn't use this amount, his blood sugar would skyrocket to dangerous levels.

When Eric attended a one-week retreat for heart patients (many of whom also had diabetes), he was advised that, because of the changes in diet and exercise, and the stress-management program that would be part of the retreat, he would need to cut his daily insulin dose in half, to make sure that he didn't end up in a coma from too-low blood sugar. He was also advised to monitor his own blood sugars six times a day with a self-administered kit, to make sure they stayed at the proper level.

I was his personal physician during this period, and so Eric reported to me daily. On day one, as instructed, he cut his insulin dosage to 22 units. His blood sugar remained normal. On day two, he cut his insulin in half again, to 11 units, and his blood sugar again remained normal. On day three, he halved his insulin again, and he still had normal blood sugar. As word got out about Eric's dramatic fall in insulin requirements, the staff became nervous and told Eric not to cut down on his insulin so fast. He responded that he was only following the dosages for what he monitored his blood sugar to be, and that they continued to stay normal. By day seven, Eric was completely off insulin. He has remained off insulin to this day, six years later, while his blood sugar continues to stay normal. He has stuck to his diet and exercise and he has continued to practice stress management. He reports his health to be better than ever.

Because he learned to cooperate with his body's healing system before it was too late, Eric was able to demonstrate what most medical experts previously thought to be impossible—he was able to get off insulin (while keeping his blood sugar values normal), something that he had depended on daily for more than 20 years.

Eric's case demonstrates that, once again, even after many years of living with such a chronic, deadly disease as diabetes, the healing system can reverse and heal such conditions. When you recognize that your body has a healing system, and that by instituting simple, natural methods that cooperate with it, your body can restore its natural state of health.

Your Healing System and Arthritis: The Story of Helen's Mother

Helen worked in my medical office and always wore a smile. Her mother, now in her late seventies and the mother of eight children, had developed a severe form of osteoarthritis in her right knee. This situation was very unsettling to her because until the previous six months, she had always walked at least one to two miles a day, and she had looked forward to this exercise time. After consulting with several doctors, she was told the only treatment that would help her would be knee-replacement surgery.

Her daughter Helen understood that sometimes I took a different approach to medicine, and she insisted that her mother see me. When I saw her mother's reports, and the X-rays, I had to agree that things did not look good for her. However, I did prescribe a simple technique that worked with the healing system; the technique improved the flow of synovial fluid inside of the knee and helped to restore mobility to the knee joint. Over the years, I have relied on this technique in my practice, and I have seen the successful rehabilitation of patients;

even those with advanced cases of arthritis improve significantly. If patients practice diligently and patiently over several months, this technique can restore joint function and promote healing in the knee.

Because the technique is so simple, and because it requires active patient participation over an extended period, I took pains to explain to Helen's mother the underlying principles of the practice to help guarantee her adherence to it. When I was satisfied that she understood how the technique worked and why it was important not to look for results right away, I made her promise me that she would practice it faithfully, regularly, and carefully for six to eight months. She agreed.

Within two weeks, Helen's mother noticed significant diminishment of pain and improved function. After one month, she began walking again. After six months, she was pain-free and walking three to four miles a day, dancing like a teenager, and praising me to the moon. To this day, seven years later, she has not missed her daily walks and has remained pain-free. No knee replacement was ever required.

There are many forms of arthritis, including *osteoarthritis*, *rheumatoid arthritis*, *gouty arthritis*, and *psoriatic arthritis*, which have as their common denominator the destruction of the joint surfaces, with increased pain and debility. Conventional medicine treats these diseases with powerful suppressive medications (many with unsatisfactory side effects), and the possibility of a joint-replacement operation, but new evidence reveals that by understanding and addressing the underlying factors that determine joint health, as in Helen's mother's case, your healing system can heal and reverse arthritis.

Your Healing System and Intestinal Diseases: Bob's Story

Bob was a pleasant, good-looking construction worker in his early twenties, with a wife and two kids. He loved baseball and was a member of an amateur league. By all outer appearances, Bob seemed completely healthy; however, if you could look inside of his intestines, you would know that he was in pain and suffering from a severe case of Crohn's disease. When I met him, Bob was a patient in the hospital in which I worked, and he was scheduled for surgery as soon as there was an opening in the operating-room schedule. He was taking high doses of Prednisone and other strong medications to control his symptoms, which included abdominal pain, weight loss, diarrhea, weakness, fatigue, and nausea.

One day, when I was making rounds at mealtime, I noticed that the food Bob was being served was rather hard to chew, rough in texture, and difficult to digest. This food just didn't seem right for someone with his condition, and because I couldn't discount the possible role that his poor diet might be playing in that condition, I asked whether his pain and related symptoms increased after he ate. He confirmed my suspicions by telling me they were definitely worse after he ate. He also told me his condition worsened when he was upset or under stress. This information did not surprise me. I then asked whether his doctor had ever talked to him about his diet or suggested special foods for his condition, or suggested relaxation or stress management. He replied, "No."

I asked Bob whether he would be willing to go on a special diet for a few days, a diet that I believed would improve his condition. I suggested clear liquids, including water, gentle soup broths, juices, herbal teas, and gelatin, and nothing solid. I told him why, explaining the mechanisms of digestion in relation to his disease. He agreed. I also showed him some simple stress-management practices, including gentle relaxation breathing to do, which would calm the nerves in his intestines.

Every day, I checked on Bob to see how he was doing. Each day, he reported remarkable improvement. After just three days, he was completely symptom free. He couldn't believe that something so simple as his diet and learning how to relax could take away the incredible pain and suffering he had been going through for the past seven years with this chronic intestinal condition. After removal of the harmful factors that created imbalance and disorder in his intestines, Bob's healing system was able to restore his body to its natural state of health.

Numerous intestinal diseases, such as *esophageal reflux, gastritis, peptic ulcer disease, irritable bowel syndrome, Crohn's disease, ulcerative colitis*, and *diverticulitis* wreak havoc on millions of people. Many of these conditions are treated with strong medications or surgical procedures, and they may be serious enough to cause death or serve as precursors to other complications, including cancer, which can be deadly. Colon cancer alone is one of the most common deadly killers in the West.

In my experience, using strong medications to attack these diseases as if they were foreign entities accomplishes temporary results at best and does nothing to address the underlying factors contributing to these diseases. Alternatively, learning to work with the healing system, as Bob did, even though doing this may take longer, also creates longer-lasting results. Working with your healing system by implementing simple, natural methods such as proper nutrition and stress management, along with other modalities that support and cooperate with your healing system, can often heal even serious, long-standing intestinal diseases.

Your Healing System and Middle-Ear Infections: Jesse's Story

Jesse was 4 years old when his parents took him to an ear specialist to consult about the possibility of having tubes surgically implanted in his ears. He had been on antibiotics almost continuously since he was 15 months old, and his ear infections were now chronic. In preschool, his teachers complained that he didn't respond to their verbal commands, and they were concerned about permanent hearing loss. After reading about the possible effects of not having the operation, which included permanent hearing loss, Jesse's parents went home thinking surgery was their only option.

When Jesse's father went for his regular chiropractic adjustment the next day, he happened to mention Jesse's situation to his chiropractor. The chiropractor told him that by adjusting the spine and removing dairy from the diets of affected children, he and many of his colleagues had reported significant successes in children with conditions similar to Jesse's. Many medical doctors, including the well-known author Dr. Andrew Weil, were now also recommending this treatment.

After postponing the conventional tube surgery, Jesse's parents brought him to the chiropractor for treatment. He gently pressed on Jesse's spine, and he educated Jesse's parents about good posture and simple breathing techniques. They also began him on the new diet that promised to decrease the amount of mucous and phlegm in the respiratory system and eustachian tubes of the ears. The chiropractic adjustments continued once a month for nine months.

Two years later, Jesse came into my office. His parents told me he hadn't had a problem with his ears since they saw the ear specialist two years earlier. Furthermore, his hearing was perfect.

Middle-ear infections are extremely common in young children and can be a nightmare for a parent. Sleepless nights, painful screaming, multiple prescriptions for antibiotics, with the eventual placement of tubes that puncture the eardrum and middle-ear chamber, along with the possibility of permanent hearing loss, are not uncommon.

When I first heard about chiropractic adjustments for middle-ear problems, I was skeptical. However, over the years, I have seen enough positive results to know that these treatments often work. Jesse's case is just one example. As remote as the connection might seem, the spinal adjustments help to improve posture and breathing, and they possibly improve the lymphatic drainage of the middle ear.

Because your healing system integrates the function of all the systems in your body, to understand and work with it requires an expanded view of how the various parts of your body are interconnected. Any healing modality or treatment that supports and cooperates with the healing system by addressing and removing the underlying factors of a disease, such as the unusual treatment just described for middle-ear problems, can result in the healing of conditions that appear to have no cure other than surgery. There is no miracle in the restoration of health and healing from any disease once you understand that your body has a healing system—and that healing is its normal, ordinary, everyday job.

Your Healing System and Multiple Sclerosis: Rachelle's Story

Rachelle was a young housewife with three children. She had been diagnosed with a severe, rapidly progressive form of *multiple sclerosis (MS)* after experiencing symptoms of loss of coordination, problems with balance, and visual disturbances. She was placed on strong, suppressive medications and referred to a specialty clinic for patients with multiple sclerosis. She was given a wheelchair and told to get used to it, because soon this would be what she would be spending the rest of her life in.

When Rachelle opened the door to the specialty clinic, she peered inside and saw hundreds of other MS patients, all in wheelchairs, and all with a look of resignation on their faces. At that moment, she had a premonition that this place would only strengthen her disease. Refusing to give up hope of overcoming her affliction, she fled the scene immediately. That moment marked the beginning of her healing journey.

Against her doctor's advice, Rachelle underwent a series of acupuncture treatments in which she experienced temporary improvement. To see her symptoms go away, even if only briefly, was all the hope she needed to continue to fight to regain her health. She decided to become an active participant in her treatment by reading, researching, and visiting doctors and healers from a wide range of alternative and complementary disciplines and traditions. She began practicing gentle yoga and took a keen interest in her thoughts and attitudes while studying the effect they had on her body. She learned that her mind and her attitude played a key role in the health of her body. She began to take better care of her nourishment, not only with her food, but also with her thoughts. She saw that loving thoughts nourished her body, whereas thoughts borne of low self-esteem and self-hatred were harmful to her body.

After 11 grueling years, Rachelle finally overcame her affliction and was declared disease free. Her classic book, *Who Said So?: A Woman's Fascinating Journey of Self Discovery and Triumph over Multiple Sclerosis*, (Rachelle Breslow, Celestial Arts, 1991) is one of the most compelling stories and critical pieces of evidence for the healing system that I have ever come across. By discovering her healing system, and learning to discard unhealthy habits and thought patterns that served as obstacles to its performance, Rachelle was able to completely reverse and heal from a disease still considered "incurable" by most so-called health experts!

Your Healing System and Kidney Stones: James' Story

James was a captain in the U.S. Air Force and a senior C-130 pilot with the 1st SOS (Special Operations Squadron) reconnaissance squadron based out of the Philippines at Clark Air Base, where I was also stationed as a flight surgeon at the USAF Regional Medical Center in the Department of Aerospace Medicine.

One day, while he was flying a low-altitude mission on a hot day over the jungles of Thailand, James began to feel a terrible pain in his back, right flank, and groin that seemed to come and go in waves. As the pain radiated from his back to his groin area, becoming stronger and more intense with each wave, it crescendoed to a steady 10 out of 10 on the Richter scale of pain and soon became unbearable. The pain became so excruciating that James, now perspiring profusely, was forced to turn over all the controls of his aircraft to the copilot while he scrambled to lie down in the back. His copilot requested clearance for an emergency landing.

After his copilot landed the plane, James was met by an ambulance that took him to the nearest hospital in Bangkok. In the hospital, he was given intravenous pain medications. He was then immediately evacuated by air ambulance and transferred to the USAF Regional Medical Center in the Philippines, where I worked.

After several hours in the emergency department of our large hospital, and numerous examinations, including X-rays, blood tests, and urine tests, James was told he had a kidney stone. Kidney stones occur as blockages in the kidneys or ureters, and they can be one of the most painful conditions ever to experience. Surgery for kidney stones is not uncommon because they can be life threatening, especially if they are large enough.

Several days later, while James was still in the hospital, after he had received voluminous amounts of intravenous fluids and pain medications, he passed a single, solitary kidney stone. He was uneventfully discharged from the hospital after a few days. At this point, everything looked good.

On follow-up examinations, however, while he was an outpatient, James' urine tests showed elevated urinary calcium, which persisted for days and weeks, and which alarmed his specialists. They suspected an underlying metabolic problem, which could lead to another kidney stone, and despite James' insistence that he felt fine and was ready to return to flying, they would not allow him back in the cockpit. They contended that he was a threat to his and others' flying safety. In the aerospace industry, and in the language of the U.S. Air Force, according to strict flight-safety policies, James was indefinitely "grounded." This meant that his flying career, within both the military and civilian worlds, was essentially over.

I believed in the intelligence and power of James' healing system, and I felt strongly that once the obstacles to its performance were removed, his healing system could correct the situation. I was convinced that his high urinary calcium was the result of the residual calcium oxalate "sand," which consisted of ultra-fine particles left over from the stone that had recently passed. This conviction was based on the information I received while I was performing a detailed medical history of the events leading up to his kidney-stone incident. Just days before the incident, James had had diarrhea, and he had become severely dehydrated at the time he was flying. While flying, he also became severely overheated in his bulky flight suit and stuffy cockpit, a condition made worse by Thailand's heat. He had also been under significant stress for six months related to an illness in the family. All of these factors predisposed him to a kidney stone.

I encouraged James to drink as much water as he could, to flush out the residual sand that I felt was responsible for his elevated urine calcium. As it turned out, simple water was all his healing system needed to reverse the dangerously high levels of calcium in his body.

Thanks to James' healing system, and his ability to cooperate with it by drinking lots of fluids, abstaining from alcohol and caffeine, and avoiding and managing his stress, about six months from the day of his kidney-stone episode, his urine calcium returned to normal, and he was permanently restored to flying status without any medications and without any waiver.

James has been flying as a senior pilot for Delta Airlines now for more than 15 years. He surfs, has three beautiful children, and hasn't missed a day of flying due to illness during this entire period. He likes to drink water, as you can imagine, and to date has never had an inkling of the kidney stone problems that almost ended his career.

Your Healing System and Cancer: Tony's Story

Tony wears his shaven head proudly, as a battlefield trophy and reminder of his successful victory over Hodgkin's disease, a malignant cancer of the lymph system, which had him down and out for several years.

Tony looks good with his shaven head and mustache. Even though he could grow his hair back if he wanted to, he prefers the look of a monk-warrior. He is in great shape, running four to five miles each day, and working full time in the automotive department of a major, national-chain department store. Although he has an air of determination about him, at the same time, he's almost always in a cheerful mood, with a little twinkle in his eyes. He is a glowing, vibrant, magnetic person. Here's a man who knows the gift of life and doesn't waste a single second feeling sorry for himself or entertaining negative thinking, in spite of all he's been through.

When I asked Tony where he thought his cancer came from, and to what he attributed his healing, the answers were simple and straightforward. "Doc," he said, "I was under a lot of stress just prior to my diagnosis. I was working too hard and worrying too much. I wasn't having fun, and I was way too serious. I never rested, and everything seemed to get to me. I had a lot of anger that I couldn't release. I felt all bottled up inside. My diet was bad. I wasn't taking good care of myself, and I knew it.

"When I received my diagnosis, I felt that it was a wake-up call," Tony continued. "In a way, it gave me an excuse to be a little selfish again and focus on the needs of my body. I changed my attitude and my ways and decided that I would turn all my troubles over to a higher power. I started taking the time to eat right, exercise, and take care of myself because I realized it was up to me.

"When I shifted gears, it's amazing how my body responded," Tony added. "While my doctors were surprised, I was not the least bit shocked over my complete reversal of cancer. I really feel it was I who brought on my own cancer, and it was I who got me out of that mess by becoming a little more aware of how my attitude, thinking, and behaviors were affecting my body. The entire process of getting ill and then being healed was completely logical to me."

When people start to realize the amazing power of their own healing systems, and start taking responsibility for their own health, as Tony did, they often become empowered to take the necessary steps to help their bodies heal. Although cancer has been and continues to be one of the most feared diseases of modern times, even cancer cannot stand up to the miraculous powers of your healing system once you learn how to remove the obstacles that interfere with its functioning. As you become more aware of the many ways your healing system strives to keep your body healthy, you will discover many more ways to support and cooperate with it to restore your health.

When you are dealing with any major, life-threatening illness and rallying your healing system to come to your support, understanding the obstacles that are interfering with the performance and function of your healing system is imperative. Some of these obstacles are obvious, such as habitual ingestion of toxic substances, poor diet, stress, and lack of exercise; others are more subtle, such as unhealthy thinking and holding onto anger. Because much unhealthy thinking and behavior is habitual and unconscious, you must first become aware of these unhealthy patterns before you can change them. As we will explore a little later in the book, you will see how your mind exerts a powerful influence on your body's healing system, and what you can do to make the mind an ally in your healing.

Closing Thoughts on Your Healing System in Action

Your body knows how to heal itself because it has a remarkably efficient and intelligent healing system. You can think of your amazing healing system as the field marshal who commands the forces of healing within your body, directing the various elements to maintain your natural state of health. I could have presented many more cases here, but it is clear from the evidence presented so far that you have a healing system that is capable of healing your body from a multitude of afflictions, even when these afflictions have become advanced and things appear pretty hopeless. As long as you are alive, you have healing power.

It is important to remember that, even though the variety of diseases and the number of afflictions you may potentially suffer from on this earth appear vast and staggering, the many ways that your healing system can heal you and keep your body healthy are, by far, infinitely greater.

To understand more thoroughly how your healing system works, and what you can do to work with it, learning about the other systems in your body with which it is allied is important. Your healing system utilizes these other systems and relies on their cooperation to initiate powerful and sophisticated healing responses whenever illness or injury threatens your natural state of health. In the next chapter, you'll learn about the critical relationship between your extraordinary healing system and the other systems in your body, and how they all work together and respond to each other in incredible ways.

CHAPTER 3

The Team Members of
Your Healing System

Your healing system is intimately connected to all of your body's other 12 systems. It is integrated within the structures and cells of these different systems so much so that when your body is in its natural state of health, the cooperation between the healing system and the other systems of the body, and the ways in which they function together, are almost flawless.

To fully understand the connections between the healing system and the other systems of the body, you first need to understand how each system functions individually and performs specialized tasks. The health of each individual system is essential to your overall health and to each system's ability to work efficiently and effectively with your healing system.

Your Skin

Your skin is the most exterior and exposed system in your body. Consisting of several layers and appearing in a variety of colors and shades, your skin is one of the most obvious features that define your body's individuality. Your skin is one continuous organ, and, much like a teddy bear or other stuffed animal's outer lining that holds its stuffing in, your skin can be looked upon as the outer covering of the body that holds in all of your internal structures. Your skin exhibits the following qualities that aid your healing system in many important ways:

- Skin is flexible. It can stretch and expand to tremendous capacities, as demonstrated during pregnancy and extreme cases of obesity. This characteristic helps your skin resist tearing and other injuries, which reduces the burden on your healing system.

- Skin can absorb sunlight. Like a chameleon, your skin can change color, depending on its exposure to the sun. Gradual increases in sun exposure result in the accumulation and deposition of a pigment known as melanin, which results in tanning. Sunlight contains vitamin D, which improves calcium absorption and helps maintain bone density. Tanning increases tolerance to sun exposure, thus allowing for greater amounts of vitamin D to be absorbed and produced. Sunlight also promotes wound healing, prevents infection, and stimulates the immune system, and so the skin's ability to absorb sunlight is a sophisticated mechanism that benefits and supports your healing system.

- Skin holds in your body's fluids. Because your body is 70 percent fluid, maintenance of proper fluid levels is necessary for optimum functioning of your healing system. When water content falls below a certain level, illness and death can ensue. Your skin prevents your body from becoming dehydrated. Dehydration also commonly occurs in burn victims. When someone sustains a severe burn to more than 50 percent of his or her body, death is a real threat as a result of the leakage of fluid out of the body through the damaged skin.

- Skin helps protect your body from infection. Intact skin is a natural barrier to most forms of microorganisms, including viruses and bacteria. When an abrasion or laceration creates a break in your skin, infection can enter into the body and penetrate into the deeper, more vulnerable tissues and cause significant disease, damage, and even death. Your skin is fairly tough and supports your healing system by keeping your body free from infection and invading organisms.

- Skin helps regulate body temperature. Your body is programmed to keep its internal temperature close to 98.6 degrees Fahrenheit, and because of your skin, it can maintain this temperature most of the time. At 98.6 degrees, all the enzyme systems in your body's internal environment function optimally, including those that work with your healing system. Any sudden or sustained reduction in this normal body temperature disrupts the health and integrity of your body. The pores in your skin also regulate body temperature by opening wider and sweating when body temperature rises too high, and by closing to retain heat when body temperature goes too low. Sweating supports your healing system by preventing your body from overheating during periods of extreme physical activity or exceptionally hot weather, when a fever is present, or when you have stress.

- Your skin is capable of absorbing moisture and other substances. Much like a frog, your skin can absorb water and literally drink from the environment. Medical scientists are now making use of the skin's absorption capabilities by creating medicines that are applied to the skin in the form of patches. These medicines include nitroglycerin for heart patients, estrogen for postmenopausal women, nicotine for people attempting to quit smoking, and scopolamine to help prevent motion sickness.

- Skin eliminates toxins and waste products. One important example of the skin's ability to rid the body of toxins is its response when the body has a fever. With a fever, sweating occurs, which helps the body eliminate the toxins caused by the infection. Until modern medicine began encouraging the use of medications to suppress fever, people with high fevers, including those fevers caused by pneumonia, were encouraged to drink lots of fluids and bundle up in heavy blankets to sweat out the toxins until the fever broke.

- Skin plays an important role in touch. Touch is a vital ingredient for physical and emotional health. Human beings require regular, compassionate touching to thrive and survive. Studies done with touching show that the cultures that advocate more touching have less heart disease and mental illness than cultures in which people don't touch very often. Babies who are not held and touched often develop a condition known as Failure to Thrive syndrome, which can have fatal consequences. Touching is essential to strengthen and fortify your healing system.

Your Hair, Your Nails, and Your Healing System

Hair helps your healing system in several ways, and although hair is usually thought of as separate from skin, your hair is a part of your skin. Each type of hair shape, color, and distribution on the body found throughout the world has been designed to aid our healing systems and keep our bodies healthy in a multitude of ways. For example, in Africa, where temperatures can become extremely hot, tightly curled hair, often referred to as "kinky" hair, serves to keep the head and body cool. Kinky hair acts like an intricately coiled refrigerator system to help trap and cool water vapors (moisture that has evaporated in the form of steam) off the top of the head. Mediterranean body hair, which is more common in warm, arid climates, protects the body from drying out, and from wind and sand. This type of hair helps to conserve fluids and regulate body temperature.

Hair also acts as a sense organ for touch. If your head begins to brush up against an overhanging object that you might not have seen, your hair will meet the object first. The movement of hair will inform you to duck your head quickly to avoid serious injury.

Toenails and fingernails are also specialized parts of your skin, and they help your healing system by protecting the delicate tips of your toes and fingers.

Wound Healing of the Skin

Your skin possesses an uncanny ability to heal itself after a laceration, abrasion, burn, or other injury. Because injuries to the skin may involve the loss of blood along with concomitant injuries to deeper structures within the body, wound healing requires the sophisticated and timely collaboration of many body systems, including the circulatory, the endocrine, the immune, and the nervous systems. Your healing system supervises and directs this remarkable collaboration.

Your Skeletal System

The skeletal system establishes the rigid framework of your body and is made up primarily of bones, which are the densest structures in your body. Intact bones that are thousands of years old can be found on archeological sites.

Your skeletal system works with your healing system in many important ways:

- Bones absorb significant stress loads and protect the body's deeper internal organs and tissues. The ribs, for example, in addition to being involved in the function of respiration, also serve to protect the heart and lungs and other vital structures in the chest cavity. The skull protects and houses the brain, the master organ in the body. The bones in the spine, known singularly as *vertebra*, and collectively as *vertebrae*, are stacked one on top of each other to form the spinal column. The vertebrae support the weight of your head; they also act like flexible conduits, encasing and protecting the delicate spinal cord, which is the main electrical, intercommunicating highway between your brain and body.

- In conjunction with your healing system, bones have an uncanny ability to mend and knit themselves back together in the case of fracture. This capability ensures that your bones will continue to protect the deeper organs and tissues of the body.

- In addition to their protective role, bones, along with muscles, are responsible for movement, which keeps your body healthy and free from disease (see the next section, "Your Muscular System"). For example, the bones of the legs are responsible for walking, running, climbing, and jumping, while the bones in the arms, hands, and fingers are responsible for movement of the upper extremities. The bones in your face participate in facial expression, chewing, and breathing; they also protect the delicate sense organs in the region, such as your eyes, ears, and nose.

- Bones serve as the body's largest pool of calcium. Calcium is required for healthy muscle contractions, heart activity, nerve transmission, and other vitally important functions that aid your healing system in keeping your body healthy.

Your Muscular System

The system that is primarily responsible for movement in your body is the muscular system. Muscles make up approximately 40 percent of your total body weight, and they alone are the heaviest and most dominant system in your body. The muscles in your body serve as key allies to your healing system in the following ways:

■ When muscles move and contract, they generate heat, which keeps your body warm. This process supports your healing system by keeping your body functioning at optimum temperatures.

■ Regular movement and exercise of the muscles improves circulation by strengthening the heart. A strong heart aids the healing system by improving the delivery of oxygen and vital nutrients throughout your body.

■ Muscles have a tremendous capacity to grow, change, and heal. They are dynamic, versatile, and highly plastic. Body builders who continually lift weights over a long period of time can add up to 100 pounds or more of solid muscle tissue to their frames, becoming powerful and strong in the process. Alternatively, yogis in India, through many years of stretching the muscles in their bodies, can mold their bodies into pretzels—they have earned the label of "rubber men" for the incredible flexibility in their joints. Muscles that are strong, flexible, and relaxed create healthy joints and ensure strength and maximum movement, which is essential for the healing system to function most efficiently.

■ Muscles also participate in important internal processes that aid your healing system in keeping your body healthy. For example, muscles of respiration participate in breathing, causing movement of the diaphragm and the rib cage, which allows air and oxygen to flow in and out of your lungs.

■ Smooth muscles, located inside various vital organs, such as the intestines, the arteries, and the bronchioles in the lungs, are critical to the functioning of these organs and the healing system. They can contract and expand the diameters of these important tubular structures, and in the process, help to direct the movement of vital body fluids and important gases such as oxygen to specific destinations within your body.

■ The following examples emphasize how indispensable the smooth muscles are to the health and performance of your healing system. When the muscles in the arteries contract, the arteries become narrower; this helps to circulate blood more quickly through your body. In the digestive system, the movement of food down the digestive tract, known as *peristalsis*, is caused by the alternating contraction and expansion of the intestinal muscles; peristalsis allows the food to pass along the length of the intestines. The same is true in the lungs, where the muscles that line the breathing tubes, known as the *bronchi* and *bronchioles*, help to regulate the flow of air in and out of your body.

Your Nervous System

The nervous system is the master communication and electrical arm of your healing system. Consisting of your brain, the spinal cord, and the peripheral nerves (like a tree with many branches), your nervous system processes information and sends and receives messages with astonishing speed and precision throughout all parts of your body.

With the help of your nervous system, your healing system knows what is going on in even the tiniest cell in the most remote region of your body. Because of your nervous system, your healing system can dispatch a concentrated, orchestrated, and effective healing response with great accuracy and speed to any area of your body.

Your nervous system consists of two main limbs:

1. The *voluntary nervous system,* which regulates the movements of such activities as standing, walking, running, jumping, sitting, swimming, and all other activities that you can consciously direct.

2. The *involuntary nervous system,* also known as the *autonomic nervous system,* which automatically controls vital body processes, such as breath, heartbeat, body temperature, visual adaptation to light, muscular reflexes, and many others.

Your healing system is exquisitely interconnected to the functioning of your entire nervous system, upon which it depends for specialized roles in communication, the regulation of vital, life-sustaining, physiological processes, and the direction of key mechanisms for the growth, repair, and maintenance of your body's natural state of health.

Sense Organs and Your Healing System

In association with your nervous system, there are highly specialized tissues and structures in your body known as *sense organs*, which include the eyes, ears, nose, tongue, and skin. Information that influences your perception and aids your healing system, and that enables you to safely move about in this world, is fed to your brain through these various sense organs. Sense organs not only allow you to avoid danger, but, more importantly, to interact with life in all its fullness. Information coming in through the senses can also directly alter your body's physiology, exerting a powerful influence on your healing system.

Your Endocrine System (Glands)

The *endocrine* system consists of the major organ-glands in your body; these organ-glands are responsible for the production, secretion, and regulation of all your hormones. *Hormones* are powerful chemical messengers that work with your healing system to influence important physiological processes and vital body functions.

The following hormones and their respective endocrine organs, commonly referred to as *glands*, make up the endocrine system and play major roles in the chemistry of your body's internal environment while they support your healing system through numerous mechanisms:

■ Adrenaline, also known as epinephrine, produced by the adrenal glands, is one of the best known of all hormones. Adrenaline is rapidly secreted during emergencies, and in response to fear, stress, or other states of excitement; it activates the "fight-or-flight" response, which causes the following changes in your body's physiology:

- increases heart rate
- increases blood pressure
- increases respiratory rate
- increases oxygen consumption
- dilates pupils
- affects many other functions that help the body direct resources to effectively deal with any emergency.

■ Adrenocorticotropic hormone, or ACTH, produced by your pituitary gland, regulates the production of cortisol from the adrenal gland. Cortisol regulates glucose metabolism, plays a key role in the immune system, and aids the healing system by acting as a powerful, natural anti-inflammatory agent.

■ Aldosterone, produced by the adrenal glands, is a powerful hormone that regulates the amount of sodium and fluid levels in the body; it also controls blood pressure.

■ Estrogen and progesterone, produced by the ovaries in women, play important roles in menstruation and pregnancy; they also have other wide-reaching effects in the body, such as bone formation, cholesterol metabolism, and the health of the skin.

■ FSH (follicle stimulating hormone) and LH (luteinizing hormone), secreted from the pituitary gland, regulate the production of ova, or eggs, in the ovaries of women, where estrogen is produced. These hormones also are involved in the process of menstruation, and they play an important role during pregnancy.

■ Growth hormone, produced by your pituitary gland, controls and regulates bone growth and overall growth in your body.

■ Insulin is produced in the pancreas and is one of the most important hormones in your body. Insulin regulates glucose metabolism and blood sugar, which are central to the health of your healing system, and to every cell and tissue in your body.

- Interstitial cell-stimulating hormone, or ICSH, stimulates the release of testosterone from the testes in males.

- Melatonin, which is strongly influenced by sunlight and plays a major role in the regulation of moods, is a powerful hormone produced by the pineal gland. Melatonin controls natural sleep and wake cycles, and the production of melanin, the pigment that helps regulate the amount of sunlight that enters into your body.

- Oxytocin, produced by the pituitary gland, regulates the process of labor by stimulating uterine contractions during childbirth. Oxytocin also aids in milk production and secretion during breast-feeding.

- Parathyroid hormone, produced by the parathyroid glands, controls bone metabolism and regulates calcium levels in your blood. Parathyroid hormone also affects calcium absorption in your intestines and calcium resorption in your kidneys. Calcium also is required for the functioning of the heart, as well as other important muscles and nerves in your body.

- Prolactin, secreted from the pituitary gland, regulates lactation and the release of breast milk following childbirth in women.

- Testosterone, produced in the testes in men, is required for testicular development, sexual maturity, the production of sperm, the development of facial and body hair, depth of voice, muscular development, and male libido.

- Thyroid hormone, produced by the thyroid gland, helps to regulate growth and development, metabolism, skin and hair growth, heart rate, body temperature, menstruation, and mood.

- Thyroid stimulating hormone, or TSH, produced by your pituitary gland, controls and regulates the function of the thyroid gland, which is one of the most important glands in your body.

- Vasopressin, or ADH (antidiuretic hormone), produced by the pituitary gland, acts on the kidneys to conserve water by inhibiting urination and also plays a role in blood-pressure regulation.

Your Digestive System

Your digestive system consists of various organs that are connected to your small and large intestines, which combine to form a continuous, hollow, twisted, tube-like structure that extends more than 30 feet from your mouth to your rectum. The following components make up the digestive system: your mouth, tongue, teeth, salivary glands, nose, throat, esophagus, stomach, small intestines, large intestines, rectum, and anus. The digestive system also includes the liver, gall bladder, pancreas, and appendix. Your digestive system, through the delivery of essential nutrients, maintains close ties with your healing system.

Your digestive system is responsible for breaking down, absorbing, and assimilating vital nutrients into your body from the foods you eat. These nutrients provide the fuel for your healing system and for your entire body, helping it grow, repair itself, and maintain its natural state of health. As your body heals from any malady, your digestive system plays a key role in delivering necessary nutrients for the purposes of rebuilding and providing new growth to damaged tissues.

Following digestion, what your body doesn't need or cannot use is eliminated through the large intestines in the form of solid wastes. Elimination aids your healing system by ridding your body of unwanted toxins and waste products.

Your Respiratory System

Your respiratory system consists of the nose, mouth, sinuses, middle ear, throat, tonsils, trachea, larynx, bronchi, bronchioles, alveoli, and lungs. Because of their role in breathing, the ribs and diaphragm are considered ancillary structures of the respiratory system. The health of each of these structures affects the health of your entire respiratory system and, ultimately, your entire body. Your respiratory system directs the flow of air in and out of your body through these various structures.

The respiratory system is responsible for delivering oxygen to your blood, which is then pumped to every cell and tissue in your body. Without oxygen, your cells and tissues cannot live. Your respiratory system is also responsible for ridding your body of *carbon dioxide*, a toxic waste product of normal cellular metabolism.

The respiratory system is connected to many other systems, including your nervous, circulatory, lymphatic, and digestive systems. When the body has an oxygen deficit, such as when a person is in shock, has a fever, or has sustained a severe trauma, illness, or injury, or when stress is significant, rates of breathing tend to automatically increase to bring more oxygen into the body. This is just one example of a critical cooperative effort between your respiratory system and your healing system.

Your Circulatory System

The circulatory system consists of your heart and blood vessels, the blood, and all the various constituents in your blood, including your red blood cells. In your heart, the *coronary arteries* are special arteries that bring the blood supply back to the heart itself. If these arteries become clogged, a heart attack can occur. Their health is critical to the health of your heart, upon whose health your healing system and entire body depend.

The circulatory system has many vital functions. It is responsible for

- Pumping and distributing blood, which contains oxygen and other vital nutrients and substances, to every cell and tissue in your body. These nutrients and substances include hormones, antibodies, enzymes, neurotransmitters, vitamins, minerals, and trace elements that are vital to the functioning of your healing system.

- Removing toxic metabolic byproducts, such as carbon dioxide and lactic acid.

- Carrying oxygen from the lungs to the various organs and tissues in your body. Hemoglobin, a very important molecule in red blood cells, accomplishes this task.

- Clotting of the blood. White blood cells, which are crucial for the functioning of the immune system, are essential for blood clotting. Blood clotting is a unique function of the circulatory system, and it occurs during times of injury to prevent excessive blood loss. Blood clotting represents one of the true miracles of the healing system.

Your Lymphatic System

You can think of your lymphatic system as the blood-purification system. The lymphatic system consists of a series of lymphatic vessels and lymph nodes that are strategically located throughout specific parts of your body. Lymph fluid circulates freely throughout the lymph system; this fluid contains white blood cells, antibodies, and important chemicals of the immune system. Your lymphatic system works closely with your circulatory, immune, and healing systems as it circulates and removes toxins and impurities from your body to keep your tissues and blood free from disease caused by bacteria, viruses, and other invaders.

Your Urinary System

Your urinary system is primarily responsible for acting as a filter for your blood to remove wastes and toxins from your body. The major organs of your urinary system include your kidneys and bladder, and they support your healing system through a number of important functions. These functions include the following:

- Your urinary system helps to conserve and regulate fluid levels in your body.
- Your urinary system filters and purifies the entire blood circulation within your body.
- Your urinary system regulates electrolyte levels, assuring that your body has proper amounts of sodium, potassium, calcium, and other key minerals and trace elements that support vital physiological processes that are essential for your healing system.
- Your urinary system monitors protein concentration in the blood, which is critical to your healing system.

Your Reproductive System

In women, the reproductive system is located in the lower abdomen and pelvic area, and it consists of the ovaries, uterus, cervix, and vagina. The breasts, located in the chest, are also included in this system. The breasts are actually dual-purpose organs, serving as nutritive, lactating glands that deliver milk immediately following childbirth; in addition, they act as attractive forces to the opposite sex, and as tissues of arousal that help promote sexual and reproductive activities. In this way, the breasts serve both an endocrine, secretory function and a reproductive one.

In men, the testes, prostate, seminal vesicles, urethra, and penis make up the reproductive system.

More than any other system in the body, the reproductive system is responsible for helping to differentiate the physical characteristics of men and women. These differences are responsible for the strongly magnetic forces that help foster the sexual attraction between the sexes. The natural result of this attraction, and the main function of your reproductive system, is reproduction and proliferation of the species. Although women can live without a uterus or ovaries, and men can live without testes and a prostate, the reproductive system is essential for the survival of the human race.

The reproductive system maintains an intimate connection with the endocrine system. In addition to having receptors for hormones produced by other organs, the reproductive system produces it own hormones, most notably estrogen in females and testosterone in males. These hormones contribute to overall health, and they can influence emotional and mental states. For instance, estrogen exerts a protective influence on the heart.

Many other systems in the body also are connected to the health and proper functioning of the reproductive system. These include the nervous, endocrine, circulatory, and lymphatic systems.

Your Immune System

Your immune system consists of a complex network of cells and organs that can produce extremely powerful chemicals known as *antibodies*. Little was known about your immune system until quite recently. Research is still discovering new facts about this amazing system, whose chief function is to defend your body against infection and other intruders.

The cellular components of your immune system consist largely of white blood cells, with highly specialized roles and functions. You can think of white blood cells as infantrymen who are programmed to destroy any invading enemy in the form of pathogenic bacteria, viruses, fungi, parasites, or other harmful organisms. The division of labor among the many types of white blood cells of your immune system is so detailed, subtle, sophisticated, and precise as to make any other army or military force in the history of the world appear primitive and impotent in comparison.

Antibodies, which are produced in direct response to specific threats and can be likened to molecular cruise missiles, are released into the bloodstream to seek out and destroy unwanted intruders with remarkable speed, accuracy, and precision. Antibodies are present in the blood, produced in large quantities upon demand. They also are in the body's mucous membranes, such as the nose, mouth, respiratory system, intestines, urethra, and other body tissues and cavities that connect to the outside environment.

Your immune system, once thought to be a completely independent system, is now known to be directly linked to your brain and nervous system, and to other systems, as well. For example, white blood cells have been discovered to possess receptors for *neurotransmitters* produced by the brain, which demonstrates a direct chemical link with your brain and nervous system. Other white blood cells have been found to have specific hormone receptors, indicating that your endocrine system communicates directly with your immune system. Even more astonishing is recent evidence that certain white blood cells can produce and secrete hormones that communicate directly with your endocrine system.

As we discussed earlier, your immune system works closely with your healing system; and although the two systems are clearly distinct, in many instances they work together to restore your body to its natural state of health.

Closing Thoughts on the
Team Members of Your Healing System

Even though an entire book could be written on each individual system presented in this chapter, I hope you now have a greater sense of appreciation for how the various systems in your body function individually and together in support of your extraordinary healing system, which orchestrates the processes that keep you healthy. In the next chapter, we will look at the many ways you can cooperate with your healing system by strengthening and fortifying it so that it can work for you most efficiently and effectively.

CHAPTER 4

Strengthening and Fortifying
Your Healing System

Your body's healing system comes prepackaged, completely installed, and fully functional, even before the first breath enters your lungs when you are born. Although the healing system is delivered to you in perfect condition, the choices you make in your everyday life can have a serious impact upon its performance and its activities. Your diet and lifestyle, home and work environment, moods and emotions, thoughts and attitudes, in addition to a multitude of other factors that are within your control, can dramatically alter the behavior and efficiency of your healing system.

You can impede your healing system's ability to perform its programmed mission, and overburden and exhaust its resources, by participating in activities that are harmful to your health. Such obstructions include the following: ignoring the basic needs of your body, putting harmful substances into your body, eating nutrient-poor foods, not drinking enough water, not getting enough sleep and rest, breathing harmful air, subjecting your body to a toxic environment, and living a lifestyle that is stressful and unhealthy.

Additional factors that can be detrimental to the intrinsic strength of your healing system include such unhealthy mental habits as chronic worrying; entertaining thoughts of fear, anger, and rage; mistrusting; holding onto resentment; maintaining a pessimistic and cynical attitude; focusing on problems and negative circumstances; depression; apathy; and giving up on life altogether. All these self-destructive tendencies exhaust your body's precious resources, interfere with your healing system's ability to do its job properly, and increase the likelihood of a serious, life-threatening illness or chronic debilitating disease taking hold of your body. These negative factors can rob you of your natural state of health and sabotage an otherwise wholesome, vibrant, rich, and rewarding life.

Alternatively, you can strengthen, nourish, and cooperate with your healing system, and even enhance its performance, by learning to listen to your body's valuable communications, understanding what is required to maintain your natural state of health. This will help you fulfill your basic physical needs of wholesome food, water, fresh air, plenty of sleep and rest, and appropriate exercise, while paying attention to your body's early warning signs when danger or illness may be approaching.

As we discussed earlier, your body, which is naturally programmed for health and vitality, can remain free of illness until your final days, which might be well over 100 years. But if you hope to come near this goal, you must cooperate with your healing system, and learn to strengthen and fortify it, to keep it in optimum condition.

Your healing system responds to your deepest intentions and most heartfelt desires. In this respect, you inwardly possess much more power than you may be aware. If you want to be happy, healthy, strong, vibrant, energetic, and active, you need to honor and take proper care of your body, and understand the intimate relationship between your body, mind, emotions, and spirit. If you do, you can make your healing system your most powerful ally in your quest for greater health and wellness.

Prevention
The Key to a Strong Healing System

From a strategic and tactical viewpoint, the best time to strengthen, fortify, and cooperate with your healing system is not when you are sick, but rather when you are healthy. So that your healing system will stand poised and ready to leap into action at the first signs of distress, it is better for it to be well prepared in advance of any anticipated calamity. As the famous case of the ill-fated Titanic demonstrates, the time to check whether there are enough lifeboats on deck for all the passengers is not when the ship is sinking, but before it leaves the port. The same is true with your healing system. Learning how to strengthen and fortify your healing system is easier when your body is not already under siege from an illness or disease. This doesn't mean that if you are now ill you will not benefit from this knowledge. On the contrary, if you are now ill, you need to focus on this important work more than ever. In fact, your very life depends on it.

Learning how to strengthen and fortify your healing system in the absence of illness or disease gives you the momentum and positive inertia to defeat any illness, should it attempt to violate the integrity and sanctity of your body. To further illustrate this point, consider the plight of a boxer vying for the heavyweight championship of the world. The time to learn how to box for such a fight is not when he steps into the ring against a formidable opponent, but rather during the many hours of preparation when he is in training for the fight. So prepared, he can then step into that ring with confidence and poise, actively calling upon his polished boxing skills to defeat his less-prepared, inferior opponent. This kind of training, preparation, and mindset is required to win. These requirements are exactly the same for your healing system. To emerge victorious from a health challenge, taking the time now to learn how to work with your healing system will give you the edge you need to defeat any condition or formidable disease that life may throw your way.

How to Be Your Own Best Doctor

I meet many people who choose not to visit doctors regularly. I am not speaking about irresponsible people who neglect their health and then, out of fear and denial, refuse to see doctors for their deteriorating health conditions. I am speaking about healthy, mature, independent people who have developed a confidence in their bodies' abilities to meet the physical challenges that face us all in this life. If they should run into a problem, instead of rushing off to the doctor, these people know how to activate their healing systems by nurturing and listening to their bodies. There is definitely a time and place to ask for help from doctors, but you can minimize these occasions when you learn to rely more on your own healing system. By learning how to listen to your body and apply some simple yet powerful principles and techniques, you will develop a deep-seated inner confidence that your body has the capacity to stay healthy and to heal itself when its health is challenged. Learning to strengthen and activate your healing system will help you prevent illness and heal yourself from any health challenge you may have to face in your life. You can learn to be your own best doctor.

Prescriptions for Strengthening and Fortifying Your Healing System

The following key ingredients constitute essential components of a healthy program aimed at strengthening and fortifying your body's healing system, whether you're focusing on prevention or on healing from an existing health problem. By paying attention to each of these factors and incorporating them into your life, you will be able to most effectively tap into your body's natural ability to heal itself and significantly improve the quality of your life.

Healing System Rx #1: Learn to Listen to Your Body

As we discussed in Chapter 2, your body comes equipped with a healing system that is constantly attempting to communicate with you, 24 hours a day, seven days a week. Through the language your healing system speaks, it sends you valuable information to help you know what its needs are.

For example, when your body is hungry, and you feel hunger pangs in your stomach, your stomach will soon begin to rumble and growl if you don't put something in your belly. When your body is tired and requires sleep, your eyes will feel heavy and you will begin to yawn. When your body needs water, you feel thirsty, which creates a strong urge to drink fluids. Similarly, when your bladder becomes full and requires emptying, you feel the urge to urinate.

In addition to these more obvious forms of communication, your body is constantly sending you other more subtle information. Depending on what kind of listener you are, you may or may not be receiving and processing these other important messages. For instance,

- When you are tense, upset, or under stress, you may notice a tight or heavy sensation in your chest, which makes your breathing slightly difficult. You may also notice your heart skipping a beat or two. You may try to ignore these sensations, as many people do; but if this is an early warning from your heart, it could lead to increased pain known as angina, which occurs when there is a lack of adequate oxygen and blood flow to the heart. These symptoms could be danger signals of an impending heart attack. Ignoring the messages could have disastrous consequences.

- You may feel queasy or notice a knot in your stomach when you are nervous, afraid, or confronted with an unpleasant situation. If the situation is not resolved and is allowed to linger, the sensations might increase, or become persistent, which could be early warning signs of an impending intestinal problem, such as an ulcer.

Even though some of us listen to our bodies some of the time, many of us don't listen until they are actually screaming at us and refusing to cooperate with us until we tend to their needs. Our bodies scream at us by causing intense pain. This pain is the body's ultimate communication strategy to try to get us to wake up to the fact that we are ignoring one or more of its vital needs. To avoid pain and to remain healthy, we need to become better listeners.

To strengthen, fortify, and cooperate with your healing system, it is critical that you first become more aware of your body's needs and learn to listen to its early warning messages, in all their myriad forms. When you become a good listener, your body will not need to shout or scream at you to get your attention, and so you will not need to experience pain, suffering, misery, illness, or disease.

How to Listen to Your Body

The following exercise is a simple yet powerful method to gain access to vitally important messages from your body's healing system:

- Allow yourself quiet alone time. Go into a safe and quiet room, close the door, and take the phone off the hook so you won't be disturbed. If you cannot find a quiet place, try using earplugs. Excuse yourself from your family duties, responsibilities, and obligations for at least 20 to 30 minutes. Make sure everyone in your home understands that you are not to be disturbed until you are finished. You may also want to put on some soft, relaxing music in the background to help set a peaceful, quiet mood.

- Find a comfortable position, preferably lying down on your back. You may place pillows under your knees, or use blankets or pillows anywhere else to help support your body so that you are comfortable. Make sure your body is comfortable before you proceed.

- Gently close your eyes and relax all the muscles in your body, as if it is melting into the surface beneath you.

- As you close your eyes and relax your body, bring your awareness to the area of your stomach and abdomen. Notice the gentle movement in that region. You can even place your hands on top of the area to help you become more aware of this movement. Feel the rhythmical, automatic movement of your breath as it flows in and out of your body. Notice that when the breath flows into your body, your stomach and abdomen gently expand and rise. Notice that when the breath flows out of your body, your stomach and abdomen gently contract and fall. Try not to control the rate or depth of this movement; rather, just let your mind be a passive observer as you watch and observe this gentle, automatic rhythm.

- Every time the breath leaves your body, feel all the muscles in your body releasing tension, and becoming more relaxed.

- Focus your awareness within, becoming aware of how your body feels from the "inside" as you continue to breathe.

- As you become more relaxed, observing the gentle, automatic movement of your breath as it flows in and out of your body, slowly and systematically scan your body, starting from the tips of your toes and moving toward the top of your head. Visit all parts in between, including your heart and chest area; your back and spine; your shoulders and neck; your groin, buttocks, and genitals; and your stomach and abdominal area.

- Notice any areas of discomfort, pain, or tension, which you may not have been aware of before, in these areas. Also notice any areas of relaxation, comfort, and feelings of vitality and health.

- After your allotted time, gently stretch your muscles, and open your eyes. Resume your normal activities. Remember to listen to your body this way regularly.

At first glance, this process may appear to be nothing more than a relaxation exercise. In reality, however, much more is going on. First, when your body is relaxed, your nervous system, which is the main communications link between your mind and body, becomes calmer and more focused. In this state, your mind also becomes quieter, more alert, and concentrated. Because your mind and body are intimately connected, when your body is relaxed, your mental powers for internal listening are also increased.

The awareness you gain from this exercise will spill over into your daily life. You will notice a heightened sensitivity to your body's inner sensations, and to its responses to your environment, the air you breathe, the food you eat, and your mental and emotional state. When you regularly practice listening to your body, you will discover important messages from it that you were unable to hear or feel before. You will become much more aware of the valuable information your body is communicating to you, and you will be better able to use this information to respond to your body's needs. Should imbalances or insults to your body occur, you will be better able to assist your healing system in correcting these imbalances as it restores your body to its natural state of health. By opening the door to better communication and cooperation, learning to listen to your body can become one of the simplest, easiest, and yet most powerful ways to strengthen and fortify your healing system.

Healing System Rx #2:
Pay Attention to Your Personal Hygiene

Your personal hygiene consists of the simple acts you perform daily to help support and care for your body. These actions include such common activities as brushing your teeth, moving your bowels, and bathing. These simple routine habits, which may seem insignificant at first, add up over the days, weeks, months, and years of an entire lifetime and, in the long run, exert a powerful influence on the performance and efficiency of your healing system. In fact, your personal hygiene can have a much greater impact on your ability to stay healthy and resist diseases than your genes, the medicine you take, or your doctor.

The elements of personal hygiene in the following sections contribute significantly to the health of your body, and they can strengthen and fortify your healing system. They can make a huge difference in the quality of your life, and in your ability to stay well and resist disease. If you want to live a long and happy, healthy life, and you are interested in preventing problems before they develop, or if you are currently struggling to regain your health, pay careful attention to the following elements of hygiene.

Dental Hygiene and Your Healing System

Good health depends on proper digestion. Digestion begins in your mouth with the chewing of food, which depends on the health of your teeth. For this reason, regularly brushing your teeth and observing good dental hygiene is important. When you brush regularly, you prevent the possibility of plaque build-up, cavity formation, and gum disease, all of which can impair digestion, interfere with proper nutrition, and adversely affect your healing system.

Bathing and Your Healing System

Bathing helps preserve the function and integrity of your skin, which is one of your body's primary defense organs. Regular bathing leaves your skin feeling fresh and clean, and it removes bacteria and germs that can accumulate on the surface of your skin. Bodies that are not washed or bathed regularly are more prone to skin infections. Microorganisms, including staph and strep bacteria, can invade your body after first appearing on your skin. Regular bathing can aid your healing system by eliminating these infections at their source.

Elimination and Your Healing System: Bowel and Bladder Hygiene

Because of normal internal metabolic processes, large amounts of toxic wastes are produced and accumulate in your body during each day. Failure to eliminate waste products and toxins promptly and efficiently contributes to the steady build-up of these materials, which can cause your healing system to bog down and become seriously impaired. Without regular elimination, you will literally drown or suffocate in your own waste. Irregular elimination can contribute to the onset of a number of serious, life-threatening diseases.

Solid, unwanted, toxic-waste products are eliminated through the large intestines in your bowel movements, while liquids are eliminated primarily through the kidneys and bladder, in the urine. Ensuring the health of these organs is essential for your healing system to operate with maximum efficiency.

Tips for Healthy Elimination

- Drink plenty of fluids, including water. Your body is approximately 70 percent fluid, and the more fluids you bring into your body, the more efficiently your healing system can eliminate and remove toxins from it. If your bowels are sluggish and need a little coaxing in the morning, a large cup of hot water or a warm beverage will usually bring fast results.

- Increase your fiber intake throughout the day and at night. Adequate fiber intake ensures more effective elimination of waste products from your intestines, thus reducing the risk of colon cancer and other intestinal diseases. The best sources of fiber include whole grains, seeds and nuts, and fruits and vegetables.

- Increase physical activity, which improves blood flow to the intestines, which helps elimination.

- Avoid low-residue foods, such as processed starches, cheeses, and prepackaged meats and other foods, which lack fiber and can cause constipation.

- Avoid excess alcohol. Alcohol can dehydrate your body, and can cause constipation along with bowel or bladder problems. Alcohol is an intestinal and bladder irritant, and chronic use can contribute to problems with these organs.

- Limit coffee, tea, and caffeinated sodas, because these usually contain tannic acids, which can serve as irritants. Caffeine stimulates the parietal cells in your stomach to produce hydrochloric acid, which, if produced in excess, can damage the lining of your stomach and intestines, and potentially lead to an ulcer or other intestinal problems.

- Eliminate foods that are highly processed or contain artificial chemical additives. These foods can also irritate and damage the delicate lining of your urinary and digestive systems.

Healing System Rx #3:
Eat a Well-Balanced Diet Consisting of Natural Foods

Food supplies the basic building blocks for the sustenance of every cell and tissue in your body, providing life-supporting energy for metabolic activities, mechanisms of defense, and the processes of repair and restoration governed by your healing system. Just as any other high-powered, performance-oriented machine requires the best fuel, your healing system requires pure and wholesome food to ensure optimum performance and functioning. Here are a few basic but critical guidelines:

- Eat a well-rounded, high-performance diet that includes adequate amounts of protein, carbohydrates, fats and oils, essential vitamins, minerals, and trace elements. Additionally, make sure you are consuming adequate amounts of fluids and fiber.
- Favor fresh fruits and vegetables, whole grains, and legumes, which contain an abundance of all of your body's basic nutritional requirements, over flesh foods. Although flesh foods are excellent sources of protein, you should minimize them in your daily diet because of their tendency toward a higher fat content, lack of fiber, and potential for higher concentration of heavy metals and environmental toxins.
- Minimize eating packaged or processed foods, which often contain preservatives and additives that, while they increase shelf life, may have harmful side effects. Packaged and processed foods generally lack the vitality, fiber, and nutrient quality that fresh and whole foods contain.
- Do not be fanatical in following a restrictive diet. Some flexibility and leniency is necessary to avoid becoming stressed when your food choices are limited or unavailable. The stress of being

too rigid in your diet detracts from whatever benefits your diet might be providing.

■ Make sure your surroundings are pleasant and enjoyable when you eat. Your healing system's ability to remain strong and active is influenced not only by the chemical constituents of the foods you eat, but by your meal patterns and the timing of your meals, in addition to many other factors surrounding food. For example, properly chewing food and the circumstances under which food is eaten also play a role in the digestion and absorption of nutrients. When you take your meals in a peaceful atmosphere, digestion and assimilation are enhanced. (In the next chapter, I'll offer more specific information on nutrition for your healing system.)

Healing System Rx #4:
Get Adequate Exercise and Physical Activity

Movement is a fundamental principle of all matter in the universe, and, along with exercise, it is an important key to a strong and healthy healing system. Movement and exercise are essential for the maintenance of healthy joints and muscles, and they are vital for your circulation and the health of your cardiovascular system. Your daily activity level is an integral part of your body's ability to stay healthy, resist illness, and maintain an active and vibrant healing system.

The Benefits of Exercise for Your Healing System

The benefits of exercise for your healing system are numerous. Because your healing system is connected to all of the other organ systems in your body, any exercise you do regularly will significantly benefit your healing system. Among its many benefits, exercise

■ Energizes and activates your healing system

■ Clears depression

■ Improves circulation to your brain, which improves clarity of thinking

■ Improves overall muscle strength in your body

■ Improves cardiac health

- Improves blood flow to stomach and intestines, which improves digestion and elimination, and reduces constipation
- Improves immune function
- Improves bone and joint health
- Improves the healing time of fractures and joint injuries
- Improves complexion and skin health by increasing blood flow to skin
- Improves blood flow to genitals, which improves sexual function

Just 30 minutes of exercise each day will bring you all of these benefits, and more.

A few of the more common types of exercise are listed in the following sections. Choose one or more, and follow the guidelines listed to strengthen and fortify your healing system.

Walking

Walking is one of the simplest and most natural ways to exercise. In traditional cultures, before the advent of the automobile and motorized transportation, people used their own two legs as their primary means of transport, in addition to their use of domesticated animals. Consequently, there was no need to set aside extra time in the day to exercise, and people in these cultures were generally more fit than those of our modern societies.

If you are extremely busy, walking is a good way to exercise and use this time to listen to music or educational tapes, socialize with friends, brainstorm ideas, or even conduct business meetings. I have often held medical meetings with several close colleagues and friends while we were walking through scenic nature trails in Hawaii, where I live. If you can find creative ways to increase the amount of time you walk, and make walking a part of your daily routine and lifestyle, your healing system will automatically benefit from an otherwise thoroughly enjoyable activity.

Tips for Walking

- Choose a time of day and specific days of the week that work best for you. Try to walk three to five days a week if this is your only exercise.

- Wear comfortable clothing, especially comfortable, supportive shoes. If you live near the beach, and it is not too cold, consider going barefoot.
- Find a safe place to walk, hopefully with interesting scenery. This place could be outside in nature or even indoors in a large mall.
- Avoid heavily trafficked areas if possible because exhaust fumes are unhealthy to breathe, and the noise and distraction of the cars may interfere with your concentration and relaxation.
- Walk with a friend or family member so you have company. Alternatively, you can use this time to be alone.
- You may want to listen to music or educational tapes with a portable tape or CD player as you walk.
- If you are out of shape and haven't done any exercise in quite a while, start with just 10 to15 minutes a day on a flat, even surface.
- Walk at a pace that's comfortable for you. Recent research indicates that it is more important to walk regularly than to walk briskly. You do not need to force or strain or be uncomfortable in any way.
- If all goes well, after one to two weeks, add 5 minutes per week so that you can eventually build up to 30 to 60 minutes each day.

Bicycling

Bicycling can be an enjoyable way to exercise while you get out and see the world. Bicycling is often considered easier on the joints than running or other exercises. This exercise helps to build up the largest muscles in your body, your legs and lower torso, while it also improves your cardiovascular health.

Tips for Bicycling

- Avoid heavily trafficked areas that have exhaust fumes.
- Start at a comfortable pace and try to ride for 15 to 30 minutes at a time.
- Make sure your bicycle and seat are adjusted to the proper height for your legs.

- Unless you are an expert, avoid strapping your feet into the pedals.
- Maintain proper posture as you ride so that your back and knees are not strained.
  - To protect your head from a fall, wear a helmet.
  - Use protective glasses or eyewear for your eyes.

Swimming

If you have access to a pool, pond, lake, or ocean, swimming can be a wonderful form of exercise that provides all of the cardiac and circulation benefits of walking. Swimming is especially beneficial if you have back or knee problems because it is a non-weight-bearing exercise that is gentle on the joints.

Tips for Swimming

- Start out slowly and increase your laps gradually, adding one lap each time you swim.
- Build up to at least 20 to 30 minutes of swimming each day.
- Alternate strokes to give different muscles in your body a more thorough workout.
- Make sure you are comfortable with your breathing as you swim, and that you are not forcing or straining.
- It is better to swim slower and longer than faster and shorter. If you make it enjoyable, the likelihood that you will continue to swim regularly is much greater.

Weight Lifting

Thanks to the many colorful characters in the world of professional bodybuilding, weight lifting has become increasingly popular. Pumping iron and weight training can increase muscle strength and improve your overall physical health. It can also relieve mental and emotional tension, and effectively strengthen and fortify your healing system.

Tips for Weight Lifting

- Start with light weights and move through the full range of motion of the exercise you're doing to ensure proper movement of the muscles being exercised.

- Balance your workout so you are not working all the same muscle groups at one time.

- Focus more on the lower body, including your legs and back, because these muscles are the largest and most important muscles in your body, and they usually are the ones most neglected.

- Stretch in-between and after weight-lifting exercises to avoid stiff muscles and joints.

- Breathe properly as you work out. It is physiologically more correct to exhale as you lift or move a weight, as if you were blowing air into the weight.

- Be smart and accept the help of a personal trainer to orient yourself on a new machine or while you are learning a new routine.

- If your muscles are sore the day after a workout, wait until the pain is completely gone before you work these same muscles again.

- Remember that muscles need rest to grow and become stronger. It is possible to overtrain and injure muscles if you do not allowing adequate rest between workouts.

- Never force or strain to the point that you feel pain. Although most gyms encourage the saying "No pain, no gain," from a medical perspective, ignoring pain in your body can result in an injury.

Aerobic Exercise

Aerobic exercise describes any sustained exercise that increases your breathing and heart rate and has the ability to make you break a sweat. Aerobic exercise requires increased air delivery to your body, which results in greater oxygenation of your tissues. You can achieve these results in numerous ways and settings, from brisk walking, running, calisthenics, hiking, biking, swimming, aerobic dancing and exercises, to sports, games, and other fun exercises. Aerobic exercise may also include the exercise you get while working on your job if you perform manual labor or are regularly involved in activities that require the steady movement of your arms or legs over a continuous period of time.

Tips for Aerobic Exercise

- Take 5 to10 minutes to stretch and warm up before and after exercising.

- If you haven't exercised in a while, start slowly and do only about 10 to15 minutes at a time for the first week.

- Make sure you are not forcing or straining your muscles or joints, and that you are not gasping for air while you are breathing.

- Slowly build up speed, distances, and length of time exercising, until you can do 30 to 60 minutes at a time.

- If you experience pain that persists in any part of your body, ease off your exercising pace and intensity. If the pain persists even with less exercise, consider stopping altogether. Trying to ignore the pain or force through the pain does not help. Doing this is how serious injuries and problems can develop.

- Remember to rest and allow some down time before you make a transition to your next activity.

Stretching

Stretching can provide tremendous support for your healing system. Stretching is becoming increasingly popular in the United States and Europe with the acceptance and introduction of traditional oriental disciplines such as yoga and tai chi into Western cultures. Even giant Sumo wrestlers in Japan stretch as part of their pre-match warm-ups and rituals. Stretching is also making its way into the medical establishment and is gradually becoming accepted as a first-line intervention in the fields of rehabilitation, sports medicine, and physical therapy for the treatment and prevention of neuromuscular disorders and injuries, including back pain, post-surgical rehabilitation, and many forms of arthritis and other joint diseases.

When done properly, stretching feels good. Stretching is something that most animals do naturally. When dogs or cats awaken from a nap, the first thing they do is stretch. Children also naturally stretch and assume all kinds of twisting, flexible, and topsy-turvy positions as they play and explore the different muscle groups in their bodies. They do this as part of the natural process of developing the coordination that is such a vital part of their normal growth and development.

As a result of the effects of stress, aging, and increasingly sedentary lifestyles, many people begin to develop severe stiffness and pain and are unable to move their joints adequately as they age. This process sets the stage for a whole host of joint diseases to set in, including arthritis. Stiffness also increases the likelihood of injuries because of the rigidity within the joints. Stretching can help reverse these harmful tendencies.

I have personally benefited from the stretching that comes from yoga, the grandfather of all stretching systems. As an introduction to proper stretching, there is no substitute for attending a gentle yoga class once or twice a week for several months or longer. Because of yoga's increasing popularity, yoga classes are now available in almost every city in the United States, Canada, Japan, and Europe. Before you start a yoga class, make sure the teacher has proper credentials and the class is not too rigorous for you, particularly in the beginning. If you have particular health needs, make sure you call this to the attention of the teacher.

Tips for Stretching

- Set aside 10 to15 minutes a day when you can be alone to do your stretching. Gradually build up to 30 to 60 minutes a day, either at one time or in divided periods, morning and evening, as your schedule permits.

- If you have never stretched before, and your muscles are stiff, start out slowly and gently. Remember not to force or strain.

- Stretch as far as you can without feeling pain. If you don't stretch far enough, your muscles will not become flexible and healthy. However, if you stretch too far, you will feel pain, and you might damage and tear your muscles.

- Do not bounce or jerk when you stretch. Again, doing this could damage your muscles.

- Breathe slowly and gently when you stretch, so that oxygen can enter into the muscle cells that you are stretching.

- Whenever possible, stretch in the morning, even though your muscles will most likely be stiffer then. This is a great way to start the day.

Healing System Rx #5: Get Enough Sleep and Rest

Sleep is one of the body's most basic physiological functions and one of the most important activities to strengthen and fortify your healing system. When you sleep, your body has a chance to recharge its batteries. Many illnesses are less symptomatic in the morning, thanks to the refreshing and regenerative properties of sleep. In fact, your healing system is most active when you are sleeping and resting, since other physiological processes are held at a minimum and cannot interfere with its work during these periods.

Alternatively, people who suffer from insomnia, or who do not get enough sleep or rest throughout their day, are at risk of becoming sick. Sleep deprivation alters the proper functioning of your healing and immune systems and predisposes you to heart disease, chronic fatigue syndrome, endocrine and metabolic disorders, nervous-system imbalances, stress-related conditions, and other serious health problems.

When you are getting adequate sleep each night, you should wake up feeling rested and refreshed. Taking a nap in the afternoon is also socially acceptable in many cultures, and many studies are now beginning to show that naps can be beneficial. Incorporating a daily 30- to 60-minute power nap into your schedule, at least on weekends, can be a great asset to your healing system.

Alone Time: An Important Form of Rest for Your Healing System

If it runs continuously, any machine or toy will eventually wear down its batteries and stop working. Your body is no different. In fact, many illnesses can be traced to the neglect of this simple, yet important, principle. Just as every ship must come in from the open seas to dock and resupply, so, too, your body must take time off from its incessant activities to allow your healing system to recharge, regenerate, and renew its energies.

Throughout our busy lives, as we give ourselves over to our work, our families, and our friends, we need to take time out to be alone and restore our precious life energies. As part of your regular routine, it is important to experience what I call "alone time" for a brief period each day.

Think of alone time as mandatory solitary confinement—not in a punitive way, but rather as a time for you to rest and heal, to quiet down your engines, to be responsible only to yourself and your body, with no phones to answer, no duties to perform, no scheduled appointments, no commitments, no burdens, no worries, no hurries. Even if your alone time is only 15 or 20 minutes a day, in this state of quiet solitude your batteries can recharge, and your healing system can work more effectively to restore health.

While this need for rejuvenation is only common sense, as a doctor, I am continually amazed at how many people expect their bodies to keep going without recharging their batteries. When these same people become sick and end up in the doctor's office because of frayed nerves, sleep deprivation, and physical exhaustion, most are shocked to learn why they became sick in the first place. They are unable to see the connection between their illnesses and their run-down state. They think their illness is caused by some misfortune or ill luck. The sad fact is that many of these folks have not yet discovered the life-sustaining practice of spending time alone with themselves. They have not learned how to tell their families or their bosses that they need time alone to recharge their batteries. In fact, it is commonly reported that people who suffer from major, chronic, debilitating diseases often complain that they have no time for themselves, that they are just following scripts that other people are constantly imposing on their lives. Insisting on alone time is one way to stand up for the needs of your body.

Learning to say "No" to excessive demands on your life energies is mandatory if you want your healing system to remain strong and healthy. Being alone allows your body time to conserve energy, and it allows your mind time to settle down and focus within so you can listen and cooperate with your healing system. When you are quiet, alone, relaxed, and peaceful, your healing system functions best. Taking the time to be alone is one of the most powerful things you can do to strengthen and fortify your body's healing system.

Healing System Rx #6:
Manage and Minimize the Stress in Your Life

In the field of engineering, stress is defined as the amount of strain experienced by a system as the result of an applied external force or load. If the system is not flexible, or if it is unable to adapt to the force or load, it can break under the strain. This description is similar to what can happen when you experience stress. If stress is prolonged or too great, your mind and your body can suffer from a breakdown in health.

Although stress can obviously be caused by major disruptive external forces such as natural disasters, political turmoil, and even war, these sources are, for most of us, far less common, less prolonged, and less dangerous than the stress caused by our own thought processes and our fast-paced, hectic lifestyles.

Stress, if not handled properly, can do considerable harm to your healing system, wasting and depleting your precious physical, mental, and emotional energy while it causes fatigue and exhaustion, which renders you susceptible to illness and disease. Stress interferes with your body's natural ability to grow, repair, and restore normal healthy tissues. Your immune system can also become damaged and inefficient with significant and prolonged stress. Stress has been linked to a number of major serious illnesses, including heart disease, high blood pressure, ulcer, stroke, and cancer, and it has been implicated as a significant contributing factor in many others.

Stress is unavoidable at times, but it is important to be able to manage it effectively and to minimize its impact. You can accomplish this through a variety of proven methods and techniques. However, you need to practice and be familiar with these techniques and methods well in advance, so that, when you do experience stress, you can easily apply them to neutralize and handle the stress more effectively. Again, all this is nothing more than sound preventive medicine.

Stress management has been shown to be a vital factor in the successful reversal of major chronic diseases such as heart disease, hypertension, diabetes, and cancer.

Learning to prevent and reduce stress in your life, in addition to managing whatever stress may be currently afflicting you, will allow you to feel much more calm and relaxed. And effectively managing stress will liberate tremendous amounts of energy in your body that your healing system can use. Fatigue will vanish, and your healing system will perform much more efficiently, enabling you to more effectively resist and eliminate illness and disease.

Many popular stress-management techniques are currently taught. All have as their common goal your ability to effectively calm and relax your mind and body, which frees up energy for healing. In Chapter 6, you will be introduced to some of these methods and techniques.

Healing System Rx #7: Enjoy Your Work

Your daily work routine, your work ethics, and your attitudes toward your work influence the functioning and performance of your healing system. For example, you might spend most of your time at work. In this setting, you may have to contend with coworker tensions, bosses, deadlines, company policies, commuting to and from work, and other issues, which require a substantial investment of your life energies. In this respect, your work and your work environment may be having a more significant effect on your physical and mental health than anything else.

Many people work at home, with less energy spent interacting with coworkers and bosses and commuting through dangerous traffic back and forth to an office, but other problems may present themselves, such as the intrusion of work into the home space, and the inability to turn off the work mode when they are interacting with their families.

Many people don't like their jobs, as numerous polls and surveys reveal, and this dissatisfaction can have a damaging effect on the healing system. Toxic emotions that have built up in the form of resentment can exhaust the immune system and deplete internal healing resources. Many people who develop chronic illnesses report feelings of long-term animosity or ambivalence for their work, often feeling hopelessly trapped in a dull and boring routine. Many other fortunate souls, having made peace with their vocation and having found their niche in the world, report that their work is like play. I discovered this positive perspective to be the case with pilots while I was working as a flight surgeon in the Air Force. They would often tell me that they couldn't believe they were being paid to fly; they felt like they should be paying the Air Force for the opportunity to fly.

Pilots and many other people who enjoy their jobs and the company of the people they work with, and of the people they serve, consistently demonstrate superior health. They feel they are part of a team, and they are uplifted by the sense of performing a valuable service to their community and fellow human beings. These positive feelings work to fortify and strengthen the integrity of their healing systems.

Many cultures consider work to be a form of worship, wherein your work and the services you provide, however humble, are an important opportunity for you to give back to the world. This perspective can enhance your self-worth, uplift your spirits, and generate positive emotions that stimulate your healing system and improve your vitality. In fact, many studies are now revealing that retirees who regularly volunteer their time in local community service enjoy much greater health and live much longer than their peers who do not participate in such activities.

If you are currently unhappy with your work, it is imperative to either change your attitude toward your work so that it can become more meaningful to you, or, if this is impossible, to find work that is more rewarding and enjoyable. Whether you work with others as part of a big company, or you work alone, learning to enjoy your work and focusing on its positive aspects will be health-enhancing, life-promoting, and a great benefit to your healing system.

Healing System Rx #8: Enjoy Your Play

One of the best ways to reduce tension and stress in your life is through play. Play represents a carefree state of mind that is vital to your overall health. This means taking the time to cultivate a sense of humor, and to be spontaneous, creative, and involved in such fun activities as sports, music, dance, the arts, or pursuing your favorite hobbies. I have met many people who did everything wrong from a health standpoint; however, because of their light-hearted attitudes, keen senses of humor, and their ability to play and have fun, they lived well beyond their life expectancy.

In nursery schools, kindergartens, and elementary schools throughout the world, play is an integral part of the daily routine and curriculum for all children. A child who does not know how to play is considered unhealthy and abnormal. This standard should also apply to adults.

Many adults become workaholics who regard play or having fun as a waste of time. On the contrary, most of humanity's greatest ideas and inventions have come from people who knew how to play and use their powers of imagination. In fact, most inventors claim their greatest ideas came to them not when they were actively pursuing them, but rather when they were involved in fun and frolic and were simply enjoying themselves. Many successful businessmen and professional people understand that, to be truly happy and healthy, it is important to know how to play.

Play is an effective way to strengthen your healing system because it helps you forget about time. In this state of timelessness, you are not worrying about the future or feeling sorrowful, grievous, or guilty about the past. Rather, you are completely absorbed and focused in the here and now. Freed from the mental and emotional forces that drain your energies and interfere with your body's internal processes of repair and regeneration, when you are playing, your healing system gets recharged. When you play, a light-hearted spirit prevails that influences brain biochemistry and causes the release of beneficial hormones, neurotransmitters, and other powerful chemicals that strengthen and support the activities of your healing system. The following story demonstrates the healing power of play.

Derek, a physician and personal friend who had been suffering from severe back pain with *sciatica*, was looking for a quick fix so he could get back to work as soon as possible. However, he couldn't find a surgeon who would operate on him promptly, so in a moment of exasperation he decided to go surfing. In his joy and enthusiasm for being in the ocean and doing something that he loved, he totally forgot about his pain and predicament. When he came out of the water, Derek was surprised to discover that his pain was gone! He became completely healed, and although his condition has not returned to this day, Derek now makes sure to take regular time out of his schedule to go surfing.

Play also encompasses the field of entertainment. Nearly every culture has made use of this aspect of play to pass on important moral, spiritual, or cultural lessons to upcoming generations, often in the forms of traditional songs, dances, poetry, or stories. While you are being entertained, you are usually in a more relaxed frame of mind, detached from your worries and problems. At these times, deep emotions can often be stirred up and released, causing laughter or tears. Again, these deep emotional responses trigger the release of beneficial hormones and chemicals that serve as powerful stimulants for your healing system. Live events such as concerts, plays, or sporting events carry an added benefit of creating intimacy and a feeling of belonging to a larger community as you share a collective, live energy that occurs when people are gathered together to focus on a common goal or activity. This sense of community can help combat the feelings of isolation and loneliness that often plague people who are struggling with health issues, lending further support to the work of the healing system.

Creativity is another important aspect of play. Pursuing hobbies, including the arts, music, singing, dancing, painting, writing, or participating in any one of a number of other activities involving the use of your hands and your more artistic side can also be a way of strengthening and fortifying your healing system. Many people have overcome life-threatening health conditions by becoming involved in creative projects that were deeply personal, meaningful, and fun for them. In fact, having your creativity stifled is now considered a major risk factor for contracting a chronic disease.

Cultivating the creative aspect of your spirit and remembering to develop a light-hearted attitude that fosters a spirit of play is important. From a health perspective, play needs to be an integral part of your daily life. Play can strengthen your basic natural energy and activate important internal mechanisms of repair and recovery that are an essential part of your healing system.

Balancing Your Work and Play

Both work and play are equally important, but balancing these important activities in your life is essential. Meaningful work lets you provide for your family and your personal needs. It also lifts your self-esteem, helps define your sense of purpose, and provides you with an opportunity to give back to the world. Play keeps you in a carefree, loving frame of mind, connected to your heart, and focused in the present. Play relaxes your body, mind, and nervous system. Maintaining a proper balance between work and play enables you to experience all these aspects of life, which helps to strengthen and fortify your healing system. Both work and play are important, and both need to be weighed and balanced with each other.

Healing System Rx #9: Develop Effective Social Skills

Since antiquity, people have lived together in families, clans, tribes, and communities to organize themselves, and to nurture and care for each other. Like bees and ants, humans are also social creatures. We depend on each other to make our lives meaningful.

Studies show that good social skills strengthen and fortify our healing systems, and that living a lonely and isolated life can be harmful to those systems.

Many people with serious illnesses have reported significant improvement in their health when they improve their socializing skills. These activities have included visiting with friends, or participating in some kind of volunteer community-support work, either at a day-care center, a senior center, a hospital, or some other charitable organization.

Well-known doctor and author Dr. Bernie Siegel tells a story to help illustrate this point. He tells of a special pass he got from God to visit both Heaven and Hell. In Hell, he saw many bowls of hot, steaming soup being served with long-necked spoons. This soup didn't look too bad until he realized that the hungry people in Hell were unable to feed themselves because the necks of their spoons were too long, and they kept missing their mouths with the spoonfuls of soup. When he got to Heaven, he was surprised to see the same bowls of soup and the same long-necked spoons. However, upon closer observation, he saw that the people in Heaven had learned to place the spoons in each others' mouths, so that everyone got fed.

Fostering a spirit of cooperation and sharing by building and developing strong social ties has been scientifically proven to improve survival. Because of the powerful biochemical effect that emotions exert on your healing system, many studies are now showing that people with inadequate social support who are lonely and socially isolated are at risk for developing serious, life-threatening physical diseases. According to the research of heart specialist Dr. Dean Ornish, social isolation and a lack of intimacy are considered top risk factors for the development of heart disease, the number-one killer in the Western world.

Good social skills begin with family and are usually learned in childhood. However, as the divorce rate continues to soar, and many families are broken apart, it is clear that many people will have to reach out beyond their families to their friends, colleagues, coworkers, and others to get the support they need to remain healthy. Doing so can strengthen their healing systems and can help to prevent physical illnesses associated with a lack of social support and intimacy.

Animals are also capable of giving and receiving unconditional love and, as pets, can serve as an important form of social support to those who may otherwise be isolated from family or friends. Senior citizens living alone who have pets have been shown to be at much lower risk for developing heart disease and other serious illnesses than those who do not have pets and are living with similar health conditions.

Developing effective social skills allows you to feel supported and connected to others. Knowing that your life counts, that you are important to others, that you make a difference, and that you have a purpose for being here create uplifting, inspiring, life-affirming emotions that help to strengthen and nourish your healing system.

Healing System Rx #10: Utilize Natural Elements That Support Your Healing System

Your body is linked to the world of nature and is dependent on certain key natural elements, including air, sun, water, and the various minerals and nutrients of the earth, for its very survival. Ancient physicians and healers understood this basic principle of health and healing. Of course, now that our medical science has advanced considerably, we have learned a great deal more about these natural elements and the complex ways in which we interact with them. And contrary to what we might expect, with all of the technological advances of modern medicine, the importance of our relationship with these natural elements to our health and healing has only increased.

Natural elements that are critical to the survival of your body can also serve as powerful therapeutic agents and medicines that aid and support your healing system when you are ill. And used preventively, these natural elements can help to keep you healthy for many years to come. Understanding and making intelligent use of these common resources from nature can significantly strengthen and fortify your healing system.

Air

As you probably know, the air you breathe contains the vital element of oxygen, which nourishes and energizes every cell and tissue in your body and is an essential ingredient to your healing system and your overall state of health. Oxygen is so important that it is the first medical agent administered to a critically ill or injured person, whether the condition is a heart attack, a gunshot wound, or any other serious life-threatening emergency. Oxygen is routinely stored for this purpose in ambulances and in all hospital emergency rooms, operating rooms, and intensive-care units.

Good, clean, fresh air, characteristically found in particular places in the world, can have life-enhancing effects on a person's health. This fact is reflected in better health statistics for those places. Generally, you can find better quality air where there is less industry and less pollution, and where steady breezes, ample water, vegetation, and mountains or hilly terrain help to purify, filter, and increase the quality of the air you breathe. Heavily forested areas usually have excellent air quality because of the voluminous oxygen so many trees produce.

Your body and your healing system deserve the best air you can find. If you find yourself indoors or in any environment with compromised air quality, walk outside or go to another place where there is good air. If you are currently battling an illness or are seeking to improve the quality of your health, pay close attention to the quality of the air you regularly breathe.

Fresh, outdoor air is almost always preferable to indoor air, which can become stale and stagnant, and which tends to attract mold, dust, and dust mites. Indoor air can also play host to toxic fumes, vapors, and other chemical aerosol irritants which, if ventilation is poor, can accumulate and concentrate. Fortunately, many indoor filters, purifiers, and humidifiers are now available to improve the quality of the indoor air you breathe.

Sunlight

In more ways than you may be aware, your health and well-being are directly linked to the sun. The sun not only fuels the reaction of photosynthesis in plants, which produces the oxygen you breathe and the food you eat, but the sun also determines the occurrence of night and day, and so influences the natural cycles that control the rhythmical ebb and flow of the chemistry in your body's internal environment. These cycles, known as *circadian rhythms*, include the most obvious cycle of sleeping and waking. Prolonged or even intermittent disruption of the sleep-wake cycle can be harmful to your healing system and can lead to disease.

The sun particularly influences your endocrine system, including your glands and hormones. Cortisol, an important hormone secreted by the adrenal glands, is markedly increased during hours of sunlight and decreased during hours of darkness. The effects of cortisol are vast and varied; it affects blood-sugar levels and immune function, which have a direct impact on your healing system. The sun also activates your pineal gland, which produces melatonin, a powerful hormone that affects the sleep-wake cycle. Melatonin also influences glucose metabolism, blood pressure, heart function, immune-system activity, and skin pigmentation, all important functions of your healing system.

Since ancient times, the therapeutic value of natural sunlight has been recognized as an essential element in healing. Physicians throughout the ages have prescribed regular sunbathing as an effective treatment for a number of common disorders. For example, the role that sunlight plays in building strong bones is well documented. Natural sunlight is the best source of vitamin D, which is required for calcium absorption in the intestines. Adding sunlight to your life can assist your healing system by ensuring that adequate calcium is absorbed to build strong bones as you grow and age.

Sunlight also aids your healing system in wound healing. It is common knowledge that wounds heal more rapidly when they are exposed to natural sunlight.

Sunshine can lift moods and improve one's outlook on the day. When people are exposed to periods of darkness or extreme lack of sunlight, depression invariably occurs. *Seasonal affective disorder (SAD)* is a common form of depression that occurs during the winter months in colder, darker climates. SAD is effectively treated with natural sunlight.

The Powerful Effects of Sunlight on Your Healing System

The sun is a powerful natural support for your healing system. Numerous studies have demonstrated the therapeutic role that sunlight plays in improving the health of those afflicted with a variety of specific illnesses and diseases. Here are a few brief examples:

- Sunlight and immune function: Sunlight stimulates immune system activity, and improves immunity.

- Sunlight and infections: Sunlight is a natural disinfectant. The ultraviolet rays in sunlight help kill pathogenic microorganisms such as viruses and bacteria. Where sunlight is scant, and darkness prevails, infections flourish. A famous example of this was the plague epidemic in the Middle Ages, also known as the Dark Ages, during which people characteristically lived in dark, crowded conditions with narrow, cobblestone streets and congested alleyways. This was the perfect breeding ground for rats infested with fleas that harbored the plague bacteria. The plague was also spread from person to person by the human body louse, which cannot tolerate direct sunlight. The plague wiped out millions, and the only people who survived the plague were those living outside of the city limits in the countryside, where they were exposed to fresh air and natural sunlight.

- Sunlight and respiratory infections: Sunlight exposure on the chest, and particularly on the back, helps speed recovery from respiratory infections, including bronchitis, pneumonia, and even tuberculosis, by drying secretions and killing microorganisms. In fact, people with TB (tuberculosis) used to be ordered by their doctors to move to Arizona for this very reason—to take advantage of the dry, sunny climate.

- Sunlight and skin infections: Skin infections, including fungal infections, staph infections, impetigo, and others improve and heal faster with natural sunlight, which acts as a disinfectant, drying agent, and natural antimicrobial agent.

- Sunlight and wound healing: Wound healing improves under the influence of direct sunlight. A wound will heal faster and resist infection more easily in the presence of sunlight.

- Sunlight and bed sores: Sunlight helps to heal bed sores and various skin ulcers.

- Sunlight and blood oxygen: Sunlight helps to oxygenate and purify the blood.

- Sunlight and jaundice: Sunlight helps to cure both neonatal and adult *jaundice,* which is a yellowing of the skin due to the accumulation of *bilirubin* in the blood, most often due to a liver problem. The standard use of hospital florescent lights in the treatment of this condition was pioneered by the discovery that babies with jaundice improved when they were exposed to natural sunlight.

- Sunlight and arthritis: Sunlight has been shown to be an effective adjunct in the treatment of arthritis, including *osteoarthritis, rheumatoid arthritis,* and other forms of arthritis.

- Sunlight and gout: Sunlight helps to break down and eliminate uric acid, lowering its concentration in the blood, and alleviating symptoms of gout.

- Sunlight and psoriasis: Sunlight helps in the treatment of *psoriasis* and helps eliminate the rash that appears as a result of this condition.

- Sunlight improves acne: Sunlight stimulates healthy renewal and regeneration of the outer layers of the skin; improves blood flow, circulation, and sweat-gland activity of the skin; improves lymphatic drainage; helps in the removal of surface oils and toxins; and helps to diminish the intensity of acne outbreaks.

- Sunlight and muscles: Sunlight increases circulation and blood flow to the skin, and improves muscle tone under the area of the skin exposed to the sun.

- Sunlight and weight loss: Regular sunbathing has been prescribed by Russian and Eastern European doctors in the treatment of obesity after it was found that sunlight stimulates thyroid-gland activity, which regulates your metabolism.

- Sunlight and peptic ulcers: Studies in Russia have also shown that sunlight affects the deep organs, including the stomach and intestines, reducing the amount of hydrochloric acid secretion, and helping to cure peptic ulcers.

- Sunlight and high blood pressure: Sunlight helps to normalize and lower blood pressure.

- Sunlight and diabetes: Sunlight normalizes blood sugar. It has been proposed that this occurs in some way through sunlight's interaction with insulin.

- Sunlight and heart disease: Sunlight reduces blood cholesterol levels. It helps to reverse plaque formation in the coronary arteries, which are the arteries that feed the heart, and it can improve blood flow to the heart. Sunlight also reduces plaque formation in the arteries going to the brain, lowering the risk of stroke. Sunlight improves oxygenation in blood and tissues, thus improving oxygen delivery to the heart and other vital organs in the body.

- Sunlight and cancer: Decreased rates of most cancers except those of the skin have been observed in animals and people exposed to regular sunlight.

- Sunlight and aging: Sunlight reduces *free radical* formation in the body; free radicals have been linked to the aging process.

- Sunlight and rickets: *Rickets* is a bone deformity of childhood caused by a lack of vitamin D, which regulates calcium absorption in the intestines. The best source of vitamin D is natural sunlight. Natural sunlight is especially important for mothers who are breast feeding, to help prevent rickets in their children.

- Sunlight and osteoporosis: *Osteoporosis* is a softening of the bones due to a loss of bone density. Increasing calcium intake is generally thought of as the solution to this problem, but regular sunbathing, with the sun being the best source of vitamin D, provides the greatest absorption of calcium in the intestines and is the most natural way to increase calcium in the blood, which leads to increased bone density.

As you can see, sunlight works with your healing system and the other organs and systems in your body in a multitude of ways to keep you healthy and strong.

Heat

Besides the sun, other forms of heat can serve as invaluable aids to your healing system. The following list is a small sampling of the applications of heat and the mechanisms by which heat provides natural support for your body's healing system:

- *Heating pads* relax muscles and improve blood flow, improve oxygenation of tissues, and help reduce swelling. Heating pads are effective in the treatment of back pain, muscle strains and spasms, joint injuries, arthritis, and many other conditions.

- *Hot water bottles* work as heating pads do and are used in similar conditions, including abdominal pain, gas, and constipation.

- *Hot foot baths* keep the feet warm and improve blood flow to the neck and chest area. They also are effective and helpful in the treatment of respiratory diseases.

- *Hot compresses* reduce swelling and help draw toxins out of affected areas. They help improve blood flow to the area being compressed, and they can be very effective in the treatment of abscesses, boils, and other skin infections and health conditions.

- *Hot water, teas, and broths* relieve congestion of mucous membranes. These liquids are often effective in the treatment of throat infections, sinus and nasal congestion, bronchitis, and other respiratory infections. They can also help to relax and soothe your colon and intestines, which aids digestion and elimination.

- *Hot showers* open and clean pores of the skin, helping to eliminate toxins while removing bacteria from skin surfaces.

- *Hot baths* relax and improve blood flow to sore or injured muscles. They are helpful for back pain, muscle pain, painful joints, and neuromuscular injuries.

- *Saunas* utilize heat to induce sweating and eliminate toxins from the body.

- *Steam baths* break up phlegm and mucous in the respiratory tract. They also relieve congestion and help to eliminate toxins from the body.

- *Jacuzzis* provide a hot-water massage to aching joints and muscles.

- *Infrared heat* relieves pain of muscle injuries, strains, sprains, bruises, and tendonitis.

Note: In using heat of any kind, it is important to remember not to overdo it and burn your body.

Water

Water is the most commonly found substance in all biosystems and arguably the most important of all natural elements. Water is so essential and integral to life that scientists exploring other planets will first look for signs of water before they declare the possibility that life exists or may have existed on that planet. You can further appreciate the importance of water when you consider that it is the dominant element in your body, constituting about 70 percent by weight and volume—not surprisingly, about the same percentage of water the surface of the earth contains.

We can look upon water, known as the universal solvent, not only as an essential nutrient for our healing systems, but also as a therapeutic agent and medicine. In addition to keeping our bodies healthy, water is almost always required in abundant amounts as a support for our healing systems when illness or disease sets in.

Maintaining adequate water intake is one of the simplest and most powerful ways to ensure good health and rapid recovery from illness or injury. Inadequate water intake can hamper the performance of your healing system and lead to dehydration, congestion, stagnation, obstruction, infection, and disease. You can determine whether you are getting enough water by monitoring the color of your urine. Dark yellow urine, which occurs when your body is trying to conserve water, invariably means that your body is low on fluids. Clear urine, like tap water, or very light yellow urine, usually indicates adequate water intake. If you are taking certain vitamins, such as the B and C vitamins, your urine can be artificially discolored; in this situation, monitoring whether or not you are getting enough water may be difficult. Also, because your urine tends to be more concentrated when you sleep, it is usually darker first thing in the morning.

When you are ill, increasing your water intake is important, to help improve the flow of fluids in and out of your body. These extra fluids assist your body's healing system to eliminate toxins, which are increased during periods of illness. Many illnesses respond dramatically if you drink only water for 48 hours or more. I have personally seen cases of many diseases, including respiratory conditions, *gastroenteritis*, gall bladder disease, gout, Crohn's disease, and many others dramatically improve by following this method. The importance of drinking plenty of water daily cannot be overstated.

In addition to drinking water, you can also employ water in many other ways as a natural and valuable support for your healing system. In fact, in Chinese medicine and the ancient medical systems of India, unique and specific internal cleansing techniques employ the use of water to help remove blockages and restore health to particular areas. In the West, water has also been used effectively in nasal douches, enemas, nebulizers, hot compresses, fomentations, Sitz baths, and simple soaking.

Minerals of the Earth and Your Healing System

The science of *nutrition* examines food sources derived from the earth and their biochemical impact on the health of the human body. Proteins, carbohydrates, fats, vitamins, minerals, and trace elements are all derivatives of the natural elements around you, without which you could not live. Scientific discoveries are now revealing that nearly every single mineral element found in the earth's crust and core, from arsenic to molybdenum, has been discovered within the human body in minute quantities. These minerals are not incidental contaminants; rather, controlled studies have determined that they are essential to the body's health.

Many of these vital mineral elements play critical roles within your body's internal environment, functioning as electrically charged chemicals known as *electrolytes*. Some of the more well known of these elements include sodium, potassium, magnesium, calcium, and phosphorous.

Electrolytes play important roles in supporting your healing system, and they participate in such diverse functions as the beating of your heart, regulation of the body's fluid levels, kidney function, brain function and the transmission of nerve impulses, bone formation, and many more. Any disturbance in the intricate balance of these minerals disrupts the flow of electricity and the transmission of electrical impulses in your body, which often causes serious illness, and possibly death. These mineral electrolytes are so important that they are routinely measured and monitored in the blood 24 hours a day in patients admitted to the intensive-care units of all major hospitals.

Salt

Salt is abundant in sea water and found throughout nature. There are many different types of salts throughout the world that consist of various combinations of minerals. However, common table salt, which consists of sodium and chloride and is used in cooking and as a seasoning, is the most well-known, most widely distributed, and biologically most important salt. Salt consisting of sodium and chloride is an essential natural ingredient in all living systems.

In addition to the necessity for a certain amount of dietary salt intake, salt is also a valuable natural support for your healing system. Sodium and chloride are arguably the most important electrolytes in your body, and they play a key role in the functioning of your healing system. Salt also has important therapeutic applications in both the prevention and treatment of various conditions and illnesses. Because of its ability to absorb water and draw fluid out, its preservative effect, and its ability to kill bacteria and other harmful microorganisms, humans have relied on salt for centuries as a valuable aid in curing and preventing infections. Learning to work with salt is a safe and effective, simple yet powerful way to assist the work of your healing system.

The following list is a small example of how salt can assist your healing system:

- *Salt packs, salt soaks, and salt fomentations* are applied externally to intact skin with warm water to help draw out unwanted fluids, swelling, and toxins from various skin and soft-tissue infections, including carbuncles, furuncles, cysts, and abscesses.

- *Salt water* also can be taken internally as an aid in various forms of intestinal cleansing, to prevent and assist in the treatment of food poisoning, diarrhea, and nausea and vomiting. (Note: When taken internally, salt water must be used under qualified medical supervision.)

- *Salt-water gargles* can be very effective in treating pharyngitis, sore throats, and tonsillitis.

- *Salt-water nose drops*, or the use of salt-water nasal douches, can be extremely effective in the treatment of nasal allergies, hay fever, rhinitis, colds, congestion, and sinus infections.

■ *Nebulized saline* is another form of salt water employed as an effective aerosol spray used in the treatment of asthma and other respiratory conditions.

Clay

The therapeutic use of clay as a natural support for the healing system among traditional indigenous cultures is well documented. Pharmaceutical-grade clay, a naturally occurring substance sometimes referred to as *bentonite*, is readily available at most drug or health food stores. Applied to the skin as a paste, clay works well as a natural drawing agent. In addition to its ability to draw off toxins and reduce swelling from infections, clay works with your healing system by supplying valuable trace elements and minerals that are absorbed into the body in minute but significant quantities. Clay applications can speed the healing of insect bites, boils, abscesses, and many other skin conditions; it can be used alone or in combination with other substances, such as aloe, salt soaks, or ginger compresses. Clay is gentle, safe, and effective, even in difficult cases.

Clay also can be taken internally as an intestinal purifier to help absorb toxins from the intestines; it has been employed like this in European folk medicine for centuries as a way to improve colon health and regulate bowel function.

Plants and Herbs and Your Healing System

Throughout the ages, man has relied on the healing properties of various plants and herbs. And although most doctors in modern countries have come to rely on medicines derived from synthetic pharmaceutical compounds, the use of plants and herbs has experienced a dramatic comeback in Western societies in recent years. Herbs and plants, when used with intelligence and discretion, can help strengthen and fortify your healing system.

Many of these natural medicines have proven track records in other countries, including China, Japan, and India. Even until recent times in our own Western medicine, *botany*, which is the study of plants, was a required course in most medical schools. In fact, many modern drugs and medicines have their origins in the natural world of plants.

Here are a few of the most common plants and herbs that are effective in supporting your healing system:

- *Aloe* grows like a succulent cactus. Its leaves contain a clear liquid gel that has healing and antiseptic qualities. Aloe can be applied topically to burns, cuts, scrapes, skin infections, and other injuries in which the raw surfaces of skin have been exposed. Aloe helps not only to fight and prevent infection but also to aid the actual healing process. It is safe and gentle, and it can even be taken internally in limited quantities to help heal ulcers in the mouth, stomach, and intestines.

- *Ashwaganda* is a traditional herbal remedy from India that has been used for thousands of years as a tonic and to enhance natural host resistance factors. Ashwaganda can be taken long term to increase one's stamina and strength.

- *Astragalus* is an ancient plant medicine from China. It is used to bolster defenses and appears to be especially effective for respiratory illnesses.

- *Bilberry* aids in wound healing and is especially effective in assisting the healing system repair damage done to small, fragile blood vessels, particularly those of the eyes and kidneys. Bilberry may also be effective in treating certain types of macular degeneration and other eye diseases, trace blood in the urine, as well as venous insufficiency and varicose veins.

- *Comfrey* is known as "knit bone" in American and European folk medicine for its ability to expedite the healing of fractures. Comfrey also aids in healing wounds of the skin, mucous membranes, respiratory system, and intestines. It can be applied externally as a poultice or taken internally. The leaves or roots of this plant can be used, although the roots are not recommended for internal use.

- *Dong Quai* is a Chinese medicine used to support the health of the female reproductive system, and it has become increasingly popular in the West. It is often used to help alleviate menstrual cramps and balance estrogen metabolism.

- *Echinacea* is a popular herb commonly used in the early stages of mild respiratory infections; it may also be helpful in wound healing and other conditions.

- *Garlic* is used as a blood purifier. Many people claim to have lowered their blood pressure with garlic. Used in soups, it is often effective for the treatment of a cold or respiratory infection.

- *Ginger* is a root that can be grated and used fresh, or dried or powdered. It can also be used in the form of a tea. Ginger helps to create heat in the body. It is offered on sea voyages as standard fare to soothe the stomach and help prevent motion sickness. As a tea, ginger is very effective in cases of pharyngitis and tonsillitis. It can often curtail the spread of strep throat if the illness is caught in its earlier stages. Ginger can also be applied to the skin in the form of a poultice; it helps to draw out toxins in cases of skin and soft-tissue infections.

- *Gingko* is derived from one of the oldest living plants on the earth. Gingko has been used in Oriental medicine for centuries, and even Western scientific research has verified that it can improve blood flow to the brain, increasing memory and mental alertness, and even eyesight. This herb is also used in the treatment of tinnitus, migraine headaches, vertigo, and as a possible agent in stroke prevention. It may also prove helpful in cases of Alzheimer's disease.

- *Ginseng* is a tonic herb traditionally valued in the Orient for its ability to prolong life, increase energy in the body, and improve sexual stamina. Some studies suggest that ginseng may improve the health of the nervous system, as well as cardiac function in the elderly, by increasing the tone and contractility of heart muscles.

- *Guggal* comes from a tree resin that grows in India. It has been used for centuries to help reduce weight. Studies have also shown guggal to be effective in lowering cholesterol.

- *Kava root* is a traditional medicine from Polynesia that helps relax the nerves. It is used as a muscle relaxant and for mild cases of insomnia and anxiety. Kava root also can be useful for back pain caused by muscle spasms. Because it can induce drowsiness, Kava root should not be used when you are driving or operating mechanical equipment.

- *Milk thistle* helps to support the health of the liver. Many patients with elevated liver enzymes resulting from chronic hepatitis and other liver conditions have reported significant improvement in their symptoms and laboratory readings of their liver enzymes after they have taken milk thistle for several months. The mechanisms by which milk thistle supports and heals the liver is still unknown, yet a growing number of conventionally trained liver specialists are now recommending it to some of their patients.

- *Neem* comes from the leaves of the Neem tree in India, which is the traditional food eaten by camels. Neem is used in Ayurvedic medicine from India as a powerful blood purifier.

- *St. John's wort* is widely prescribed in Europe as an antidepressant. You might need to take this herb for several weeks to notice its effects, and you should not take it with any other conventional psychiatric medication. By itself, St. John's wort is generally quite safe and often effective.

- *Turmeric* comes from the ginger family. The dried, powdered root is the part of the plant most often used. Turmeric gives curry powder its characteristic yellow color. Turmeric applied to the skin as a paste is often effective in a variety of skin disorders. Taken internally, it helps to improve the health of the liver and eyes. It also is now being used as an adjunct in the treatment and prevention of certain cancers and liver disease.

- *Valerian* has been used in folk medicine as an aid to anxiety and insomnia, and it is quite effective in mild cases of these conditions. Valerian is also sometimes recommended as a gentle muscle relaxant.

Many natural medicines are quite potent, so it is important to be careful that they do not conflict with any other medicine you are currently taking. As with any new substance you take into your body, if you experience untoward effects, discontinue its use and seek the advice of a qualified health professional for further recommendations.

Closing Thoughts on Strengthening and Fortifying Your Healing System

In time, falling raindrops carve deep canyons and valleys out of mountains. Added to other grains of sand, a tiny grain of sand can make a large beach or vast desert. Similarly, individual health factors, which may seem insignificant and unworthy of our attention when considered alone, form the very foundation for strengthening, fortifying, and activating your healing system when they are added together. In combination, these factors also can substantially improve your overall health and the quality of your life. These factors include listening to your body; paying attention to your personal hygiene; maintaining a healthy diet; doing regular exercise, stretching, and stress management; balancing work and play; developing good social skills; and incorporating healthy natural elements into your daily routine, such as drinking plenty of water, breathing fresh air, getting adequate sunshine, and using natural herbs and minerals when appropriate.

In the next chapter, we will look more closely at the critical role diet and nutrition play in strengthening and fortifying your healing system. By following a few simple dietary and nutritional guidelines, you will not only greatly improve your overall health, but you'll also gain the maximum benefits from your extraordinary healing system.

CHAPTER 5

Fueling Your Healing System

High-performance machines, from racing cars to rocket ships, all require specialized fuels to make them go. Your body is no different. In fact, your body is the greatest of all high-performance machines on this earth, created to last up to 100 years or more. Your body is an engineering masterpiece of nature, more complex, sophisticated, durable, and intelligent than anything ever crafted by man. Your body is adaptable to a variety of climates, environments, and life situations, capable of moving in an infinite number of ways, and of enduring and surviving conditions of extreme hardship and deprivation.

As you already know, your body has been designed with such skill, precision, and expertise that it comes equipped with its own healing system. This extraordinary system is self-contained, self-monitoring, and highly intelligent, and is capable of supervising and initiating mechanisms of repair, restoration, and recovery from a huge assortment of illnesses, injuries, and insults. To accomplish these tasks, your healing system mobilizes specialized cells and stimulates powerful biochemical reactions that can rapidly mend damaged tissues when you are ill or injured. It also maintains a balanced and highly ordered natural state of health when you are not sick or injured. No other machine on this earth can boast of such a system. And just as with any other high-performance machine, your healing system performs best when it receives special, high-performance fuel. The fuel your healing system requires is wholesome, nutritious food.

A Wholesome Diet for a Strong Healing System

The best way to keep your healing system strong is to eat a balanced, wholesome, simple, natural diet. Such a diet consists of a well-rounded blend of all essential nutrients. These nutrients include adequate amounts of proteins, fats, carbohydrates, vitamins, minerals, trace elements, fiber, fluids, and other vital nutrients such as *phytochemicals* (special health-promoting molecules found in fruits and vegetables). Your daily requirements of these substances will vary according to where you live, what you do, and your basic metabolic requirements.

The Best Fuel for Your Healing System

Fruits, vegetables, grains, legumes, nuts, and seeds provide the purest energy source for your healing system, and these foods are essential for strengthening and fortifying this most important system in your body. In addition, fruits, vegetables, grains, legumes, nuts, and seeds

- Constitute the nutritional foundation for most other mammals, including those with much larger muscle mass than humans. Our primate cousins, including gorillas, chimpanzees, orangutans, baboons, and monkeys, also eat foods almost exclusively from these categories.

- Are generally easier to digest than most flesh foods, and, again, represent the purest energy source for the metabolic demands of your healing system.

- Are lower on the food chain and contain far fewer toxins and environmental pollutants than most foods that are derived from the flesh of other animals.

- Take less time to cook, and are generally safe enough to be consumed raw.

- Have less chance of spoiling and putrefying than animal products do. As a result, the possibility of contamination and food poisoning from these foods is much less.

- Are usually less expensive, and don't require the extensive and continuous refrigeration for transport and storage that flesh foods need.

These simple, wholesome, natural foods are the keys to the health of your healing system. All nutrients are ultimately derived from the soil and atmosphere of the earth, and eating a wide variety of these foods will ensure the best chance of a complete diet.

Use the following list as a guide to the foods that serve as the best fuel for your healing system. Depending on where you live and what is available, you may have many more food choices within these categories of fruits, vegetables, grains, legumes, nuts, and seeds.

- Whole grains, including rice, wheat, oats, rye, corn, and barley

- Leafy greens, including lettuce, spinach, and cabbage

- Roots and stems, including carrots, turnips, potatoes, and onions

- Beans and legumes, including soy beans, pinto beans, sweet peas, black-eyed peas, chickpeas, mung beans, lentils, and peanuts

- Seeds and nuts, including walnuts, pecans, cashews, hazelnuts, and almonds

- Fruits, including apples, oranges, bananas, pineapples, cherries, berries, grapes, apricots, peaches, and watermelon

- Other vegetables, including bell peppers, broccoli, cauliflower, cabbage, squash, tomatoes, chili peppers, okra, and mushrooms

Essential Nutrients for Your Healing System

Before we go on, it is important to discuss briefly the essential nutrients that we mentioned earlier—protein, carbohydrates, fats and oils, vitamins, minerals, trace elements, and phytochemicals—and how they affect your healing system. Doing so will give you a greater understanding of the rationale behind the practical ways to fuel your healing system.

Protein and Your Healing System

Protein provides the structural elements for growth and repair of your bodily tissues, and it is one of the most important nutrients for your healing system. Protein is also the primary nutrient building block for your muscles which, at 40 percent of normal body weight, are the largest and most dynamic, energy-dependent structures in your body. In addition to its predominance in muscle tissue, protein is found in nearly all cells and tissues of your body, including your blood.

Adequate dietary protein intake is required for growth in children; if it is not taken in required amounts, it can result in muscle-wasting disorders in children. But because the daily requirement for protein is only about an ounce a day, a lack of protein today in Western countries is rare. In spite of this, unfortunately, a lingering fear of not getting enough protein drives much of the unhealthy dietary practices currently in vogue in Western countries. This fear results in overeating, which can lead to obesity and can be very harmful to your healing system.

Many people in Western countries have come to depend on meats and animal products as convenient sources of protein. Unfortunately, these foods contain highly saturated animal fats with no fiber, which creates an unnecessary burden on the healing system. Learning to incorporate protein from non-meat sources in your daily diet is a much healthier and safer approach for your healing system.

Carbohydrates and Your Healing System

Carbohydrates are derived from plants. Carbohydrates constitute the major fuel source for your healing system. The old, common name for carbohydrates was *starch*, which we sometimes attribute to the heavier, denser carbohydrates, such as potatoes and certain grain flours that make bread. Starch was erroneously thought to contain "empty calories," but today we know differently. Because carbohydrates provide the greatest overall return of energy of all foods, marathon runners and triathletes typically "carbohydrate load" before a major race by eating lots of pasta and breads. They know from experience that this is the best long term, high-performance fuel for their dynamic bodies.

Grains such as rice, wheat, oats, corn, barley, and millet, in addition to potatoes, are the largest staple food crops in the world, and these have served as traditional sources of carbohydrate nutrient energy for the majority of the world's population for many years. These foods, which contain "complex" carbohydrates, are the longest lasting, slowest burning, and most efficient of all fuel sources for your healing system. Additionally, they usually contain lots of fiber, and so are extremely beneficial to the health of your colon and heart. Foods with complex carbohydrates also are valuable sources of essential vitamins, minerals, and trace elements, and other nutrients such as phytochemicals. To strengthen and fortify your healing system and keep it running smoothly and efficiently, your diet should consist of about 60 percent complex carbohydrates.

Fats and Oils and Your Healing System

Fats and oils are essential for the performance of your healing system. Specifically, they promote healthy skin and nails, and they contribute to the structural integrity of cell membranes in your body, which aids your healing system in preventing infection. Fats and oils also help to protect and coat nerve sheaths, which improves the health of your body's communications. As you know, your healing system depends on an efficient and accurate communications system. Fats and oils also pad and cushion internal organs in your body, protecting them from injury while they insulate and keep your body warm. Because fats are lighter than water and are high-energy nutrients, they are also a convenient way to store fuel that your healing system can use when food intake is inadequate or scarce.

For these reasons, a small amount of fats and oils in your daily diet is necessary for your health. Additionally, some fat-soluble vitamins and other nutrients can be absorbed only with fats and oils. For example, omega-3 fatty acids, found in flaxseed oil and certain fish oils, help the healing system with blood clotting and can be absorbed only with fats and oils.

There are, no doubt, other beneficial nutrients in certain fats and oils that have not yet been discovered. But because fats and oils represent the densest and most concentrated forms of food energy, their over-consumption can contribute to obesity and other health problems, including heart disease, the number-one killer in the Western hemisphere. Fat intake should be restricted to 10 percent to 25 percent of your total daily calories, depending on your activity level and current health status. For example, Dr. Ornish, at the University of California in San Francisco, found that a 10-percent daily fat intake works best to aid your healing system in reversing heart disease.

Cholesterol is an important type of structural fat that supports the health and integrity of your healing system and, in particular, your cell membranes. In addition to the cholesterol it obtains from your diet, your body can manufacture its own cholesterol from other fats and oils. A diet that exceeds your body's basic daily caloric requirements, however, will create more cholesterol in your body than is needed, and, if this occurs, the excess cholesterol can form blockages that clog arteries and lead to heart disease. Reducing total fat intake, or restricting total calories, while increasing daily activity levels can help lower cholesterol levels and aid your healing system to dissolve blockages, open up clogged arteries, and improve blood flow to your heart.

Vitamins and Your Healing System

Vitamins are naturally occurring compounds that are essential to the healthy functioning of your healing system. They work with your body's various enzyme systems and are critical to the performance of important, life-sustaining processes involved in the growth, repair, and regeneration of healthy as well as damaged tissues. Although vitamins are usually required in much smaller quantities than other basic nutritional elements, such as proteins, fats and oils, and carbohydrates, a diet that doesn't include them at all can impair the functioning of your healing system and result in illness.

Vitamin requirements often change over time, they vary slightly for males and females, and they increase during pregnancy and lactation. Athletic training and recovery from illness and injuries may increase the body's requirements for one or more vitamins. Because the body's biochemical pathways and metabolic processes are complex, subtle, and still remain largely unexplored, it is certain that more vitamins than we currently know about will be discovered in the future and recognized as essential to our healing systems.

The best way to ensure adequate vitamin intake for your healing system is to eat a well-rounded, wholesome diet with plenty of whole grains, nuts, seeds, fruits, vegetables, and a certain limited amount of fats and oils (again, specific vitamins require fat for absorption). When a problem occurs in a specific area of your body, you may need to supplement normal dietary sources with a specific vitamin, or concentrate on eating foods that contain higher quantities of a specific vitamin, to support the work of your healing system in that area.

Vitamins That Strengthen and Fortify Your Healing System

The list that follows describes the various vitamins that are essential to the health of your healing system. This list is a guide and is not all-inclusive; new vitamins are currently being researched, and many more are still to be discovered. The recommended dietary allowances (RDAs) listed are per-day estimates, based on the findings of the Food and Nutrition Board, National Academy of Sciences, National Research Council. The RDAs are for people 14 years of age and older. They vary slightly for males and females, with requirements changing during pregnancy and lactation, athletic training, and recovery from illness and injuries.

- *Vitamin A* aids your healing system in protecting the health of your eyes; it also promotes healthy skin growth. A lack of vitamin A can cause poor night vision and blindness, as well as skin problems. Recent research suggests that vitamin A also helps prevent certain cancers. Good sources of vitamin A are foods that contain beta carotene, including most orange and yellow fruits and vegetables such as mango, papaya, squash, yams, and carrots. The recommended dietary allowance of vitamin A is 800 micrograms (mcg) to 1,000 micrograms (mcg).

- *Vitamin B₁ (thiamin)* aids your healing system in maintaining the health of your nervous system. A lack of vitamin B_1 can cause beriberi and other disorders of the nervous system and brain. Good sources of vitamin B_1 include whole grains, legumes, vegetables, fruits, and milk. The recommended dietary allowance of vitamin B_1 is 1.1 milligrams (mg) to 1.5 milligrams (mg).

- *Vitamin B₂ (riboflavin)* supports your healing system by protecting the health of your skin and nervous system. A lack of vitamin B_2 has been linked to dermatological and neurological problems. Good sources of vitamin B_2 include most vegetables, cereals, and grains. The recommended dietary allowance of vitamin B_2 is 1.3mg to 1.7mg.

■ *Vitamin B_3 (niacin)* supports your healing system's role in maintaining healthy skin, nerves, and gastrointestinal health. A lack of vitamin B_3, or niacin, can cause *pellagra*, a serious disease. Good sources of vitamin B_3 include grains, nuts, most vegetables, and legumes. The recommended dietary allowance is 15mg to19mg.

■ *Vitamin B_5 (pantothenic acid)* participates in a variety of physiological processes that support your healing system. These include energy metabolism, blood-sugar regulation, and production of antibodies, cholesterol, hemoglobin, and hormones. The recommended dietary allowance is 4mg to 7mg.

■ *Vitamin B_6 (pyridoxine)* is used by your healing system to protect the health of your nervous system, blood, and urinary system. A lack of vitamin B_6 has been linked to nervous-system disorders, anemia, and bladder stones. Good sources of vitamin B_6 include whole grains, cereals, nuts, and most vegetables. The recommended dietary allowance is 1.6mg to 2mg.

■ *Vitamin B_{12} (cyanocobalamine)* aids your healing system in supporting the health of your central nervous system, and in the production of red blood cells. A lack of vitamin B_{12} causes anemia and nervous-system disorders. Good sources include milk and dairy products, most animal products, and fermented soy products. Because vitamin B_{12} is one of the most potent substances known to mankind, and because your liver has a tremendous capacity to store this vitamin for up to five years, the recommended dietary allowance is very small, at only 2mcg.

■ *Folic acid* works in conjunction with vitamin B_{12} to support your healing system's role in maintaining healthy nerves and red blood cells. A lack of folic acid, sometimes seen during pregnancy and alcoholism, can lead to anemia and nervous system disorders. Good sources of folic acid include grains, cereals, dark green vegetables, and fruits. The recommended dietary allowance is 180mcg to 200mcg.

■ *Biotin* aids your healing system in maintaining healthy skin and nerves. A lack of biotin has been implicated in skin and nervous-system problems and may affect cholesterol metabolism. Good sources are soybeans and grains. The recommended dietary allowance of biotin is 30mcg to 100mcg.

■ *Vitamin C (ascorbic acid)* aids your healing system by playing an important role in wound healing, collagen formation, immune defense, inflammation, and cancer prevention. Vitamin C deficiency can cause *scurvy*, a disease characterized by fragile blood vessels and impaired wound healing. The best natural source of vitamin C is most fruits, including citrus. Certain vegetables, including red chili peppers, are also good sources of vitamin C. The recommended dietary allowance is 60mg.

■ *Vitamin D* aids your healing system by playing a key role in calcium metabolism and bone formation. A lack of vitamin D causes rickets and can contribute to osteoporosis and other disorders. Natural sunlight is the best source of vitamin D. Naturally occurring substances in the skin absorb sunlight and are converted into the active form of vitamin D. Vitamin D is now added to milk, cheese, and butter. The recommended dietary allowance is 5mcg.

■ *Vitamin E* (d-alpha-tocopherol) supports your healing system by playing a key role in wound healing. When applied topically, vitamin E aids in scar formation and helps keep skin healthy and strong. When taken internally, it also acts as an antioxidant, important in the prevention of heart disease and cancer. Good sources of vitamin E include the oil of many seeds and nuts, vegetable oils, and wheat grains. The recommended dietary allowance is 8mg to10mg.

■ *Vitamin K* supports your healing system as an essential component of your body's blood-clotting mechanisms. Vitamin K is naturally produced by a specific strain of bacteria that live within your own intestines, where the vitamin is absorbed. Good dietary sources of vitamin K include green tea, spinach, cabbage, and other leafy green vegetables. The recommended dietary allowance is 65mcg to 80mcg.

You can see from these descriptions how important vitamins are to the optimum functioning of your healing system. Be sure you include vitamins in your daily diet, and that you get at least the minimum daily requirements for each one.

Minerals, Trace Elements, and Your Healing System

In addition to vitamins, minerals are also powerful essential nutrients that aid and support your healing system. They are required for growth, repair, and regeneration of tissues, to keep your body healthy and free from disease. Minerals are derived directly from the earth's core, and they have unique properties. They are integral to the structure and function of important enzymes, hormones, and they transport molecules, such as hemoglobin, within the body. As noted earlier, almost every mineral element that exists in the core of the earth has been found to exist in minute quantities in the human body. Even arsenic, generally considered to be a poison, is required in trace amounts by your body.

Trace elements are chemically related to minerals and usually classified in the same nutritional category. The difference between trace elements and minerals is that minerals are required in slightly greater amounts than trace elements, and their functions are a little better understood. We know that trace elements are required for good nutrition and health, but we don't know exactly how much of each one is needed and exactly what each one does. We do know, however, that a deficiency of trace elements in your body results in a failure to thrive, increased susceptibility to disease, and even death. So although they are required in very small amounts, trace elements are absolutely critical to the optimum functioning of your healing system.

Minerals and Trace Elements That Support Your Healing System

Following are the most important minerals and trace elements for the health and functioning of your healing system.

Important Key Minerals

■ *Calcium* plays a key role in helping your healing system with bone formation, blood clotting, nerve conduction, and muscle contraction, including the muscles of your heart. Sources of calcium include dairy products, broccoli, leafy green vegetables, and some fruits. Osteoporosis can result from a lack of calcium and increased parathyroid hormone secretion. The

RDA for most men is 800mg/day. For premenopausal women, the RDA is 1000mg/day, and for postmenopausal women and elderly men it is 1500mg/day.

- *Copper* is important for your healing system to regulate cell metabolism, collagen formation, and tissue repair. Sources of copper include fruits, grains, seeds, and nuts. The RDA has not yet been established.

- *Fluoride* supports your healing system and is important in tooth and bone formation. Sources include mineral water, plants, and fruits. Many dentists and pediatricians recommend supplementing with fluoride for children if you are living in an area where the water supply may not be fluoridated. The RDA for fluoride has not yet been established.

- *Iodine* is a key element of thyroid hormones and plays a critical role for your healing system in energy metabolism, including the regulation of body temperature. Iodine deficiency results in the well-known condition of goiter, which produces a large swelling in the neck that is the result of an enlarged thyroid gland. Good sources of iodine include sea water, sea salt, algae, and sea foods. The RDA is 150mcg.

- *Iron* is a central part of the hemoglobin molecule and functions in oxygen transport, which is essential for your healing system to repair and restore the health of organ tissues. In addition to red meats, sources of iron are all red fruits and vegetables, including beets, watermelon, raspberries, cherries, strawberries; dried fruits, including raisins, dates, and figs; beans; and certain leafy vegetables, including spinach. Vitamin C enhances the absorption of iron in your body. The RDA for iron is 10mg.

- *Magnesium* is important for your healing system to regulate energy metabolism and blood pressure. Sources of magnesium include leafy green vegetables and fruits. The RDA for magnesium is 280mg to 350mg.

- *Phosphorous* is important for helping your healing system support bone metabolism. Good sources of phosphorus include fruits, vegetables, and whole grains. The RDA is 800mg to 1200mg.

- *Potassium* is important for your healing system to support the functioning of your heart while helping to conduct nerve impulses in your body. Potassium, along with sodium, also helps your healing system by facilitating water movement in and out of your cells, and by directing water flow in and out of your body. Good sources of potassium are most fruits and vegetables, including green leaves as well as roots and tubers. The RDA for potassium has not been established.

■ *Sodium* is an important electrical ion in your body that aids your healing system by playing a key role in nerve conduction while regulating the movement of water across cell membranes and tissues. The most common source of sodium is table salt. Keep in mind that too much sodium for certain people has been linked to excess water retention, which can be a problem if you have congestive heart failure, hypertension, and kidney disorders. The RDA for sodium has not yet been established.

■ *Sulfur* is important for helping your healing system aid and support the formation and structural integrity of proteins and other compounds in your body. Good sources of sulfur include both plant and animal proteins. The RDA has not yet been established.

Important Key Trace Elements
Other important minerals, called trace elements, are essential to the health of your body and your healing system, but they are required in minute amounts. These minerals include: arsenic, bromine, boron, chromium, cobalt, manganese, molybdenum, selenium, silicon, tellurium, vanadium, zinc, and quite possibly many others, including cadmium, lithium, silver, and gold. Good sources of trace elements include rich and varied plant life grown in natural, volcanic-derived, organic soil, which is the most fertile source of all minerals on this earth. Even though they are critical to the health of your body and healing system, in general, trace elements are present in the body in such small amounts that determining exactly how much you need every day is difficult.

Vitamin and Mineral Supplements

Research shows that you are better off getting your vitamins, minerals, and trace elements in their most natural form, the foods that you eat, rather than from supplements. This is because vitamins, minerals, and trace elements are better absorbed when they are bound to other natural nutritional elements digested and assimilated by your body. For instance, iron is better absorbed in your intestines in the presence of vitamin C. For this reason, I generally don't recommend vitamin or mineral supplementation unless you are suffering from a specific vitamin deficiency or a health condition that could be significantly improved through vitamin therapy, or your diet is incomplete in one way or another.

If you choose to supplement your diet, do so with discretion and care. Supplemental vitamins and minerals are concentrated and not in their natural state, and if you take them in excess, they can cause serious health problems. Vitamins and other supplements should never replace a good, wholesome diet. I frequently encounter people who do not focus enough time and thought on their diets but instead rely on their supplemental vitamins and minerals to make up for any deficit in their diets. When it comes to selecting healthy, nourishing foods for your healing system, it is of paramount importance that you take time to listen to and work with your body. When you are just starting out, it is also a good idea to work with your doctor and preferably a reliable nutritionist to help you determine the best nutritional program for your individual health needs.

Phytochemicals: Nature's Medicines

Phytochemicals are naturally occurring chemicals in plants that have both nutritional and health-enhancing effects, and they support your healing system in many ways. Phytochemicals facilitate the processes of growth, repair, and tissue regeneration. They also help prevent certain chronic, degenerative diseases, including cancer and heart disease. Among the better-known phytochemicals are the *carotenoids*, including beta carotene, a parent compound to vitamin A, found in yellow- and orange-colored fruits and vegetables. Carotenoids prevent heart disease and are beneficial in the prevention of certain cancers. *Lycopenes*, found in tomatoes, are also helpful in the prevention of certain cancers, heart disease, and other chronic conditions. Many health experts feel that Italians have such low rates of heart disease and cancer because of their steady diet of tomatoes, which contain lycopenes.

Other phytochemicals play a significant role in supporting your healing system and can help overcome a wide variety of diseases, particularly the prevention and healing of certain cancers, heart disease, and even macular degeneration, the leading cause of blindness in the elderly. Because these important phytochemicals come from a wide variety of plant sources, it is important to eat a wide variety of colorful fruits and vegetables to make sure your healing system is getting enough of these natural chemicals.

Probiotics and Your Healing System

Probiotics represent another class of compounds important in the nutrition and health of your healing system. Probiotics are produced by certain strains of bacteria that naturally live in your intestinal tract, and they also occur in nature. These strains of bacteria can aid your healing system in combating illness, restoring health, and maintaining proper biochemical balance in your body. More than 500 different strains of bacteria have been discovered to live in your intestines, helping to break down ingested foods while producing valuable metabolic byproducts that are then absorbed and carried to the various cells and tissues in your body. One of these products is vitamin K, which your healing system utilizes as an essential ingredient in blood clotting.

Scientists have discovered, for example, that ingesting *lactobacillus* bacteria, commonly called *acidophilus*, which occurs naturally in yogurt and is now available in supplemented commercial milk preparations and other products, reduces childhood diarrhea, decreases the likelihood of intestinal side-effects while people are taking antibiotics, and prevents yeast infections in women. Probiotics often can successfully combat infections, especially those of the intestinal tract, and possibly those of the respiratory system. They may also reduce the required dosages and possible toxicity of childhood immunizations. Probiotics appear naturally in many traditionally fermented foods, such as vinegar, wine, cheese, yogurt, tempeh, and soy sauce.

Twelve Essential Tips for Fueling Your Healing System

To help strengthen and fortify your healing system with the right fuel, you need to follow a few simple nutritional guidelines. Keep in mind, however, that we all are unique individuals with different nutritional needs that can change and evolve as we grow, age, or modify our activities or environment. It is important, therefore, that you not cling blindly to any one set of stringent nutritional or dietary formulas that may not be appropriate for you. As a general rule, listen to your body, trust in its inherent wisdom and natural state of health, and respond intelligently to its ever-changing nutritional needs and demands.

Tip #1: Eat a Simple Diet Rich in Fruits, Vegetables, Whole Grains, Seeds, Nuts, Beans, and Legumes

For the sake of high-performance nutrition, most experts are now recommending a simple diet predominantly based on foods obtained from fruits, vegetables, whole grains, beans, legumes, nuts, and seeds. These foods are more balanced and contain a much higher concentration of vitamins, minerals, trace elements, and other valuable nutrients than flesh- and meat-based foods. Plant-based foods also contain more beneficial complex carbohydrates, more unsaturated fats and oils, and, contrary to popular opinion, they are also excellent sources of protein. Numerous studies have clearly established a link between a greater intake of fruits and vegetables and greater health and longevity. Under most conditions, these are the best fuels for your healing system. These foods are also an excellent source of fiber, which is essential for optimal intestinal health. Fiber has been shown to prevent colon cancer as well as heart disease. We also obtain valuable fats and oils from these foods. Plant-based foods contain less saturated fat, and they also contain fewer toxins and less pesticide residues than other foods. Plant-derived proteins, which are plentiful in beans, legumes, nuts, seeds, and grains, are generally more beneficial than protein from meats and animal flesh. When you consume meats or animal products, try to eat less, and try to eat these foods only as condiments or flavorings, as the Chinese and Japanese do. And if you feel so inclined, eat them during special occasions, such as holidays or birthdays, as a form of celebration, as the early hunting-gathering societies did.

The trend toward a healthier diet consisting of simpler, more wholesome, natural foods and fewer flesh foods is supported by the health data from the countries with the largest populations in the world, including China and India, in addition to other countries where people derive the majority of their nutritional requirements from fruits, vegetables, grains and legumes. In these countries, there is far less heart disease, hypertension and stroke, cancer, diabetes, arthritis, and other chronic degenerative diseases—the so-called "diseases of civilization"—than in countries that derive more of their nutritional requirements from flesh foods and animal products.

Meat and flesh-based foods are convenient sources of protein, which helps maintain the growth and health of muscles, but most studies now reveal that these diets have greater disadvantages than advantages. Most meat-based diets contain harmful substances, such as saturated fats that can clog the arteries in your heart and brain, and environmental toxins, including heavy metals and pesticide residues, which are stored and concentrated in animal tissues. When we compare them to other simple, wholesome, natural foods, meats also lack sufficient fiber and other essential nutrients, such as vitamins, minerals, and trace elements.

Although many people erroneously assume that plant-based diets are lacking in protein, their fear of not getting enough protein from plant sources is not scientifically valid. Studies have proven that it is easy to get abundant protein from a diet that combines grains and legumes with other fruits and vegetables. Other studies have shown that traditional cultures around the world that have survived for centuries on these simple, wholesome, natural foods show little to no evidence of heart disease and cancer.

Many excellent meat substitutes are now available that are derived from soy, legumes, and other vegetable-protein sources. In the more progressive cities in America and Europe, many restaurants now offer these products on their menus, as do most supermarkets and grocery stores.

The average daily protein requirement for most adults is less than 40 grams, which is a little more than an ounce. Whenever there is a question of adequate protein intake, daily protein requirements can be met by combining beans (legumes) or seeds with grains. An example would be eating beans and tortillas, as we commonly do when we eat Mexican food. An even simpler example would be a peanut-butter sandwich on whole-wheat bread. Tofu is also an excellent complete protein, and it can be prepared in many ways. Dairy products, including milk, cheese, butter, and yogurt, are also excellent sources of protein. Many excellent nutrition plans and cookbooks for healthy eating based on a diet that incorporates more fruits and vegetables are available.

Tip #2: Consume More Fluids, Including Soups, Juices, Herbal Teas, and Water

Your healing system requires adequate fluid intake to function optimally. Because your body is 70 percent fluid, all metabolic processes in your body occur predominantly in a liquid internal environment. For this reason, it is important to drink lots of water throughout the day. The more liquids you consume, the more effectively fluids can circulate in your body, and the more rapidly your body can eliminate toxins. Fluids also aid in the healing of infections and many other congestive and degenerative conditions. Many illnesses can be traced to chronic dehydration resulting from a lack of fluid or water intake. Fresh fruits and vegetables, many of which are more than 95 percent water, are excellent sources of fluid.

Tip #3: Consume More Fiber in Your Diet

Fiber is an essential fuel additive for the health of your colon, heart, and healing system. Adequate fiber intake ensures your ability to eliminate unwanted waste and toxins from your intestines, and it can help prevent cancer and degenerative diseases. Because meat doesn't have fiber, and because most Americans eat more meat than any other food, they usually don't get enough fiber in their diets. This lack of fiber causes problems with elimination, which results in the steady buildup of toxic waste in the body. Waste buildup puts an extra burden and strain on the healing system and can set the stage for illness. The best sources of fiber are predominantly fruits, whole grains, and other plant-derived vegetables, including beans and legumes, nuts and seeds.

Tip #4: Eat Food That Is Prepared Fresh

Consume food that is prepared fresh each day. Don't eat food that is stored in freezers for long periods of time, has been sitting on shelves for a long time, or was prepared months to years in advance and then prepackaged. This food often has lost its vitality and nourishment, and it also may be harmful to your body. Also avoid refined foods, including refined flours, which are devoid of fiber and often contain harmful additives and preservatives. If you eat breads and pasta, try to eat those made with whole-grain flours. Eat less artificial and refined sugars. Instead, when you crave sweets, eat more fresh fruits and natural sweeteners, such as honey and fruit-derived sweets, including juices and dried fruits. Processed, refined, and packaged foods lack the vitality, freshness, and fiber that your healing system requires to function optimally, and they may cause it to work overtime by creating unhealthy conditions in your body.

Tip #5: Include Raw Foods in Your Daily Diet

Eat at least one portion a day of raw foods, including fresh vegetables and fruits. This raw food could be in the form of a salad with fresh sprouts, or fresh fruits and vegetables, such as carrot sticks or fresh apple pieces. Raw fruits and vegetables are loaded with vitamins, minerals, and trace elements, and they contain a high fiber and fluid content. Make sure, however, that you chew raw foods well because they can be difficult to digest if they're not chewed adequately. Raw fruits and vegetables, with their high fluid and fiber content, assure efficient circulation and elimination in the body, while they provide essential vitamins, minerals, trace elements, and natural sugars for your healing system.

Tip #6: Eat Regular Meals, at Regular Times

Your body's digestive system is set up to handle regular meals. Going all day without eating, and then overeating for dinner, is a common habit that can contribute to digestive problems, overburdening your body and making your healing system sluggish. A steady flow of nutrients works best for your healing system, not starving it all day long and then overloading. Graze on healthy snacks if you get hungry, or if your blood sugar gets low. However, make sure not to spoil your appetite for your meals. Eat more toward the earlier part of the day and less in the evenings.

Tip #7: Take the Time to Plan and Cook Your Meals

Proper nutrition is essential for your health. Although preparing healthy, wholesome food might take a little extra thought and time, just remember that your healing system deserves and requires the best fuel you can give it. Like anything that's worthwhile, proper nutrition takes planning and preparation. If you wait until you are hungry to decide what you are going to eat, you will most likely grab the nearest food available, which could be fast food or convenient junk food. Take the time to shop for and cook healthy, wholesome foods.

Tip #8: Create a Pleasant Ambiance When You Eat

Eating your food under pleasant circumstances, in a calm, quiet environment, enhances the smell and taste of the food and improves digestion. While eating, use pleasant settings, including quality plates, silverware, and serving utensils. Light a candle or use soft lights at the table. Avoid watching TV while you eat, or eating with the stereo or radio blasting, which can interfere with proper digestion and the assimilation of vital nutrients. Avoid arguing or getting upset for any reason while you eat. If you are upset, it is best to wait until you are calm to eat because emotional upheaval can adversely affect body chemistry and have a negative impact on digestion and your health. Cultivate a spirit of gratitude for the food that you consume. Many cultures around the world consider the ambiance surrounding food, such as how it is prepared, and how it is received, to be equally important to, if not more important than, the biochemical composition of the food.

Tip #9: Chew Your Food Slowly and Thoroughly

The process of digestion begins in your mouth, aided by digestive enzymes secreted by your salivary glands. So chewing your food slowly and thoroughly is important. Doing this makes digestion easier and more efficient for your stomach and intestines.

Most healthy, fresh, wholesome food requires thorough chewing before you swallow it. Proper chewing depends on good teeth, which is why dental hygiene is also an important part of your overall physical health and personal hygiene. Not chewing your food slowly and thoroughly because you are eating when you are in a hurry or upset can cause indigestion and rob your healing system of necessary vital nutrients.

Tip #10: Eat a Wide Variety of Foods

Do your best to satisfy your body's nutritional requirements by eating a wide variety of foods. This variety will ensure the opportunity for a greater selection and utilization of nature's essential nutrients. In the past, populations that were confined to limited choices in their diets often came down with severe nutritional deficiencies.

Because many vitamins, minerals, trace elements, and other nutritional substances are associated with natural pigments and dyes that contribute to the specific colors of certain fruits and vegetables, many nutritional experts recommend eating as wide a variety of fruits and vegetables as possible, including every color in the rainbow in your diet at least weekly. For all practical and scientific purposes, this approach represents the safest and most reliable way to ensure the highest-octane fuel for your high-performance healing system.

Tip #11: Eat Fewer Rich, Heavy Foods

Rich, heavy foods taken in excess can clog your digestive, lymphatic, and circulatory systems, draining your body of healing energy. Such foods have been linked to a number of diseases, including gout, gall bladder disease, heart disease, diverticulitis, and many others, including cancer.

Rich, heavy foods, which contain a lot of fat, oil, and protein, represent the most difficult of all foods to digest, often taking at least four or five hours, and sometimes even longer. The time and energy required to break down and digest these foods will interfere with the performance of your healing system. The process of digestion can redirect blood flow and energy away from the work your healing system is doing. If you are healing, and you are not undernourished, it is important to keep your diet light. Avoid or minimize rich and heavy foods.

Tip #12: Minimize the Use of Alcohol and Stimulants

Minimize or reduce alcohol intake. Consider eliminating it altogether or saving its use for special, festive occasions. Alcohol, which is a nervous-system depressant and also has negative effects on the liver, can make your healing system sluggish and incompetent.

In addition, minimize or eliminate the use of stimulants, including caffeine, which is commonly found in coffee, tea, and caffeinated sodas. Caffeine stimulates the nervous system and can increase mental agitation and cause stress. Stress constricts your blood vessels and promotes the fight-or-flight response, which interferes with the performance of your healing system.

Closing Thoughts on
Fueling Your Healing System

It is important to remember that your body is a high-performance machine, with an extraordinary healing system that requires the highest-performance fuels available from the purest sources. Repair and restoration of damaged tissues require energy, and the energy you consume in the form of food will have a tremendous influence on your healing system and your overall state of health and well-being.

Remember to eat foods that are wholesome and nutritious, fresh and balanced, and that contain plenty of vitamins, minerals, trace elements, fluids, and fiber. These foods include most fruits and vegetables, whole grains, nuts, seeds, soups, herbal teas, juices, and water. Make sure you are getting adequate protein, carbohydrates, fats, and oils in your diet. Eat natural foods that represent every color in the rainbow at least once in a week's time to get enough phytochemicals. Take time to prepare your meals thoughtfully, eat regularly, avoid unhealthy snacking, and chew your food well. If you are attempting to heal yourself from a chronic illness or condition, reduce the amount of flesh food in your diet, or eliminate it altogether. Avoid rich and heavy foods unless you need to put on weight. Also be careful with alcohol and caffeine intake.

There are many excellent resources for nutrition. When it comes to fueling your healing system, respect your individuality, remember to keep an open mind about trying and learning new things, and don't be too rigid or fanatical about following a stringent dietary regimen that has worked for others but may not be right for you. Above all, stay informed, and listen to your body as you focus on fulfilling its ever-changing nutritional needs.

CHAPTER 6

The Power of Your Mind and Your Healing System

Your mind is your healing system's most powerful ally. Working through your brain and nervous system, your mind can send powerful messages to your body that can dramatically influence the performance of your healing system. Through these mechanisms, a sophisticated communication feedback system sends precise, split-second information from your body back to your brain. Your mind remains in intimate contact with your body's ever-changing internal environment while it works side by side with your healing system. In the words of well-known physician and author Dr. Andrew Weil, "Wherever nerves are, activities of the mind can travel."

All mental activity, whether conscious or unconscious, has a powerful influence on your healing system and can enhance or interfere with its performance. For example, when your mind is in a positive state, immersed in thoughts of love and affection, caring and compassion, enthusiasm, health, happiness, joy, and peace, beneficial chemicals known as *neurotransmitters* or *neuropeptides* that are secreted by your brain can actually infuse your body with positive energy, strengthening your healing system and improving your health. Alternatively, when your mind is in a negative state, with thoughts of pessimism, cynicism, jealousy, anger, hatred, fear, revenge, self-criticism, blame, shame, guilt, and despair, you are sending negative messages to your body via equally powerful neuro-chemicals that can weaken your healing system and interfere with its ability to do its job effectively. In the words of Robert Eliot, M.D., "The brain writes prescriptions for the body."

When you understand the power of your mind, and its enormous ability to work either for you or against you, you will no longer waste valuable time or energy blaming outside forces, including "fate," "bad genes," "evil microbes," a polluted environment, or other people for your illnesses, diseases, or lack of good health. Outside forces can certainly play a role in disease processes, but, in the final analysis, your health is based more on the personal choices you make for yourself, moment by moment, each day of your life, and your ability to optimize the incredible power of your mind to aid your healing system. You are the one who is ultimately responsible for your health, and so it is imperative that you understand this principle. More than any other power or force in this world, your own mind can serve as your healing system's most qualified and capable partner.

How Your Mind Affects Your Healing System

Your mind works through your brain and nervous system, generating thoughts that are converted into electrical impulses. These electrical impulses travel through the many nerves that are distributed to the various organs and tissues of your body, in much the same way as electricity moves through wires.

For example, when you want to move your arm, before the actual movement, a thought is first generated in your mind that causes electrical impulses to stimulate specific nerves that will in turn direct the muscles in your arm to contract. This sequence of events results in movement in your arm. The part of your nervous system that is responsible for this type of movement is known as the *voluntary nervous system* because the movement is voluntarily brought into action by your own conscious thinking.

Another part of your nervous system, however, known as the *involuntary nervous system, or autonomic nervous system,* is more wide-reaching in its distribution and more powerful in its influence over your body's internal environment. The autonomic nervous system regulates such critical biological functions as your heart beat, your breathing, your blood pressure, your digestive processes, your perspiration, your vision, your elimination of waste products, and many others.

Within the autonomic nervous system are the *sympathetic* and *parasympathetic* branches. The sympathetic branch increases activity and movement in your body; this branch is responsible for the well-known fight-or-flight response. The fight-or-flight response occurs when you are feeling threatened or are experiencing stress, and it can be initiated by thoughts of fear, worry, anxiety, panic, and anger. It can be measured by an increase in heart rate, oxygen consumption, breathing, blood pressure, and blood flow to the large muscles of locomotion in your legs and arms. These physiological changes are beneficial to help you "fight or flee" during a crisis or emergency, but they also serve to inhibit the activities of your healing system, which generally requires a more quiet and relaxed internal environment within which to operate. Additionally, when the fight-or-flight response is elicited repeatedly, or prolonged over a lengthy period, it can prove harmful and damaging to your body because it creates too much work for your healing system.

The parasympathetic branch of the autonomic nervous system counterbalances the sympathetic nervous system and the fight-or-flight response by producing a calming effect on your body. This branch is associated with states of rest, relaxation, repair, regeneration, and healing. Thoughts that activate the parasympathetic nervous system include those of relaxation, peace, love, serenity, harmony, and tranquility.

In these ways, your mind plays a pivotal role not just in directing the movement of certain muscles in your body, but, far more importantly, in influencing and modifying the physiological processes of your internal environment in ways that have a direct effect on your healing system. Because your brain can process approximately 600 to 800 thoughts every minute, you can see what an enormous impact your thinking and mental activity can have on the health of your body.

Mind as Healer, Mind as Killer

You can use your mind for your body's ultimate health and healing, or you can use it in a way that turns against you to the detriment of your health. Your mind and your thoughts can cause real physiological changes in your body, as the *placebo effect* demonstrates. If you learn to use your mind to cooperate with your body's healing system, it can be your healing system's most powerful ally, a loyal servant and friend. If you do not use them properly, your mind and thoughts, through the release of powerful neuropeptides, hormones, and electrical nerve stimulation, can weaken and damage your body's health, interfere with your healing system, and cause premature physical deterioration, disease, and even your ultimate demise. If it is not properly trained and used, your mind can become a definite liability, prove to be your worst enemy, and even kill you. The following story about Jerry, one of my patients, demonstrates the crucial principle that learning how to use your mind for the benefit of your body's health and well-being can literally mean the difference between life and death.

Jerry was a tire salesman from a small town in Texas. He was in his early sixties and had already suffered from one near-fatal heart attack just a year earlier. He was lucky to be alive. His cardiologist had placed him on restricted activities until further notice. However, Jerry could not resist the offer of spending the weekend with his buddies in a small hunting cabin in the mountains of Colorado. Even though he had decided to go on the trip without letting his doctor know, he told himself he would take it easy and not disobey his doctor's orders. He would not push himself or do anything strenuous that might injure his heart.

However, because of the increased altitude in the mountains where Jerry was staying, the oxygen was a little thinner than he was used to—something he had forgotten to take into account. As he was returning to his cabin one evening after an uphill stroll, he began to feel the familiar chest pain and pressure that signaled another heart attack coming on.

At that moment, Jerry made a conscious decision to use the power of his mind to avert a possible heart attack. He simply told himself, "I refuse to have another heart attack!" His mind was so absolutely committed to avoiding the dreaded experience of having a heart attack again that his symptoms subsided, and his pain went away. He has never had another problem with his heart since that day. Of that day, Jerry told me, "Doc, I just made up my mind that it wasn't going to happen to me again! I simply refused to have another heart attack!"

Stories like Jerry's are not uncommon, and they demonstrate that, when constructively applied, your mind can be a powerful ally of your body's healing system. Your healing system is programmed to listen to your mind, so it is important to be conscious of the thoughts and messages you may be sending.

The Merry-Go-Round and the Sorry-Go-Round

Every day, researchers are discovering more ways that your mind and body are connected and influence each other. The intimate relationship between your mind and your body affects your health in many ways. For example, people who are happy, emotionally balanced, and socially well-adjusted enjoy better health and are sick less often. When you are in a good mood and feeling good about yourself, you will most likely want to take better care of your body; eat wholesome, nourishing food; take time to exercise; get enough sleep and rest; and participate in other life-promoting activities that will contribute to your body's overall health. Alternatively, if you become depressed, or if your spirits are low, you will not have the energy to take very good care of yourself. You may not feel like exercising regularly, which can weaken your cardiovascular system and possibly cause you to gain weight as a result of inactivity. All this can put you at risk for heart disease, diabetes, high blood pressure, and other diseases. Or you may not eat healthily or drink enough fluids, which can lead to excessive weight loss and vitamin, mineral, and other nutrient deficiencies, leaving you weak and dehydrated, vulnerable to disease. You may not bathe as regularly as you should, which can lead to skin infections, and the possibility of other infections, as well. Depression can create stress and anxiety, which can have a further negative impact on your health. All of these factors have a negative influence on your healing system.

In the same way that your body is powerfully influenced by your mind, your mind is also influenced by your body. For example, when you are feeling physically fit, exercising regularly, eating good food, getting adequate sleep and rest, and feeling relaxed, your mental faculties will be sharper and clearer, and your attitude and outlook on life will be inspired and enthusiastic. Conversely, certain physical ailments such as anemia, thyroid dysfunction, nutritional deficiencies, and insomnia are known to cause mental fatigue, lethargy, anxiety, and altered mood states. Hallucinations and mental psychosis can occur with electrolyte imbalance caused by extreme dehydration, heat stroke, or kidney dysfunction. That chronic pain can lead to mental depression is also well-known. Even a cold, cough, or flu can make you feel low and affect your attitude. Additionally, when you feel bad physically, you can easily become frightened and anxious. Under conditions of impaired physical health, mental health is adversely affected, and it is not uncommon for thoughts of impending doom, prolonged suffering, and even death to accompany such illnesses, especially if the illnesses are more severe or prolonged.

Whether you begin with poor physical health that creates poor mental health, or poor mental health that creates poor physical health, you can get caught in a harmful cycle without even realizing what is happening, a cycle that can be difficult to break. With the poor health of your body pulling your mind down, and your lowered mood and depressed mental health adversely affecting your body, you can tumble down, down, down in a continuing spiral of increased suffering on both mental and physical levels, into worsening physical and mental health.

This cycle is known as the Sorry-Go-Round. The Sorry-Go-Round is a term I like to use to describe the downward spiraling cycle that occurs when poor physical health affects your mental health, which affects your physical health, which affects your mental health, and so on. But this cycle also can first begin with your mental health affecting your physical health. The point is not which came first—the physical or mental problem. It is that they feed off each other and create a harmful downward-spiraling cycle that is difficult to break.

Through the power of your mind, you can become aware of this harmful cycle when it afflicts you, and, once you are aware of it, you can successfully break it by implementing positive, beneficial changes on both physical and mental levels in a two-pronged approach (both physical and mental) that will lead you to what I call the "Merry-Go-Round."

The Merry-Go-Round describes the opposite state, in which your mind and body are cooperating with each other in a positive way for your optimum health. Contrary to the Sorry-Go-Round, in which a downward spiraling effect of continued negative mental attitudes and degenerating physical health occurs, in the Merry-Go-Round, an upward spiraling effect of positive mental and enhanced physical health perpetuates itself. When your body feels healthy, your mind feels good. When your mind feels good, your body is also likely to feel healthier. When you feel good physically, this uplifts your mood and contributes to a positive mental state. A positive mental state helps to inspire life-affirming, positive, optimistic thoughts that will have beneficial effects on your body's physiology. This kind of positive interaction is what your healing system thrives on.

The Merry-Go-Round strengthens and nourishes your healing system so that it can perform at maximum capacity. This is one of the most obvious reasons you want to ride on the Merry-Go-Round, or, if you have fallen off, to get back on as soon as you can. You can take definite measures to ensure that you ride on the Merry-Go-Round. A few are suggested here to get you started. Remember, a two-pronged approach that implements both mental and physical strategies works best.

- Exercise can be an important strategy to help you get back on the Merry-Go-Round if your mental health and spirits are currently low and slumping. If you or a loved one suffers from depression, studies have shown that exercise can help overcome this problem. This is just one example to demonstrate that the improvement in physical health often results in the improvement of mental health.

- Stress-management techniques, which you will be reading about shortly, can help you avoid the knee-jerk tendency to become fearful, anxious, and scatterbrained in the face of daily problems, and they are another powerful way to stay on the Merry-Go-Round.

- Positively programming your mind for health and healing is another important method to help you get on the Merry-Go-Round. This chapter describes several practical strategies that are based on this important principle.

The health of your healing system depends on your ability and determination to get off the Sorry-Go-Round and get on the Merry-Go-Round. In this chapter, you'll learn various ways to do this, and to enhance and strengthen your healing system so it can do its job effectively and efficiently.

Psychoneuroimmunology and Your Healing System

Psychoneuroimmunology, known as *PNI* for short, is an important new field of medical science that studies the interaction between your mind and your immune system. New findings in this field have a direct bearing on understanding how your healing system works because, as you know, your immune system is linked to your healing system in the defense of your body. Your healing system collaborates with your immune system and depends on the health of your immune system to function at its best.

You may recall that your healing system and your immune system are decidedly different, and they also have certain similarities. One similarity is that they both are affected by your thoughts, emotions, attitudes, and the activities of your mind.

Rigorous and innovative scientific investigation in psychoneuroimmunology is helping us to understand more about the wonderful healing resources that exist within us. It also is helping us to lay to rest several key, erroneous myths about how our bodies function in relation to our minds. One myth was that what goes on in the mind has absolutely nothing whatsoever to do with what goes on in the body, which was taught to young doctors in medical schools for several hundred years. To support this erroneous notion, it was further believed that the immune system, which manages the body's defenses, functioned completely independent of the brain. But, thanks to several important discoveries by researchers working in the field of psychoneuroimmunology, these outdated beliefs have finally been proven wrong. There is now unequivocal proof that your mind talks directly to your immune system. This new understanding is based on the following findings:

- Specialized receptor sites for *neurotransmitters,* which are chemicals produced by the brain, are now known to exist on specific white blood cells.
- Tiny nerves have been discovered that are connected to the lymph nodes. This discovery provides concrete evidence that the immune system and

lymph nodes, which contain white blood cells, are directly connected to the nervous system and the brain.

- Powerful hormones have been discovered that are produced and secreted by specific white blood cells. This means that the immune system talks to the endocrine system and directly participates in one's emotional experience.

These advances in psychoneuroimmunology lend further scientific evidence to what Hippocrates and other ancient physicians and healers have been telling us for thousands of years: that a positive mental and emotional state can improve the body's ability to heal itself.

Practical Strategies for Using Your Mind to Strengthen Your Healing System

Your mind is your healing system's most valuable and powerful ally, and so it is important to learn how to maximize your mind's incredible power. The following techniques and strategies can help you focus and direct your mind to strengthen your healing system.

Positive Mental Programming

Pilots have one of the most dangerous, difficult, responsibility-laden jobs in the world. Because the lives of many people are in their hands, their sound physical and mental health is of the utmost importance. As a consequence, both the psychological and physical exams for pilots are among the most meticulous and closely scrutinized of any occupation in the world. When pilots are trained, they go through a form of mental training that includes programming their minds into a specific, success-oriented mode. Pilots must focus their thought processes on creating strategic, action-oriented behaviors that will result in a positive outcome and nothing else. Pilots do not have the luxury of entertaining thoughts that will contribute to a negative outcome during the flying mission. Airplanes move fast. If pilots make mistakes, even small ones, in the blink of an eye those mistakes can be fatal, not only for the pilots, but for the flight crew and passengers, as well.

Nowhere is the importance of this mental training for pilots more apparent than during landing. Landing a plane is one of the most challenging and difficult aspects of flying any aircraft. Upon descent and before landing, pilots set their sights for the runway while they are communicating with the control tower. Just as they will line up their airplanes along a certain approach to the runway, they have already focused their minds on a specific train of thoughts that entertain only a preselected sequence of decisions and actions that will produce a successful landing. Some flexibility is required, of course, but all thoughts during this period must be focused on the positive outcome of a safe and successful landing. Pilots cannot entertain any unproductive thoughts that could possibly result in a negative outcome. If pilots were to entertain such foolish thoughts, the sheer weight of their distractive powers would most likely result in a crash. A kind of self-fulfilling prophecy would most likely ensue. Entertaining negative thoughts would prevent the pilots from focusing on the constructive thoughts that are necessary to execute the precise skillful movements required for successful landings.

In the world of health and healing, as in flying, the key role that your mind plays in determining a positive, successful outcome cannot be overstated. When it comes to your health, you simply do not have the luxury of entertaining negative thoughts or negative outcomes. Just like a pilot, you need to set your sights on a positive outcome, believe that outcome is possible for you, and then act on that belief, refusing to allow any unhealthy thoughts of disease and suffering to distract you from your goal. Your healing system needs this positive thinking to function at its best and keep your body and all its systems running smoothly. Without the nourishment and fuel of positive thinking, your healing system will become "distracted" from its critical role in maintaining your health and well-being, and it will not be able to function properly.

For example, If you come down with a respiratory infection or any other illness, and you want to get better, focus your mind on being healthy again by implementing the following mental strategies:

- Set your sights firmly on the goal of being healthy again.
- Mentally repeat that you will get better, and continue to do so until the belief is firmly ingrained in your mind.

- Make a mental checklist of things you can do to get better soon. For instance, if you have a respiratory infection with a fever, your checklist may look something like this:

  Call in sick for work.

  Contact your doctor.

  Get plenty of rest.

  Drink fluids.

  Avoid rich, fatty foods.

  Keep warm.

  Take medicines as needed.

  Continue to set your sights on your goal of being healthy, mentally repeating this goal as often as you can.

- If you cut your finger and are bleeding profusely, the same mental programming would apply, only the checklist would differ somewhat:

  Find a clean cloth, cotton ball, or bandage, and apply direct pressure to the wound.

  Place your hand above your heart to reduce blood pressure and bleeding.

  Once bleeding has stabilized, contact family members or friends to inform them of your injury.

  If the wound needs professional attention, seek immediate medical care.

  If you are seen by a health professional, follow his/her orders concerning wound care, cleansing and bathing of the wound, and medical follow-up.

  Restrict activities as needed to assist the process of wound healing.

  Continue to set your sights on the healing of your wound and the restoration of your health. Mentally repeat this goal as often as you can.

Adapt your positive mental programming to fit the needs of your particular situation and condition. Many people have used positive mental programming successfully to overcome even serious health conditions, including cancer, heart disease, multiple sclerosis, and HIV. The following story is a good example of the powerful effects of positive mental programming.

Jan's Story

Jan was diagnosed with breast cancer, and even though she went through the grueling treatments of a radical mastectomy, chemotherapy, and radiation, she was given only six months to live.

Rather than giving up all hope and becoming another cancer statistic, Jan decided to enlist the help of her mind to rid her body of this dreaded condition. She had read about other people overcoming insurmountable odds to defeat their diseases, and she thought that, if it was possible for them, she might be able to do it, too. Because her life was on the line, she plunged headfirst into researching how she could possibly turn her health around. She committed herself to programming her mind in a positive way.

While Jan was deciding to concentrate on nutrition and natural supplements that could build up her strength and resistance, she also began reading books on how her thoughts and attitudes could stimulate healing mechanisms deep within her body, even though at that time the idea of a healing system was virtually unknown. Practicing several mental techniques that helped her relax, slow down, stop worrying, and develop a better sense of humor, Jan began to focus more on a positive outcome. After several months, she began to feel more energy, vitality, and stamina coming into her body. With these obvious physical signs of improvement, her attitude improved, and she began to actually believe she might be able to follow in the footsteps of others who had similarly overcome cancer. She did all this in spite of the mastectomy she had and the odds that were weighing heavily against her.

Today, 30 years later, Jan is totally cancer free and radiates a spirit of calm reassurance and optimism that is obvious to anyone who meets her. She has long outlived the doctors who first pronounced her death sentence. Through her difficult journey, Jan has come to realize the tremendous healing power of her own mind. She selflessly volunteers her time in assisting other women with breast cancer, encouraging them not to give in to hopelessness and despair, but, rather, to use the body's greatest ally in healing, the mind, to strengthen and fortify their healing systems through the cultivation of life-affirming, constructive thoughts and positive mental attitudes.

Infusing Your Healing System with Positive Beliefs

Beliefs are powerful thoughts that we hold onto and invest with great energy as if they were true, even though they might not be true. Your beliefs help to shape the way you think and view the world, and often they are backed by the collective support of many people, including family and friends. Your beliefs are also reinforced and influenced by many factors, including your education, the books you read, the media, your colleagues, peers, community, religious preferences, gender, and age, and your own personal thoughts and unique life experiences.

Beliefs can be passed down from one generation to the next. They can extend far back in time, covering centuries, and even millennia. Beliefs often gain strength over time. The more people who share in a similar, common belief, the more powerful that belief becomes. When beliefs become heavily invested with a lot of time and energy, letting go of them and changing them is difficult, even when they are wrong. For example, in medieval Europe, before Christopher Columbus's historic voyage in 1492, the belief was that the world was flat, and that if you sailed too far out to sea, you would fall off the edge of the world. Of course, we now know that this belief was not true, but for hundreds of years, many peoples' lives were affected by this limited view.

Beliefs are constructed of powerful thoughts, and as such they can play a major role in determining your health. Beliefs can significantly influence the performance of your body's healing system through the powerful messages they send to every organ, tissue, and cell in your body. If your beliefs are positive, healthy, and life sustaining, they can work to your advantage. For example, in a well-known study that looked at Harvard University graduates over a 25-year period, those who believed their health was good or excellent at the beginning of the study had significantly fewer illnesses and diseases, far better survival statistics, and reported enjoying much better health at the end of the 25-year study period than those who reported their health as only fair or poor.

The following approaches will help you infuse your healing system with positive beliefs:

- Choose a positive belief that supports your goals of improved health. Examples might be "I believe I can be healed," or "I am becoming strong and healthy."

- Refuse to entertain beliefs that oppose your positive belief about your health.

- Write down your positive belief and repeat it, first saying it out loud to yourself, then whispering it, and then mentally repeating it over and over again as often as you can, whenever you can.

- Read books, watch movies, and participate in activities that nurture, support, and reinforce your positive belief about your health. Such activities might include eating healthy food, getting adequate sleep and rest, going for regular exercise, receiving massages once a week, and so on.

- Seek out and surround yourself with positive, optimistic people who reinforce your positive belief about your health.

- Avoid people who oppose your positive belief. If you have a pessimistic, unsupportive doctor, find one who can be more optimistic and encouraging.

- You may choose as many positive health beliefs as you desire.

Negative beliefs, which are based on fear and pessimistic projections concerning your health, can actually interfere with the performance of your body's healing system and can result in harm to your body. If you sustain such beliefs over a sufficient time period, they can even become self-fulfilling prophecies. Again, recalling Dr. Eliot's famous words, "The brain writes prescriptions for the body," this is only common sense. For example, if you think long and hard about getting cancer, you may be contributing to the physiological processes that will create a toxic internal cellular environment that can actually cause cells to mutate and manifest in cancer. If you think long and hard about getting a heart attack, your thoughts and beliefs can create the internal chemistry within your body that constricts the coronary arteries in your heart and shuts down the blood supply to your heart muscles, which can contribute to an actual heart attack.

Even though scientific research in these mind-body interactions is still relatively new, a large number of studies already in the medical literature confirm the reality of these destructive mental processes. The good news is that many new studies are now showing that you can transform and overcome these negative influences by focusing more on positive, life-enhancing beliefs and incorporating an optimistic view of the world into your beliefs.

An example of the power of positive beliefs is evident in the story of AIDS. When AIDS was first discovered, just the diagnosis of being HIV positive was enough to kill a person. More than the actual virulence of the virus, this result was due largely to the fear and dread these individuals associated with the mysterious elements of the virus and the disease. Now, people are better informed and not so fearful about HIV and AIDS. Not only has HIV lost its diagnostic shock value, but the long-term survival rates and quality of life also have improved dramatically among people who are HIV positive. For the most part, this change has come about not so much through breakthroughs in miraculous medications, but rather through people becoming empowered to fight back and reclaim their health through a change in their beliefs about HIV. Basketball superstar Magic Johnson is one such example, and there are many others.

Transforming Negative
Beliefs into Positive Beliefs

Entertaining and holding onto beliefs that will enhance your health may not be easy, especially if you were raised in a family or environment that taught and encouraged negative beliefs. However, you can succeed by following the strategies described in this chapter.

In fact, many people who have overcome serious, life-threatening afflictions did so by discovering that the roots of their physical suffering were anchored in the muck of unhealthy, negative beliefs they had harbored about themselves and their bodies since childhood. Some of the more commonly reported of these negative beliefs are these: "You are a bad person," "You do not deserve love," "You do not deserve to be happy," "You need to be punished for your sins," "You deserve to suffer and have pain," or "The only way you can receive attention or love is if you get ill."

For many people who have overcome serious illnesses, healing from the physical aspects of their diseases meant expunging the disease at its psychological roots. They needed to let go of the deeply ingrained, negative beliefs that led to a lifetime pattern of unhealthy, self-destructive thoughts and related behaviors such as smoking, overeating, drinking, drug abuse, staying in abusive relationships, having unsafe sex, and taking unnecessary risks that lead to accidents and injuries. These negative beliefs and behaviors are not unlike those that would cause people to end their lives by putting a bullet in their brains or jumping off of a bridge.

Of those who have successfully healed themselves, many have been able to look back on their diseases as gifts that helped them transform mentally, emotionally, and spiritually into more vibrant, stronger, healthier individuals. The physical cures were merely side benefits they enjoyed along the route of the deeper healing that occurred. The following story is a dramatic example of the power of the mind and how one person healed himself by transforming and overcoming his negative beliefs.

Josh's Story

In his sophomore year of college, Josh was diagnosed with a rare, malignant brain tumor. His type of tumor carried a poor prognosis. Fewer than 12 people in the entire world had had this type of tumor, and no one had lived longer than a year after the diagnosis was made, even with the best treatment that conventional medicine had to offer.

Although Josh was initially devastated by the news, something in his mind refused to buy into his death sentence. He believed in his heart that his body could heal itself. He did not say much to others, but, secretly inside, Josh vowed to defy the statistics. As he set about changing his diet and lifestyle, reducing his stress, and taking the time to listen to his intuition, Josh took a leave of absence from school to concentrate on his deeper healing. After just 4 months, a CT brain scan showed that his tumor had indeed grown a little smaller. His doctors were amazed and told him to keep doing whatever he was doing. After 9 months, the tumor had shrunk to less than one-third of its original size. After 18 months, 6 months after he should have been dead, Josh's tumor was no longer detectable on the CT scan. Three years later, the tumor still had not recurred. Josh was elated, but he wasn't surprised. Now a doctor himself, Josh counsels his patients on their attitudes while he educates them about their mind and the power of their beliefs to improve the quality of their health. Josh is not against conventional medical treatment to increase the odds of a successful outcome when a patient is faced with a difficult diagnosis, but he believes that the transformation of negative beliefs into positive, healthy ones is imperative. He is living proof that optimistic beliefs can activate internal healing mechanisms and overcome incurable diseases.

Because your body is programmed to obey your mental commands, it is imperative to begin now to program your mind to embrace positive, life-affirming beliefs, as Josh and many others have done. Many methods and techniques are available to help you do this, including self-improvement books and tapes, motivational videos, inspirational TV programs, prayers, mantras, uplifting quotes and sayings, genuinely helpful friends and supportive peer groups, compassionate and wise counselors, and supportive doctors and healers.

Four Basic Positive Beliefs

Whenever you find yourself falling prey to negative beliefs, gently but firmly shift your focus to four core beliefs. (Note: You may want to substitute your own positive beliefs, rather than what is suggested here. In the beginning, however, keep it simple by using no more than four.) You need to reinforce these four basic beliefs and drive them deep into your subconscious mind and body, like driving a railroad spike solidly into the ground with a sledge hammer. Once these beliefs are solidly embedded, they will attract other positive beliefs to your mind and, in turn, infuse your healing system with the positive energy it needs to function at its best.

Belief #1: I am lovable just as I am.
Belief #2: I deserve to be happy, healthy, and fulfilled in my life.

Belief #3: My body has a healing system, and it knows how to heal itself.

Belief #4: My body wants to be healthy.

- Begin repeating these beliefs to yourself, first out loud, and then silently throughout the day.

- Write the beliefs down on a small card. Keep them on your bathroom mirror, in your car, at your office, or in any place where you'll see them several times a day.

- Record the beliefs on a tape recorder or on a message machine.

- Memorize the beliefs, so that whenever you catch your mind in a fearful, doubting, pessimistic, or negative mode, or if your mind strays from your goal of improved physical and mental health, you can bring it back on a constructive track that will strengthen and nourish your healing system.

If you follow this strategy faithfully, you will see how vibrant and alive your body will feel as it responds to your new mental commands. Through these positive, life-affirming beliefs, your healing system will awaken, arise, and shift into high gear to perform smoothly and efficiently for you.

Stimulate Your Healing System with Positive Self-Talk

You probably have seen and heard homeless people in the streets of our cities, talking out loud to themselves. Upon seeing them, the first thought that probably pops into your head is that they are crazy!

The irony is that you and I also talk to ourselves, every day of our lives. The only difference is that when we talk to ourselves, we usually do so quietly, in the silent chambers of our own minds. Our internal dialogues, unlike those of "crazy street people," are generally kept strictly personal and private. These private dialogues are known collectively as *self-talk*. Examples of self-talk include the times when you mentally pat yourself on the back and say, "Good job! well done!" or when you criticize yourself and say, "You jerk! You messed up again!"

Your self-talk can have a huge impact on the health of your body and your healing system. Self-talk generates thoughts that create nerve impulses that alter and modify the physiological workings and internal chemistry of your body. Negative self-talk, which focuses on negative thoughts and what is wrong with your life, can be very destructive; it can create both physical and mental problems. Alternatively, positive self-talk, which is based on an optimistic mental attitude that sees problems as challenges and fosters a more positive outlook on life, can create and maintain a strong, resilient healing system and robust good health.

Positive self-talk, on the one hand, centers on such themes as hope, enthusiasm, inspiration, compassion, creativity, beauty, appreciation, optimism, love, generosity, health, and healing, and it exerts a positive, uplifting, life-enhancing influence on your healing system. While you are engaging in positive self-talk, you are your own cheerleader, your own corner man in the heavyweight boxing championship fight for your life.

Negative self-talk, on the other hand, is usually based on the following themes: anger, resentment, revenge, jealousy, hatred, guilt, blame, shame, self-criticism, low self-esteem, pessimism, cynicism, sarcasm, hopelessness, futility, fear, sadness, grief, sorrow, worry, illness, and suffering. By sending unhealthy messages to your body, negative self-talk interferes with the performance of your healing system. Negative self-talk creates tension and a feeling of heaviness in your body; when it becomes habitual or continuous, it tears down your body's health.

More dangerous than most external agents of disease, negative self-talk can sabotage and weaken your body's defenses from the inside as it creates toxic chemical imbalances that can lead to chronic, degenerative diseases. Negative self-talk contributes to poor personal hygiene, and unhealthy diets and lifestyles. Most importantly, negative self-talk sends self-destructive messages to your body that interfere with your healing system.

You are in control of your thoughts and the master of your own internal dialogues. Therefore, you can stimulate your healing system and improve the quality of your health and life by carefully censoring negative, unhealthy thoughts while reinforcing positive, healthy, life-affirming thoughts.

Numerous techniques, strategies, and activities are available to help you program your mind into the language of positive self-talk.

Here are a few of the more well-known techniques that have worked for many of my patients:

- *Affirmations:* These are positive, life-affirming statements that you can verbally or mentally repeat continuously until they become deeply ingrained in your subconscious. With continuous repetition and practice, affirmations eventually become automatic and easily accessible to you when you need them. An example of a rather well-known affirmation is "Every day, in every way, I am getting better and better!" Affirmations are not only life affirming and health enhancing when practiced over time, but they can be comforting and reassuring in the short run, as well.

- *Art and literature:* Being around great works of art, including paintings, writings, and sculpture, can help get you out of the rut of negative self-talk and make you realize that there is more to life than pain, suffering, and sorrow. Participating in the arts can help bring you one step further into the positive realm.

- *Audiotapes:* Books on tape and recordings from inspirational authors can be powerful tools to help you reprogram your mind to focus more on positive self-talk. You can listen to affirmations in tape form while you are driving in your car or while you are at home, until they are deeply ingrained in your psyche.

- *Chanting:* Chants are uplifting and inspiring affirmations or prayers that are rhythmical and melodic in form. They are similar to songs, but simpler and more focused in their purpose. Chants for health and healing can help you shift out of unhealthy negative self-talk into the beneficial realm of positive self-talk. There are many wonderful uplifting and inspiring chants from nearly every culture, including Native American, African, Aboriginal, Sufi, Christian, Muslim, Hindu, Jewish, and Buddhist.

- *Friends and family:* Spending quality time with friends, family, and trusted elders and wise people in whom you can confide also can be very helpful to inspire positive self-talk. Being around people with whom you feel safe, in an environment where you feel warmth, affection, and acceptance, and with those you can look up to and admire, knowing they care for you, can uplift and inspire your self-talk to be more positive.

- *Gratitude journal:* Writing down all your thoughts and feelings about the things in your life you are grateful for can be an effective way to help you shift your focus from seeing a glass that is half empty to one that is half full, and to reroute your thoughts and feelings away from what is *not* working in your life to what *is* working. Many successful people, including Oprah Winfrey, keep a gratitude journal.

- *Hobbies and entertainment:* These enjoyable activities will help you forget about time; they will allow your mind to be absorbed in constructive thought and positive self-talk. It is difficult to talk negatively to yourself when you are engaged in a creative activity that you truly enjoy.

- *Hypnosis:* Hypnosis is another tool that many people have successfully applied to aid their mental reprogramming of habitual, negative self-talk into an internal dialogue that is much more positive and helpful. Many people have found hypnosis to be one of the safest and most effective methods available for quitting smoking. Contrary to popular fears and myths, hypnosis is safe and does not allow another person to take over or control your mind. Rather, most therapists teach self-hypnosis, a technique that shows you how to tap into the hidden powers of your own subconscious mind so that your mind can align itself with your body and work with your healing system.

- *Mantras:* We can liken mantras to prayers and chants that are repeated continuously, either silently or out loud. Most mantras come from the East Indian tradition, but you can adapt any phrase or expression that has meaning for you from your own native language. Effective mantras for healing should be short, rhythmical, and melodic, to facilitate easy repetition. Some mantras are known to be very powerful because they not only help infuse your mind with positive energy through contemplation of their meaning, but, through repetition, their sounds can activate certain life-enhancing vibratory energies in your brain and nervous system. You can use mantras for specific occasions and circumstances; specialized mantras that can be very effective also exist for health and healing. An excellent resource for mantras is *Healing Mantras* by Thomas Ashley-Farrand.

- *Music:* Singing, listening to and playing music, and dancing— especially when it accompanies chanting and singing uplifting songs and sacred music—can help uplift your mind while they improve your self-talk. Engaging in negative self-talk is difficult when your mind is occupied in positive musical activities.

- *Nature:* Immersing yourself and your senses in the beauty and mystery of nature can have a dramatically positive effect on your self-talk.

- *Prayer:* Norman Vincent Peale, in his classic book *The Power of Positive Thinking,* describes the positive impact that prayer has on our thoughts and minds, as well as on our health. In every tradition of the world, prayer is universally recognized for its ability to lift people out of the mundane quagmire of hopelessness and despair, futility and depression. In his two books, *Healing Words* and *Prayer is Good Medicine,* Dr. Larry Dossey cites numerous scientific studies that document the health-enhancing benefits and effectiveness of prayer, even in the face of devastating terminal illness and major life-threatening events. By providing a "senior partner" or "higher authority" to consult with, prayer can serve as a vehicle to take the pressure off your life, remove your fears and worries, manage your stress, and shift your self-talk into a more positive mode.

- *Reading:* Reading uplifting, inspirational books, including autobiographies of great people who struggled against adversity and overcame major obstacles, can help you focus your self-talk more on the positive aspects of your life. Self-improvement books can also be of great help.

- *Sports and games:* These can help you develop confidence in your body's ability to move and perform like an athlete. Even people with serious handicaps such as amputations of both legs, or people who are wheelchair bound, are now competing on an international level to demonstrate that disease, illness, limitation, and activity restrictions are more a state of mind and can often be overcome with the help of positive self-talk.

- *Visualization and imagery:* These are mental techniques with scientifically proven benefits not only for health and healing, but also in the high-performance, physically demanding world of professional sports and international athletic competition. By using the visual and imaginative powers of your mind, you can help produce a significant positive shift in your internal dialogues, stimulate your healing system, and promote measurable improvement in your physical health.

The Placebo Effect

The *placebo effect* is a scientific principle that demonstrates just how powerful an influence your mind has on your body. The placebo effect is a unique phenomenon observed during clinical trials for new, potentially useful drugs.

When a study is launched to test the usefulness of a new drug, half of the patients, known as the *experimental group*, will receive a pill that contains the new drug, while the other half, known as the *control group*, will receive a *placebo*, which is a pill that contains no drug at all. Both groups are told what to expect from the new drug, and both groups believe their pill contains the new drug. In nearly every study of this type, a large percentage of those receiving the *placebo*, the pill without the drug, will report physical changes consistent with those expected from the new drug being tested. These changes can be measured and are real; they are not just a figment of the imagination. There is no possible way to explain the placebo effect other than by acknowledging that the mind has the power to make these changes happen in the body.

Emotions and Your Healing System

Emotions are packets of mental and physical energy that move through and attempt to move out of your body, much like a river whose water steadily moves toward its greater destiny of the ocean. The word *emotion* comes from the root *emote*, which means *to move out*.

Your emotions have a profound impact on your physical health, and they play an integral role in the functioning of your healing system. Your emotions are connected to your endocrine system, which includes your pineal, pituitary, thyroid, parathyroid, and adrenal glands, as well as your pancreas and reproductive organs. During emotional experiences, powerful hormones are released into your bloodstream from these various organs, and these hormones have far-reaching effects on your body and your healing system.

For example, when you are in a highly excitable state, either feeling exuberant joy or intense fear, your adrenal glands release *epinephrine* (*adrenaline*), which can constrict blood vessels, accelerate heart rate, increase blood pressure, and affect lung and kidney function. *Cortisol*, which can suppress your immune function, is also released at these times. All of these functions are critical to your healing system. *Insulin*, which regulates sugar metabolism, is also produced in response to certain emotions, especially when you are feeling frightened, angry, or under stress. These are just a few of the more commonly known hormones associated with your emotions, but you can see what a profound effect they can have on your healing system.

Being in touch with your feelings, understanding what they are and what they mean, is important for the health of your healing system. When you are in touch with how you feel, you usually feel energized and alive. When you are out of touch with your emotions, you tend to feel separated from life, isolated and lonely. Feelings of loneliness and isolation create stress, which, if sustained, can have harmful repercussions on your healing system.

Clear evidence now exists that suppressing emotions can be damaging to your health and your body's healing system. Repressing emotions goes against the natural laws of the universe that require the natural energy of emotions to move out of your body to seek conscious expression. Numerous studies have shown that people who continuously suppress their emotions are more likely to fall prey to serious illnesses, including heart disease, hypertension, diabetes, cancer, autoimmune diseases, and other chronic conditions. Other studies have shown that people who are able to access their feelings and express themselves enjoy better health and greater longevity. Rather than suppressing your feelings and emotions, most medical experts are now recommending that, to prevent illness, it is important to get in touch with your feelings, whatever they are, and then learn to express them in healthy ways.

Healthy feelings create sensations of comfort and ease in your body. Some healthy feelings are joy, happiness, peace, contentment, serenity, satisfaction, and love. Because they release powerful hormones, these feelings are extremely beneficial to the health of your body's internal environment, and they can keep your healing system vibrant and strong for many years. Of course, the most powerful healthy feeling of all is love.

Because feelings are located in our bodies, there are really no negative feelings or emotions, though this probably sounds like a contradiction. Feelings just are, and they cannot be judged on any level by anyone. Even anger, pain, and sadness, generally considered to be "negative" emotions, can be appropriate and beneficial, especially when we acknowledge and release them from our bodies in a timely and sensible manner. The problem occurs when we do not release these emotions, but rather, as we discussed before, we hold onto and contain or suppress them. Under these circumstances, suppression of so-called negative emotions can be harmful. Healing often occurs when the roots of these unhealthy emotions are exposed and then released from your body.

Getting Rid of Emotional Baggage

Unhealthy emotions that are not released from your body can pile up and cause a big mess. Like lugging around too much baggage, or having a backflow of garbage that begins to smell and fester, unhealthy emotions that are not released from your body can create toxic chemistry in your body's internal environment that interferes with your healing system's performance. Releasing your emotional baggage by learning to let go of stored up negative feelings, such as old resentment and anger, will help to lighten the burden that may be dragging down your body and making it sick.

Anger is the most notorious aspect of emotional baggage that, if not released from your body, can be detrimental to your health. Anger leads to resentment, jealousy, hostility, hatred, and rage; if it is suppressed and allowed to build up over time, anger can cause damage to your body's internal environment, particularly your blood vessels and cardiovascular system. Many people have experienced fatal heart attacks or strokes because of their intense anger. Anger that has piled up for years and not been appropriately released can also erupt explosively and violently at the drop of a hat, causing great harm to yourself or others. Seemingly insignificant events can often trigger this stored-up anger. Many of the horrendous crimes and wars in the world can be traced back to this inappropriate expression of anger. Prolonged, continuous anger disturbs the mind, creating emotional volatility as well as mental instability. When you are angry, you are mad, and it is not by coincidence that insane people were, and still are, referred to as "madmen." Anger that is buried deep and never allowed to come out, so-called "frozen anger," has been implicated in severe forms of depression and mental illness.

Anger wastes energy and may cause actual damage to your body, creating a double burden to your healing system. This is why it is imperative to release anger appropriately and prevent its unhealthy buildup. Once anger is expressed and released appropriately, other emotions are often discovered, most notably, pain. If you can release your anger, feel the pain, and move through the pain, you can discover the most important emotion of all, love.

Here are a few tips for releasing unhealthy emotional baggage:

- Close your eyes and notice any sensation of discomfort in your chest, stomach and abdomen, or in any other part of your body.
- Do your best to put a name that relates to a feeling, such as sadness ("I feel sad"), anger ("I feel angry"), and so on, on this sensation.
- Allow yourself to feel the full extent of your feelings, whether they are anger, resentment, jealousy, guilt, shame, sadness, or sorrow. (There is a saying among behavioral scientists: "You cannot heal what you cannot feel.")
- Speak aloud or write down the name of this sensation or feeling. Try to understand what caused it. See whether there might be other feelings underneath this one that may be encouraging the expression of this feeling.

To further help you release anger and emotional baggage, you might want to try the following activities:

- Write down all you want about your negative emotional experience until you feel you have expressed all you need to say.
- Shout out loud at the top of your lungs everything related to your negative emotional experience while you are driving in your car with the windows rolled up (so nobody can hear you).

- Take a plastic baseball bat and strike a pillow as often and as hard as you like, or punch or kick a punching bag, while repeating out loud an angry, emotionally charged phrase that is appropriate to your anger. (I suggest you do this in a room or area where no one can disturb you, and vice versa.)

- Perform any other physical activity, including lifting weights or aerobics, while you focus on releasing anger and other unhealthy emotions. This process can be cathartic and healing. Remember that the word *emotion* comes from the word *emote*, which means *to move out*. Moving your body can often help anger and other emotional baggage to move out of your body and be released.

- Seek professional counseling or therapy.

- If you've gone beyond the anger to feel your pain, you may notice tears flowing automatically from your eyes as you feel and release your pain. Under these circumstances, the release of pain while you cry can be extremely beneficial for your healing system.

Love: The Most Powerful Emotion of All

Love is the most powerful and important emotion in the world. It is the greatest source of nourishment, strength, and energy for your healing system. Love can be awakened by outside forces, but its true origins emanate from the mysterious depths of your own heart. Love is connected to the creative forces of the universe, and for this reason it can exist beyond the borders of your mind and body, and extend to every human heart. Where there is love, there is healing, even in the face of devastating disease and life's most horrendous trials, tribulations, and suffering.

Since the dawn of civilization, wise men and sages, mystics and philosophers, poets, artists, and healers have all declared that love is the most powerful healing force in the world. Thanks to new medical research, scientists and doctors are now beginning to acknowledge the accuracy of this view. Studies now show that people who report having more love in their lives, even if that love is coming only from their pet dog or cat, live longer and suffer from fewer diseases. In the words of Dr. Bernie Siegel, "Love is the most powerful known stimulant of the human immune system." In the words of The American Holistic Medical Association's charter declaration, "Love is the most powerful medicine in the world!"

Love is stronger than fear. In fact, love overcomes all fears and doubts. Whenever fears and doubts get the better of you, immediately shift your attention to loving thoughts. Start entertaining thoughts of love for yourself, your family and friends, your pets, and whoever and whatever is near and dear to you. Continue to focus on that which you love. If you can't find anything, it's time to get out your emotional shovel and start digging through the layers of garbage that may be covering up your heart. Keep digging until you reach it. There you will find love as it has always been: ever comforting, ever healing, powerful, generous, timeless, and eternal.

Love is the essential nature of your soul. When you are in pain and feeling bad, either in body, mind, or spirit, remember this. If you have tried everything else and nothing has helped you so far, try love. It will heal you!

Laughter and Humor Are the Best Medicine

When you are laughing, you feel happy and joyful. This positive mental and emotional state has been clinically and scientifically proven to have tremendous health-enhancing effects on your body, working like an elixir on your healing system.

I've met people well into their eighties, nineties, and beyond, who, from a health standpoint, did everything wrong. They smoked, they drank, they overate, and they didn't exercise. What they did right, however, was learn how to laugh and not take life or themselves too seriously. This was the case with Norman Cousins, well-known author of *Anatomy of an Illness*, who, while suffering from a painful, incurable condition, discovered that after just 15 minutes of solid belly laughter while he watched comedy movies, he got two hours of pain-free sleep. He eventually went on to completely heal himself, eradicating all traces of illness from his body by following this prescription of laughter.

Humor and laughter also activate the body's natural pain-control mechanisms that release *endorphins* and *enkephalins*, powerful opiate-like neurochemicals produced by the brain. Laughter can relax the mind and body and not only neutralize the effects of the fight-or-flight response, but energize and activate your healing system, as well. This is why well-known physicians such as Drs. Patch Adams and Bernie Siegel advocate the health-enhancing benefits of laughing regularly and cultivating a sense of humor in your life.

A Humorous Rx

To increase your laughter and fun, and to strengthen your sense of humor, try the following prescription:

- Watch comedy movies or comedy television shows one to two times a week. If you haven't seen the movie *Patch Adams*, starring Robin Williams, I highly recommend it.
- Watch standup comedians, either in person or on TV.
- Read the comic section or "funnies" regularly in the newspaper, and comedy books and magazines.
- Watch cartoon shows with your children, grandchildren, or friends, or rent a Disney animated movie to watch by yourself if you live alone. Go to Disneyland or Disney World, or to your local amusement or theme park as often as possible.
- Play with children as often as possible.
- Remember to let out the child within you.

Stress and Your Healing System

Stress interferes significantly with the performance of your body's healing system. Stress stimulates and activates your sympathetic nervous system, which initiates the fight-or-flight response. Recall that when the fight-or-flight response is activated, adrenaline is released, which causes excitation and increased activity in your body. Blood flow, nutrients, and energy are shunted away from your body's internal organs and dispatched to the large muscles of movement in your arms and legs so you can fight or flee. Under these conditions, healing and repair mechanisms are put on hold, and with diminished blood flow, nutrients, and energy, your healing system tends to bog down and function poorly. Repeated stress can have damaging effects on your body such as elevating blood pressure to dangerous levels, restricting blood flow to the heart, and creating inflammatory lesions in the stomach and intestines. Stress creates more work for your healing system and can overtax your body's healing resources.

One definition of stress is *information overload*—too much information coming into our lives too quickly, which can overwhelm us. Although there has always been stress associated with the human condition, today far more information is coming at us from more directions, and at a much faster rate than in the past. It is difficult to decide which information is important and which is not. Your life often depends on taking prompt and responsible action based on correct information, and too much information complicates and confuses this process. Information overload is creating more stress for more people than ever before.

Stress also seems to increase as the pace of life increases around us, resulting in hurried and frenzied activity. The increased speed and pace of our modern lifestyles contributes to more tension and stress around us as we rush to meet more deadlines for an increasing number of responsibilities and activities.

Another definition of stress is a sense of isolation: isolation from friends, family, community, the world, your self, or your higher Self. This isolation may have nothing to do with physical location. Even in the middle of a sprawling metropolis such as New York City, people can feel isolated, disconnected, and lonely. We can perhaps better understand the stress of isolation by examining the popular saying "No man is an island." Because man is inherently a social creature, to remain alone or isolated for long periods is stressful. Prisons apply this principle when they subject troublesome prisoners to solitary confinement as the ultimate form of discipline and punishment.

Because of the potentially damaging effects and negative influence of stress on your healing system, learning how to rest, relax, and manage stress effectively is critical to your health. Stress-management techniques activate the "relaxation response," which completely neutralizes and disarms the fight-or-flight response. These techniques work with your healing system to help activate repair mechanisms that can reverse the effects of chronic, stress-related diseases. Stress-management techniques and strategies can help your body regain and maintain its natural state of health and vigor. The following story demonstrates the effectiveness of stress management in stimulating the healing system.

Conrad's Story

Conrad was a highly ambitious young man who had always done well in school. He was class valedictorian in high school and earned excellent grades in college. Upon graduation from college, Conrad was placed in a progressive telecommunications company as a junior executive, a position in which he received an excellent salary with many benefits. He worked long hours at his new job because he liked the work and wanted to make a good impression on his bosses.

However, since high school, Conrad had experienced increasingly disturbing digestive-system symptoms of gas and diarrhea. Sometimes he had abdominal pain that woke him from his sleep. These symptoms intensified after he graduated from college. By the time Conrad came to see me on his twenty-eighth birthday, three specialists had already diagnosed him with *inflammatory bowel disease*. He had been placed on a regimen of *corticosteroids*, pain medications, and *gastrointestinal antispasmodics*. These medications initially seemed to help, but now they were losing their effectiveness and made him feel drugged and out-of-sorts. These symptoms interfered with his job performance and his personal life.

When I saw Conrad, I noticed that he appeared very agitated and restless, in addition to his physical symptoms. He told me that, for as long as he could remember, he had always been tense and couldn't relax. I recommended several lifestyle changes to Conrad, including a change in his diet, and I also taught him a simple technique to help him relax and manage his stress.

After just six weeks of relaxation training and practice, Conrad reported marked improvement in his condition. One year later, he was off all medications and had only an occasional flare-up. Four years later, Conrad is essentially symptom free, except when life becomes particularly tense at home or at work. Having made the connection between his mind and his body and how stress can contribute to his inflammatory bowel disease, Conrad knows that relaxation and stress management are not an option, but rather a necessity for his continued good health.

Acceptance and Assertiveness to Reduce Stress

One key to reducing stress in your life can be summed up in the famous serenity prayer that many 12-step programs use: "God grant me the serenity to accept the things I cannot change, courage to change the things I can, and wisdom to know the difference." This wish involves both the acceptance of certain limitations and realities in your life, and the determination to improve those aspects of your life that can be changed. Living by this philosophy can take a tremendous weight off your shoulders, and it can empower you to better your life in myriad ways.

Rather than running away from problems, difficulties, or conflicts, or escaping through various unhealthy distractions such as alcohol, drugs, food, sex, or other self-destructive and irresponsible behavior, be assertive and face your problems head on to help reduce stress. Being assertive requires thinking positively, using your resources, and heeding the advice of those you trust to effectively discover and implement the best solutions for your problems.

Assertiveness and acceptance are powerful ways for you to reduce the stress in your life. They encourage a more creative, solution-oriented approach to life by enabling you to view problems and difficulties as challenges, educational opportunities, and necessary growth experiences for your higher good.

Stress-Management Methods and Techniques

The following proven stress-management methods are simple, powerful, and effective, particularly when you practice them regularly.

Deep Relaxation to Reduce Your Stress

One of the most powerful ways to fortify your healing system is to neutralize the effects of stress by learning how to relax your mind and body. Because none of us were ever taught this skill, however, very few of us know how to do it. Instead, to gain temporary relief from the tensions and pressures around us, most of us have learned to resort to artificial means of relaxing, such as drugs or alcohol. These substances create dependence, have side effects, and ultimately can be harmful to our bodies.

Relaxation is one of the most, if not the most, important first steps on the road to healing. Relaxation neutralizes and reverses the effects of stress and allows your mind, your nervous system, and all the systems in your body to cooperate with your healing system. Relaxation helps to initiate healing mechanisms that operate deep within the organ tissues of your body.

Relaxation has many proven benefits, including the ability to reduce stress, lower blood pressure, improve immune functioning, and calm and stabilize nervous-system activity, and so it is important to learn this invaluable, essential skill. Relaxation goes far beyond sitting back with a six-pack of Budweiser and watching a Monday-night football game. While doing that might be enjoyable, there are other, more powerful ways to relax that naturally calm and soothe both your mind and your body.

Relaxation is the foundation of other powerful mind-body techniques that can support and nurture your body's healing system. Learning how to relax is as easy as learning how to drive a car. In the beginning, all it takes is a little practice.

Here's a deep relaxation technique that is easy and effective:

- Secure a 15- to 20-minute time slot for yourself during which you can be quiet and alone.

- Make sure you won't be disturbed during this 15- to 20-minute period, and that you have no responsibilities to attend to—no phone or pager to answer, no diapers to change, no stove or oven to turn off. Find a room where you can close the door and be free from all distractions. (You might need to wear earplugs or headphones if it is noisy.)

- Lie down on a bed or on the floor, making sure you are in a comfortable position on your back. You may need to place blankets or pillows under your knees, head, and back. Make sure you are not cold.

Note: Before you proceed, you will find it helpful to get a small tape recorder and record your voice as you read the remaining instructions out loud, slowly and calmly. After you have recorded this exercise, you will have your own relaxation tape. You can lie down and let your own words guide you through deep relaxation any time you wish.

- Keep your hands along the side of your body, with your palms facing up, or fold your hands on top of your stomach and abdomen. Gently close your eyes and bring your awareness inside of your body.

- Notice in the area of your stomach and abdomen the slight up-and-down movement that occurs with the movement of your breath as it flows in and out of your body. When the breath flows into your body, your stomach and abdomen gently rise, gently expand. When the breath flows out of your body, your stomach and abdomen gently fall, gently contract.

- Without trying to control the rate or depth of this movement, allow your mind to be a passive observer of the rhythmical flow of your breath as it moves in and out of your body, causing your stomach and abdomen to rise and fall.

- Every time the breath leaves your body, feel all the muscles in your body releasing tension and becoming more relaxed. (Note: A natural relaxation phase occurs in your body during each exhalation of the breath. When you pay close attention to your body and its breathing processes, you can feel this relaxation phase quite distinctly.)

- Now bring your awareness down to your feet and toes. Using your breath and the natural relaxation phase that occurs during each exhalation, gently relax all the muscles in your feet and toes.

- Relax all the muscles in your ankles, lower legs, knees, thighs, hips, pelvic area, buttocks, and lower spine.

- Relax all the muscles in your stomach, abdomen, and chest, as well as the muscles in your middle and upper back, including the area between your shoulder blades.

- Relax all the muscles in your shoulders, arms, forearms, wrists, hands, fingers, and fingertips.

- Relax all the muscles in the back of your neck and head, and those on the top of your head.

- Relax your forehead, and all the muscles around your eyes, ears, and jaws, and all the muscles in your face.

- Relax all the muscles in your body.

- Now slowly bring your awareness to the tip of your nose, where the breath is flowing in and out of your body through your nostrils.

- Without trying to control the rate or depth or the movement, notice the gentle flowing movement of your breath as it comes in and out of your body at this point.

- Observe the breath as if it were separate from you.

- As you continue to observe your breathing for at least 5 to10 minutes, let your mind and body relax completely.

After you complete this exercise, gently open your eyes and stretch your entire body. Make sure not to rush to your next activity. Take the time to savor the calm and relaxed state you have just experienced. Know that this is not an artificial or contrived state, but rather your natural state of being. Focus on remaining in this calm and relaxed natural state throughout the day, until the next time you are able to do this exercise. Practicing this exercise regularly brings the most effective benefits.

How Deep Relaxation Strengthens and Recharges Your Healing System

Deep relaxation quiets down the nervous system and slows metabolic processes in the body so that the healing system can do its work unimpeded. With these obstacles removed, your healing system can perform more efficiently and effectively. Because the healing system functions best in a quiet, calm environment, deep relaxation is one of the most powerful techniques for strengthening your healing system. Other benefits of deep relaxation include the following:

- You will feel more relaxed throughout each day, and you will feel more peaceful from within, even during difficult and stressful situations.

- You will become much more aware of stressful situations and their effects on your body. You will learn how to avoid unnecessary stress and how to manage stress more effectively by remembering your natural relaxed state.

- You will become much more aware of the harmful consequences of such emotions as fear and anger in your body, and you will be able to move through and release fear and anger much more effectively and swiftly through your ability to relax.

- You will have more energy throughout your day. Stress wastes energy and causes fatigue in your body. The more relaxed you are, the less fatigue you will experience in your life. Releasing tension and becoming more relaxed frees up tremendous amounts of natural energy in your body.

- Relaxation eliminates tension and decreases pain. If you have a chronic medical problem that causes persistent pain, you will experience less pain through the practice of regular relaxation.

- If you suffer from anxiety, phobias, or even depression, you will most likely see improvement in these areas in a relatively short period of time.

- Deep relaxation stimulates your healing system and activates deep internal processes of healing.

As you can see, deep relaxation will benefit you in many ways, physically, mentally, and emotionally.

Breathing to Reduce Your Stress

Because your breath is the link between your mind and your body, working with your breath is one of the most powerful stress-management modalities known. When you are mentally agitated, anxious, or under stress of any kind, your breathing is disturbed and becomes more shallow and rapid. When you are relaxed, your breathing becomes slower and deeper.

Normally, we go about our activities without any awareness of our breathing. However, without your breath, you couldn't live. Your existence depends on the continuous flow of oxygen that comes into your body from the air you breathe.

Improvement in your health occurs when you can breathe in a more relaxed and easy way, which will result from practicing the simple yet powerful breathing techniques in this section. Deep breathing increases lung capacity and builds up the strength of your respiratory system, creating more efficient breathing. Efficient, relaxed breathing brings in more energy for healing and regeneration for these two critical reasons:

1. With improved breathing comes increased oxygenation of the blood. Increased oxygenation of the blood means greater oxygen delivery to every cell, organ, and tissue in your body.

2. As your breath becomes more efficient, smooth, and relaxed, there is a calming effect on your brain and nervous system, which reduces overall mental and physical tension.

In a powerful way, both of these factors work synergistically to relieve fatigue and create more energy in your body, improving the functioning and performance of your healing system.

Breathing Exercise #1: Breath Awareness

- Find a quiet place where you can be alone for 10 to 15 minutes. Make sure you are absolutely free of all obligations and responsibilities during this time slot.

- You can lie down on your back as in deep relaxation, or you can sit in a chair or on any comfortable, firm surface. Make sure you are in a comfortable position.

- Close your eyes and bring your awareness inside of your body. Notice the gentle movement in your stomach and abdomen. (You obviously will need to keep your eyes open to read the instructions for this exercise. For maximum benefits, however, keep your eyes closed after you have read and familiarized yourself with this technique.)

- Notice that when the breath flows into your body, your stomach and abdomen gently expand and rise.

- Notice that when the breath flows out of your body, your stomach and abdomen gently contract and fall.

- Without trying to control the rate or depth of this movement, continue to observe this automatic movement in your stomach and abdomen as your breath flows in and out of your body.

- Every time the breath flows into your body, feel the oxygen from your blood entering into the cells and tissues of your body, energizing and strengthening your healing system and entire body.

- Every time the breath leaves your body, feel all the muscles in your body becoming more relaxed.

- Now direct your awareness to the tip of your nose. Watch the breath as it flows in and out of your body. Again, without trying to control the rate or depth of the movement of your breath, focus on seeing the breath as separate from you.

- Every time the breath leaves your body, feel your entire body becoming more relaxed, and your mind becoming more calm, serene, and peaceful. Feel the power of this natural state of calmness and tranquility in your entire body.

- Feel the healing energy from your breath flowing into every cell and tissue of your body, as your body becomes more healthy, vibrant, and alive with each breath your take.

- After breathing like this for 10 to15 minutes, slowly open your eyes. Before you resume your normal activities, appreciate the power of your breath. Notice its calming influence on your mind and its energizing effect on your body. Know that your breath is always available to you should you begin to feel stressed, anxious, or fatigued at any time. Keep this awareness of breath with you as often as possible. Have as your goal to practice this breathing exercise every day for at least 5 to10 minutes. If your schedule permits, build up to 30 minutes per day. The best time to do this exercise is in the mornings or evenings, when it is usually more quiet.

Breathing Exercise #2: Breathing with Sound

- Find a quiet place where you can be alone for 10 to15 minutes. Make sure you are absolutely free of all obligations and responsibilities during this time.

- You can lie down on your back, as in deep relaxation, or you can sit in a chair, on the floor, or on any firm surface. Make sure you are in a comfortable position.

- Gently close your eyes and bring your awareness inside of your body. (You obviously will need to keep your eyes open to read the instructions for this exercise. For maximum benefits, how-ever, keep your eyes closed after you have read and familiarized yourself with this technique.)

■ Open your mouth and breathe in and out slowly. Every time you breathe out, make the sound "aahh," which is the sound that the doctor asks you to make when he or she examines your throat. Make sure this sound is coming from your throat. You can place one hand on the front of your neck in the throat area to check whether your vocal chords are vibrating.

■ Next, whisper this same sound as you breathe, making it softer and gentler.

■ Next, close your mouth while you continue to make this same gentle, whispering sound; allow the breath to flow in and out of your nose, yet continue to focus on the sound coming from your throat area and vocal cords.

■ Gently lengthen and deepen the flow of your breath, but make sure you are comfortable with your breathing.

■ Make your breath smooth and flowing as you make this soft, gentle sound, which should feel like a gentle grating sensation in your throat. Make this sound on both inhalation and exhala-tion. Continue to gently lengthen your breathing.

■ Make this sound softer as you continue to breathe in this manner. In fact, make this sound barely audible, so that some-one sitting next to you wouldn't be able to hear it.

■ Continue to gently lengthen and slow your breathing as much as you can, making sure your breath is smooth and flowing as you make this soft, gentle, grating sound. Make sure you are comfortable with your breathing, and that you are not experi-encing any sensations whatsoever of forcing or straining or dis-comfort.

■ Keeping your eyes closed, continue to "breathe with sound" in this fashion.

■ If you are doing this technique correctly, you will begin to feel more relaxed, peaceful, and focused in your mind and more energetic in your body.

▪ Stay with this technique and these sensations for as long as you like, gradually increasing to a maximum of 15 to 30 minutes at a time.

This is a powerful yogic breathing technique from ancient India known as *Ujjayi Breathing*. The technique not only combats stress by helping to keep the mind calm and focused, but it also improves lung capacity and respiratory function as it brings more energy into your body. Ujjayi Breathing purifies the nervous system and enhances the performance capabilities of your healing system.

Meditation to Reduce Your Stress

Meditation is a simple yet powerful way to manage your stress. It can calm your mind and rejuvenate your body, and in so doing help strengthen your healing system. Meditation is not mystical or magical. It is natural and ordinary, and when done correctly, it can have a tremendous effect on your physical and mental well being.

In the early 1970s, Dr. Herbert Benson at Harvard University documented the beneficial therapeutic effects of meditation and its ability to lower blood pressure. Since then, numerous other studies have demonstrated the wide-reaching, therapeutic benefits of meditation and its ability to help heal many other serious conditions, including heart disease, cancer, and AIDS.

Meditation occurs when you are not thinking about the past or the future, and you are just aware of what is happening in the here and now. We have all experienced a meditative state at one time or another, even if only for a few brief moments. As children, we experience this state of mind much more frequently. Children like to play a lot, and, when they play, they are so intent on their playing that they are often not aware of anything else. They may be hungry, but they will completely forget about food because of their total absorption in their play. This focused state is very much like meditation.

Meditation can help bring back the energy and enjoyment of life that you experienced as a young child. By relaxing your mind and helping focus your awareness in the present moment, meditation lightens the burdens of your past and future, releasing pent-up energies and precious internal resources that are now available for your healing system to use.

There are many techniques for meditation. For meditation to work for you, it is important to find a style or technique that suits your own personal tastes and needs. The following meditation is offered as a sample of what is available to you. Meditating regularly for just 10 to 15 minutes a day, or more if your schedule permits, will result in tremendous improvement in your health.

Drifting Thought-Clouds Meditation

This is a simple meditation technique that takes only a few minutes:

- Find a quiet place where you can be alone for 10 to15 minutes. Make sure you are absolutely free of all obligations and responsibilities during this time.

- You can lie down on your back, as in deep relaxation, or you can sit in a chair, on the floor, or on any firm surface. Make sure you are in a comfortable position.

- Gently close your eyes and bring your awareness inside of your body. (You obviously will need to keep your eyes open to read the instructions for this exercise. For maximum benefits, however, keep your eyes closed after you have read and familiarized yourself with this technique.)

- Observe your breathing and the gentle movement of your breath as it flows in and out of your body, as described with the previous breathing exercises.

- As you continue to relax and observe your breathing, imagine that you are in a room with very high windows on either side.

- As you breathe and continue to relax, it will be inevitable that certain thoughts may come into your mind. Rather than holding onto these thoughts or reacting to them, just imagine that these thoughts are soft and fluffy clouds gently passing in and out of the windows in the room.

- Continue to relax and observe your breathing, letting any thought that comes into your mind be like a soft and fluffy cloud, gently drifting in and out of the windows in your room.

- Do not let any thought disturb your peaceful, relaxed state of mind; rather, let it go on its way like a soft, fluffy cloud drifting by.

You can do this meditation whenever you feel yourself becoming anxious or tense, or when you are experiencing disturbing thoughts of any kind. When you become proficient at it, you can even do this with your eyes open, in the midst of other activities.

Visualization/Guided Imagery to Help Manage Your Stress and Strengthen Your Healing System

From the Wright Brothers to Alexander Graham Bell and Thomas Edison, all great inventors in the history of the world began with an imaginative idea that came from their minds. Imagination sows the seeds of reality, and it can play a huge role in influencing the performance of your healing system while it helps your body maintain its natural state of health.

Your mind is a powerful force, and whatever imaginative thoughts you dwell on can become a reality in your life. This is especially true for thoughts about your health. Your brain is a powerful, metabolically active transformer of pure electrical energy; as a result, thoughts generated in your brain and directed to certain areas of your body can exert a powerful effect on the physiology of that part of your body. By recognizing the tremendous imaginative power of your mind, you can learn to harness this power and focus the energy it generates to fortify and boost the effectiveness of your body's healing system.

Guided imagery and visualization are powerful techniques that have helped many people overcome such serious life-threatening illnesses as cancer and heart disease by making use of the connection between their minds and bodies, and using the power of their imaginations for healing purposes. For example, pioneer cancer specialist and radiation oncologist Dr. O. Carl Simonton showed that many of his patients were able to successfully increase their immune system activity, stimulate repair and regeneration of damaged tissues, and demonstrate reversal of their diseases by using their minds to imagine their white blood cells removing the tumor cells in their bodies. In his classic book *Love, Medicine and Miracles*, Dr. Bernie Siegel shares the stories of many of his cancer patients who also overcame their diseases through the successful application and use of visualization and imagery techniques. Dr. Marty Rossman, in his book *Healing Yourself*, also shares stories of numerous patients of his who healed themselves through the use of these specific techniques.

You've no doubt heard the saying "A picture is worth a thousand words." Because your mind thinks in terms of pictures or images, it continually processes information by visualizing and imagining anticipated scenarios as you project yourself into the future. This is how your mind thinks and makes plans, and it is one of the most natural and powerful things you do. Your body is influenced by your mental activities, and by this same process you can influence the state of your own health. However, this influence can work for you or against you. Consider, for example, the case of worrying.

Worry is the negative application of your imagination, fearfully projecting your mind into the future and visually imagining worst-case scenarios of events to come. This process causes anxiety, which increases stress. Stress results in the constriction of blood vessels and inhibits the flow of vital bodily fluids, which can result in congestion and accumulation of toxins in various parts of your body. In addition to high blood pressure and heart disease, chronic worrying has been shown to contribute to the formation of ulcers and numerous other illnesses and diseases.

Conversely, numerous studies have also shown that when people learn to harness the constructive forces of their minds and overcome the harmful habit of persistent worrying, their health will invariably improve. For this reason, it is vital that you learn how to use your mind and the power of your imagination to improve your health and the quality of your life. Visualizing or imaging can be an important ally for your healing system as it directs healing energies to specific areas of your body.

How to Begin Guided-Imagery and Visualization Techniques

Guided-imagery and visualization techniques are best performed with your eyes closed and when you are in a relaxed state. Begin as you would with the deep relaxation methods, and the breathing techniques that you just read about in this section. Make sure you are in a comfortable position and your breathing is slow and relaxed. When you feel your mind becoming calm and your body relaxed, introduce the specific imagery and visualization techniques that best suit your needs. Please do not feel limited or restricted in any way by the few suggested techniques listed here. Many wonderful styles of imagery and visualization techniques are available from trained teachers and professional therapists, from the books listed in the reference section of this book, and from your own creative imagination.

If you are currently trying to heal from any affliction in your body, you will realize the best results by practicing imagery and visualization techniques regularly over an extended period of time, until you are completely healed. For serious, life-threatening conditions, set aside at least 15 to 30 minutes, twice a day, for the practice of imagery and visualization techniques. For illnesses that are not life threatening and are less severe, practicing these techniques once a day for 15 to 30 minutes will be helpful.

Positive Imaging for Activating Your Healing System

- While you are in a relaxed and serene state, keep your eyes closed and your awareness focused within.

- See yourself as very small, standing in the interior of your body.

- See yourself with a clipboard and pencil in hand, and a hard hat on your head, as you monitor and make notes of your body's various internal organ systems.

- Allow an image of your healing system to form in your mind. Without judging, notice the first shape or form that appears.

- See yourself speaking to your healing system. Hear its gentle and confident voice answer back to you. Spend time carrying on a conversation with it, just as you would with any other person. Ask your healing system any question, and tell it anything you wish. Try to get to know it. Make sure you listen carefully to responses to your questions and dialogue. You might want to ask it whether it has a personal name and whether you could use this name in future communications with it.

- After dialoguing and becoming familiar with your healing system on a more personal level, see yourself gently directing your healing system to any area of your body that needs healing or about which you are concerned.

- See yourself calmly and persistently speaking words of encouragement to your healing system and the other systems in your body under its supervision, to make sure your body is functioning optimally and harmoniously.

- See yourself making notes of your healing system's progress as you continue to encourage it to perform its tasks of repair and restoration where they are needed in your body.

- Ask your healing system what it needs from you so that it can continue to do its job most efficiently.

- Thank your healing system for the work it is doing on your behalf.

- Make a point to meet again in the near future.

- Breathe life into these feelings and into your body as you complete this exercise, maintaining positive feelings about what you have just visualized.

- Relax and take a deep breath as you finish this exercise.

- Open your eyes when you are done.

- Write down any insights or thoughts about your experience.

This visualization/guided-imagery technique is only a small sampling of what is available to you. You can modify and apply this technique to suit any health condition that you would like to improve. The beauty of visualization and guided imagery is that they can enable you to gain incredible insights and access key information about the state of your health. Further information about visualization and guided imagery is given in the resource section in the back of this book.

Pray to Reduce Your Stress

Prayer serves as a powerful stress-management tool, perhaps one of the most powerful known to man. Prayer can open a channel of communication for you to dialogue with the wise and infinite powers of our sacred universe that exist outside as well as within you. In this capacity, prayer offers you a way to hand over your problems and worries to a higher power, relieving a lot of tension and stress in the process. Prayer is one of the oldest, most universal, and most effective methods of stress reduction. However, for prayer to work for you, you have to be comfortable with the type of prayer you use, as well as the context, style, and method with which you choose to pray.

Many scientific studies have now been conducted that demonstrate the therapeutic efficacy of prayer. One study even showed clinical improvement in people who were prayed for from a distance and didn't know it. Many of these people didn't even believe in God. In Dr. Larry Dossey's best-selling book *Healing Words*, this fascinating study and others are discussed in great detail.

No matter how embittered or cynical you might have become during your life's journey, it is never too late to attempt to contact this divine source through honest and sincere prayer. Miracles can occur when you do. In fact, consider how you got on this earth and the fact that you are alive right now. Those are in themselves miracles!

Whether or not you have a particular religious or spiritual affiliation, or even if you are an agnostic or an atheist, you can still learn to open your heart and contact the loving, intelligent force and power that created you and sustains your very life.

When you do take the time to unburden your troubles to a higher power, sharing all your pain, sorrow, problems, fears, and disappointments, make sure that you take a few moments to wait for wise counsel in response to your prayers when you have finished. You can often obtain tremendous insights and wisdom in this process. However, higher powers are known to speak very softly and quietly, so to enhance your ability to receive a response to your prayers, first calm your mind by practicing relaxation, breathing, meditation, or all three of these in sequence before you initiate the act of prayer.

Alternatively, you might find it helpful to release your pain, worries, tensions, and fears to the ocean, the sky, the stars, a mountain, or some other special entity, force, or place in nature that comforts and reassures you. You may do the same with a trusted friend, loved one, or wise counsel, or the great unknown mystery of the universe that remains open and receptive to creative ideas, insights, and the healing force of love that exists in your heart.

Peace of Mind and Your Healing System

Your body does not operate in a vacuum. To a large degree, its state of health registers and reflects what is going on in your life, which in turn is a product of your mental habits and thoughts. A crazy, chaotic, troublesome life, born of a disturbed mind, creates a stressful life, creates chronic physical tension, depletes the body's energies, depresses the immune system, repeatedly triggers the fight-or-flight response, and interferes with the performance of your healing system while it renders the body susceptible to illnesses and diseases from both internal and external agents.

When your mind is disturbed, like an out-of-control roller coaster or a furious tempest, it can create violent mood swings that can upset your body's internal balance. These mood swings cause the release of potent hormones and strong chemical modulators that can wreak havoc on your body's internal organs and tissues. A disturbed mind opens the door for a plethora of diseases to enter your body, creating opportunities for a smorgasbord of potentially dangerous disorders that can make your life miserable and quite possibly take you to an early grave. Your healing system cannot possibly operate efficiently under these conditions.

A peaceful mind, conversely, creates a relaxed, healthy body and contributes to a more harmonious internal environment in which your healing system can work smoothly and efficiently. When your mind is at peace, and you are relaxed and tranquil, feelings of love, contentment, happiness, and gratitude naturally and spontaneously arise. These feelings produce powerful hormones and gentle, soothing nerve impulses that bathe and nourish your healing system in a flood of loving, life-giving energy. Just as a calm sea makes for smoother travel for any ship, so too a peaceful and tranquil mind makes for a calmer, smoother, more harmonious internal environment for your body's healing system.

Just as your body's natural state is one of health, so, too, your mind's natural state is one of peace. Keeping your mind calm and relaxed may take some training if you have forgotten what it is like to be peaceful, but it will be well worth the effort. A peaceful mind is essential for a healthy body. If you want to effectively promote the work of your healing system, one of the most important things you can do is to actively recruit your mind in this process by keeping it peaceful and calm. The stress-management techniques described in this chapter, along with the chapter's other prescriptive elements, provide the most powerful, time-proven methods to help you achieve and maintain this most valuable of all possessions.

Closing Thoughts on the Power
of Your Mind and Your Healing System

You have seen in this chapter the powerful influence your mind has over your healing system. Every thought that is registered in your mind has the potential to create powerful chemical changes in your body, changes that affect the processes of healing and repair. Staying calm and relaxed, positive, optimistic, and enthusiastic is vital to maximize the incredible ability of your mind to cooperate with, support, nourish, and strengthen your healing system.

The practical strategies, techniques, and exercises prescribed in this chapter are based on proven clinical experience, but to reap their benefits, just reading them is not enough. Set aside time as suggested to practice one or more of these extremely helpful techniques, so they will become a part of your daily routine and lifestyle, just like brushing your teeth is. If you or a loved one is currently battling a major, life-threatening illness, doing this is not an option; it is a necessity.

The next chapter will reinforce the importance of minimizing stress in your life as we explore how a strong and healthy healing system has enabled many people to achieve great longevity. You'll learn how these people were able to reach the age of 100 or more, and how, by harnessing the energy and power of your extraordinary healing system, you can, too.

CHAPTER 7

Aging, Long-Lasting Health,
and Your Healing System

Your ability to live longer is not a matter of mere chance, but is, for the most part, a systematic, self-determined process. Your body comes equipped with its own healing system and can last, on average, 100 years. Of course the choices you make in your everyday life can shorten or lengthen this time. The point of living longer, however, is not just to extend your life, but to enjoy a higher quality of life as you age, and to participate fully in life, remaining enthusiastic and active to the very end of your days. Doing this requires you to be healthy. The process of achieving a long life while remaining healthy is what I call *long-lasting health*.

If you carefully study the lives of people who have enjoyed long-lasting health, you will discover primarily personal health habits, diets, lifestyles, and attitudes that are consistent with the ideas and methods that work with their bodies' healing systems and that have been presented in this book. Understanding and applying these ideas and methods will help you enjoy long lasting health, as well. But you must also be prepared for certain challenges you might have to face as you age. The following story illustrates my point.

An elderly woman was suffering from a painful knee condition that had been troubling her for some time. The pain was only in her right knee, but it was severe enough to make walking difficult. She couldn't figure out what was causing the pain. Her friends all told her it was the result of old age, and to stop worrying about it. However, because the pain interfered with the quality of her life, she refused to accept this explanation, and she eventually made an appointment with her doctor to find out what was going on.

When this woman went to the doctor's office, the doctor examined her knees thoroughly. He first bent her knees one way and then the other. Then he banged them with a rubber hammer to check their reflexes. She was asked to stand on one leg at a time, and then hop up and down, first with both feet on the floor, then with just the right leg, and then with the left. The doctor also thoroughly examined the other parts of her body. At the conclusion of his exam, he shrugged his shoulders and replied, "I'm sorry, ma'am; I can find nothing seriously wrong with your knee. I'm afraid it's just due to old age."

The woman, by now completely fed up with this type of explanation, replied, "I'm sorry to disagree with you doctor, but there must be another reason, because my other knee is the exact same age and it is perfectly fine. Thank you and have a good day!"

This story illustrates two very simple, yet important points that I want to clarify and emphasize here at the outset of this chapter. Understanding them now will help you to better grasp the challenges of working with your healing system as you age.

First, there is an unhealthy, yet common tendency in our society, and among our medical professionals, to attribute most forms of chronic illness to advancing age. As you age and develop symptoms of one kind or another, it is all too easy to blame these symptoms on old age.

Second, if you want to remain healthy as you age, you will need to educate yourself and learn to ignore negative, pessimistic, fearful, and erroneous ideas about what causes illness. Instead, focus on the important task at hand: working with your healing system to help you achieve long-lasting health, incorporating all the methods, strategies, and techniques that you have learned so far.

Advancing Age Does Not Cause Illness

Even though advancing age and illness are often linked, if you examine the facts and pay careful attention to the underlying causes of most diseases, you will discover that *old age and illness have nothing to do with each other.* The majority of the diseases that afflict us as we grow older are caused by factors that have nothing to do with age. Let me explain.

If you look around the world and peruse the international public health data, you'll see that the majority of the diseases that afflict us as we age in the Western industrialized societies are virtually absent in poor, developing countries. These diseases include heart disease (the world's number-one killer), high blood pressure, diabetes, emphysema, arthritis, cancer, and many other conditions that are rampant in North America and Europe, but that are rare in places such as Africa and Asia. These diseases, referred to by the late Dr. Albert Schweitzer as "diseases of civilization," have been shown to be directly linked to factors under our own control, such as our diet, lifestyle, and personal health habits. These factors accumulate over a lifetime, and their cumulative effects become increasingly harmful as we age, *but they are not caused by age.* Eventually, they just take their toll.

For example, a person who continually smokes two packs of cigarettes a day for 25 years or more is likely to develop emphysema or lung cancer when he or she reaches 60 or 70 years of age. Does this mean that emphysema and lung cancer are diseases of old age? Absolutely not. It means that these conditions are more likely to occur in people whose bodies have been abused over a long period of time and, for this reason, are more commonly seen with advancing years. If you continually harm your body and fail to respect or cooperate with your healing system, it is a simple fact that, in time, you will most likely become ill. The abuse factor, rather than the age factor, causes the majority of these illnesses.

If you carefully examine other major illnesses, including diabetes, heart disease, arthritis, and cancer, among others, you will almost invariably discover similar underlying factors and mechanisms at play, factors and mechanisms that are much more related to unhealthy diets, lifestyles, and personal health habits than to old age. So I will repeat myself by stating that old age and illness have nothing to do with each other.

As you work with your healing system, remember the importance of adopting an attitude similar to the lady in the story with the painful knee. Make use of the power of your mind and your own personal health choices to directly influence your healing system, and concentrate your energies on creating positive health for yourself. As long as you are alive, no matter how compromised your health might currently be, your healing system has the capacity to heal your illnesses and improve your health.

How Your Mind Affects Your Healing System As You Age

"You are as old as you think you are" is a common saying in many cultures and folk traditions around the world. According to our modern scientific understanding, this dictum appears to contain much truth. Your attitude about your health and your life has a direct effect on your healing system.

Your mental attitude, and your expectations about your health and health outcomes, which reflect healing-system functioning, are strongly linked. Many studies have demonstrated that a healthy mental attitude not only creates healthier biochemistry in the brain and body, but also is more likely to support a healthy, active lifestyle. Both factors directly benefit your healing system, producing a healthier, disease-free body and a longer life span. A positive attitude will strengthen your healing system, whether you are 30 years old or 103 years old, and it will literally add years to your life.

In his book, *RealAge*, Michael Roizen, M.D., makes clear that, based on scientific studies, your mental attitude can affect your physical health and your body's healing system in two ways: 1) Your mental attitude determines how well you treat your body through your daily personal health habits, and 2) your mental attitude can directly influence your physical health through the brain-body connection, wherein neurochemicals and electrical impulses produced by your brain can cause powerful physical changes in every organ and tissue in your body. These factors have a direct impact on the vitality of your healing system and how you age.

As a consequence of these findings, Dr. Roizen discovered that how old you are in biological years can be very different from how old you are in chronological years. For example, people in their twenties and thirties who abuse their bodies with tobacco, drugs, or alcohol; live high-stress lives; have poor diets; practice unsafe sex; do not exercise; reflect unhealthy mental attitudes; and exhaust the resources of their healing systems often wear their bodies out by the time they are 40 or 50 years of age. These people often become sick and disabled, dying prematurely from unnatural causes. At any point in time, these people appear much older than their actual age, and, in biological terms, they are much older. These people have not learned how to honor and work with their healing systems, and in the end (which usually comes much sooner than need be), having become old before their time, they pay with their lives. Conversely, other people in their seventies, eighties, nineties, and even hundreds are biologically much younger than their birth dates indicate. They exhibit not only bodies that are far more youthful than their chronological age, but mental attitudes and thinking that are similarly youthful. They have mastered the art of learning how to cooperate with their healing systems, and they are perfect examples of how, by doing so, the rewards of superior and long-lasting health have become theirs.

Elizabeth's Story

The story of Elizabeth, one of my patients, is a good example of how your attitude about your age significantly affects your healing system. Elizabeth, 83 years of age, had regularly practiced yoga for several years, but she had not come to class for about six months. When I asked her why, she said that she had been traveling for an extended period and had neglected to stretch and move her body. She felt embarrassed by how stiff she had become in the interim, especially in her hands and fingers, which had become quite painful. Because of the pain, she decided to see another doctor while she was traveling. He diagnosed her as having arthritis of her hands and fingers. This diagnosis further discouraged her and sent her into a mild depression. She said she was feeling disabled, handicapped, and old, and she commented that she was afraid she could no longer keep up with the younger students.

I urged Elizabeth to return to class. She sheepishly appeared the following morning. I told her to take it easy and not push herself. She did fine. After the class, Elizabeth thanked me for insisting that she return. Since that day, more than three years ago, she hasn't missed a class. Not only has her mental attitude improved and her depression lifted, but her physical flexibility has improved as well, especially in her hands and fingers. Today, there is no evidence of any arthritis in her hands. By changing her mental outlook about her age and learning to work with her healing system, she was able to regain her health. Elizabeth now appears and behaves much younger than her 83 years, and there's no sign of "old age" setting in any time soon.

Bill's Story: One Among Many

Bill was a patient I met through my work with Dr. Dean Ornish. Bill demonstrated the importance of cultivating a healthy mental attitude about his age while he successfully overcame and reversed his heart disease. At the age of 85, after he had succeeded in winning back his health, Bill was interviewed by a reporter who inquired about his secret to a healthy, vibrant life, which he obviously demonstrated by regularly traveling around the world, hiking in alpine altitudes, and practicing yoga every day. To this question, Bill replied, "Old age is something that happens to someone who is at least 15 years older than me!" This is the kind of attitude that improves the performance of your healing system and contributes to long-lasting health.

In my 10 years of work with Dr. Ornish, I had the opportunity to work with many other wonderful patients. Like Bill, these folks demonstrated remarkably optimistic mental attitudes about their lives and their ages, in spite of their histories of severe, advanced, life-threatening disease. In fact, it turned out that an optimistic mental attitude was critical to strengthening and fortifying their healing systems in their quests to successfully reverse their heart disease, one of the world's most dangerous and deadly of all diseases. An interesting finding that surfaced early on in Dr. Ornish's research supported this observation about the relationship between their attitude and their success in overcoming heart disease.

Before Dr. Ornish's research, numerous studies had concluded that heart disease was an irreversible and incurable disease. These studies had repeatedly demonstrated that once a person developed heart disease, it would continue to progress and get worse as the person got older, eventually killing him or her. Again, this is exactly what would be predicted based on our society's current views about aging and disease. In the early stages of Dr. Ornish's groundbreaking research, which uncovered new evidence about how the heart could heal itself, the general expectation, based on these beliefs, was that if reversal of heart disease was possible, it would be seen in those patients who were younger and had less severe disease.

Contrary to what was predicted, however, the opposite turned out to be the case: The oldest and sickest patients showed the greatest improvement in the shortest time. These results ran completely counter to what the experts had predicted. Everyone, including Dr. Ornish, was stumped.

Upon further inspection, however, the results began to make sense. The oldest patients with the most advanced heart disease had tried all the latest high-tech interventions, including surgery, without success. Having exhausted their options, they turned to Dr. Ornish out of desperation. Because their lives were on the line, these people were highly motivated to improve their health, much more so than their younger, less-ill peers. They also recognized the need to enlist a positive mental attitude in their quest to overcome their illnesses. Because of their motivation and attitude, regardless of their advanced age, these people demonstrated the greatest adherence to all the elements of Dr. Ornish's program, and they showed the greatest reversal of disease and the most improvement in health in the shortest period of time. Once again, this story illustrates that regardless of your age or the severity of your illness, your healing system is ready to heal you when you start to work with it.

I know of many people with other diseases, including hypertension, diabetes, arthritis, and cancer, who have similar stories. The evidence seems clear. When you harbor a negative mental attitude about your life and fail to take good care of yourself, you impede the function of your healing system and are more likely to age faster, succumb to illness more easily, and die sooner. Conversely, when you learn to positively align your mental attitude and personal health habits with your healing system, you are much more likely to enjoy greater health as you age . . . and to live longer, as well.

How Your Beliefs Affect Aging and Your Healing System

Your attitudes, thoughts, and beliefs about your age and health powerfully influence the performance of your healing system. These beliefs are strongly shaped by your culture and the society in which you live. For example, if the society in which you live says that old age begins when you reach your fortieth or fiftieth birthday, you will probably start to feel old when you approach this age. If people around you also start telling you that you look old, this will reinforce your inner belief that indeed you are getting old. When you start feeling older, any ache or pain or feeling of discomfort in your body will reinforce this unhealthy belief, which in turn will undermine the work of your healing system and accelerate the aging process.

As I discussed earlier, to wrongly believe that as you grow older your health will continue to deteriorate with each passing day is also common in Western cultures. Further, it is generally believed that there are diseases specific to old age, and that, as you become older, you are destined to contract one or more of these illnesses. Attached to these beliefs is the fear that old age is a natural progression of illnesses and maladies in preparation for the final act of human life, which is death, also considered to be the most painful, tortuous, and terrifying experience of all. (As we shall see later, this scenario needn't be the case.)

These beliefs and attitudes create fearful expectations concerning what kind of fate awaits you as you get older. For example, in the West, particularly in America, older people are looked upon as a burden to society, and old age is considered an illness. Elderly people are often sequestered and farmed out to nursing homes to live out their lives. No one wants to spend his or her final days lonely and isolated, surrounded by four walls, cut off from family, friends, and loved ones, and so the aging view old age as a curse and a punishment. These factors conspire to create a tremendous amount of underlying anxiety about growing old that can interfere with the function of the healing system and accelerate an elderly person's demise.

Because of these negative beliefs and fears about old age, people in the West often try to avoid and deny the aging process altogether. To escape the terrible curse of growing older, people will desperately try to turn back the clock and reclaim their youthful appearance with superficial cover-ups. Coloring their hair when it begins to show gray; using drugs; using hairpieces or surgically transplanted hair to compensate for hair loss; undergoing face lifts, chin lifts, and tummy tucks; receiving hormone injections; overdoing vitamins and supplements; and taking prescription medications to revive sexual vigor are just a few examples that, while they initially might appear to be good ideas, often represent attempts to run away from the deeper fears of growing old. Attempting to look younger on the outside while being terrified about growing older on the inside only feeds into the dehumanizing illusion that your body is all you are and all you have. As long as you fear growing old, a fear that causes mental and physical tensions that interfere with the functioning of your healing system, you will not age gracefully or be able to extend your lifespan in a way that improves the overall quality of your life.

To resolve this internal strife, learning how to relax and accept yourself as you are, in spite of your advancing age, will be helpful. Doing this will set in motion the processes of cooperation between your mind, body, and healing system, and will allow you to enjoy natural, long-lasting health for many years to come. To help you relax and accept yourself as you are, begin regularly practicing the relaxation and stress-management techniques that are recommended in this book. These methods work from the inside out and will prove to be invaluable aids to help you not only look younger, but feel younger, as well.

Expectations and Longevity

By studying people who consistently remain healthy while enjoying great longevity, we can learn a lot about how cultural beliefs and attitudes about aging can benefit our healing systems and contribute to long-lasting health. For example, among the Hunza, who dwell in the mountains of Central Asia and consistently live beyond the age of 100 years, there is considerable lack of disease. His peers consider a 70-year-old Hunza man to be a youngster, and they expect him to remain healthy, active, and productive until well beyond this age. Because of the powerful impact the mind has on the body, the cultural mindset and expectations of the Hunza exert a positive influence on their healing systems, contributing to less illness, greater overall health, and increased longevity. If you expect to be working in the fields and riding your horse when you are 100 years old, as the Hunza typically do, you will have a much greater likelihood of remaining disease free and performing these activities at that age. The Hunza are able to age gracefully, stay healthy, and live longer because they have a much healthier outlook on life at all stages, including old age.

Even in the West, now that people are living longer, what once was considered old age clearly no longer applies to today's standards. As I've previously mentioned, centenarians, people who live to 100 years or more, currently make up the fastest growing segment of the U.S. population. Considering this statistic, there is no medical reason why a 70-year-old person cannot fully participate in an active life, including running a farm, driving a tractor, owning a business, working as a doctor or a mailman, playing tennis, snow skiing, water skiing, surfing, or even hang-gliding or bungee-jumping. In fact, because of these increasing longevity statistics (the average American male now lives to 74 years, the American female to 79 years), the U.S. federal government's Social Security program is presently encouraging senior citizens to continue working past the age of 65, until age 70, before they begin collecting retirement benefits. These longevity statistics create changes in expectations about our health and our capacity for aging as a nation. These changes will, in turn, create better cooperation and support of our healing systems, which will contribute to healthier people, fewer diseases, and still-greater longevity across the board.

The Myth of Age-Related Diseases and Your Healing System

When comparing disease trends around the world, one is struck by the remarkable absence in non-Western countries of diseases that are looked upon as naturally endemic to the West, especially those diseases that are associated with genetics and aging, such as heart disease, diabetes, arthritis, emphysema, cancer, and others. If these diseases were truly due to "old age" and genetics, then we should be seeing widespread prevalence of these diseases in the elderly on a global scale; but we are not. These diseases are specific to Western societies and cultures, and they are due to causes that are anything but natural. As we discussed earlier, unhealthy diets, lifestyles, and mental-emotional factors that cause stress and create chemical imbalances in the body's internal environment are the root causes of these diseases.

One of the better-known studies that demonstrates this fact compared rates of diabetes in older Japanese men who lived in Japan with those who had moved to Hawaii, and with those who had immigrated to the U.S. mainland. The study observed very low rates of diabetes in the older men living in Japan, where diabetes is quite rare. Rates of diabetes were twice as high in the group that had moved to Hawaii. In the third group that had immigrated to the U.S. mainland, where the men had adopted Western diets and lifestyles, the rates of diabetes were so high that they were identical to those of other Americans of the same age group. This study provided strong evidence that diet, lifestyle, and personal health habits, not age or genetics, were responsible for the increasing rates of diabetes observed in these Japanese men. Other studies have shown similar increases of other common diseases in immigrant populations who left their native countries to settle in North America and Europe.

I share this information so that you will not be fooled by the conventional myths about aging and illness that abound in our society. I don't want you to fall prey to the illusion that there are diseases "out there" that are more powerful than you are. Instead, I want you to understand that the underlying causes of most major diseases are simple factors such as diet, lifestyle, personal health habits, and attitudes that neglect, ignore, and work against your healing system. These factors, which are the ultimate forces in determining whether you will remain healthy or become ill, are within your control. When these factors are aligned in support of your healing system, you can feel confident in knowing that, even as you age, you will be able to conquer and defeat almost every illness and disease that life may throw your way.

Contrary to popular belief, the following major categories of illnesses, often associated with advancing age, are not caused by age-related factors at all. (For specific recommendations for learning to work with your healing system to prevent and overcome these illnesses, refer to Part Two and to earlier chapters.)

Alzheimer's disease is prevalent in the elderly and is associated with memory loss and progressive *dementia*, or loss of intellectual function. Alzheimer's is common in senior citizens who have been neglected and have not received ongoing, adequate intellectual stimulation, or, for one reason or another, have withdrawn from social interaction. Alzheimer's appears to be more of a functional neurological problem than related to a specific anatomical defect. For instance, when the brain becomes overloaded with information, and stress and tension are present, symptoms worsen. Although experts are trying to discover a genetic link or determine another underlying factor to its cause, a recent 13-year study concluded that social factors are the most significant contributing causes to Alzheimer's disease.

In many cases, symptoms of Alzheimer's can improve through adequate social contact, learning how to relax while calming down the nervous system, practicing regular stress management, and paying closer attention to all of the factors that improve the health of the healing system. Proper diet, along with natural remedies, including gingko, which improves blood flow to the brain, may also be helpful.

Arthritis is a general category of common joint diseases. Arthritis encompasses several different illnesses that have as their common denominator progressive stiffness, swelling, and pain in one or more joints. These illnesses, although more common in old age, often show up in joint areas of the body that have been neglected, have not been used because of previous injury or lack of movement, or have been overused. The most common joints affected include the hands and fingers, toes, knees, hips, and spine. But often more than just physical factors contribute to arthritis; these conditions usually become worse during times of stress, emotional upheaval, or dietary imbalances, or from other causes. The good news is new evidence that, like heart disease, many different forms of arthritis are reversible and curable. Of course, this evidence is not surprising when you understand that your body has a healing system.

Cancer is often erroneously attributed to the aging process by health experts who cite diminished immune function in the elderly as a primary contributing factor. Cancer can affect all age groups, and although certain cancers may occur more frequently in the elderly, other more closely associated risk factors, if avoided, can significantly lower cancer risk. In working with your healing system, preventing cancer is easier than treating it. For this reason, it is better to incorporate early preventive measures that include a healthy diet and lifestyle. If cancer occurs, treating it is easier if it is caught early, and many cases have been arrested and cured in the early stages. Even in advanced stages, however, cancer can be successfully defeated if you enlist the help of your healing system and cooperate with it on every level. There are many case reports of people who have successfully overcome cancer, even in its advanced stages. Doctors Bernie Siegel and O. Carl Simonton are two cancer doctors who have shared many of these inspirational and courageous stories in their books. The more you learn, the clearer it becomes that advancing age does not cause cancer, and not only the young, but people of all ages who have a strong and effective healing system, conquer it.

Depression is more commonly seen in the elderly, but it can strike at any age. In the elderly for whom a lack of meaning or purpose in life has become pronounced, circumstances are ripe for depression to set in. The danger of depression is that in its more advanced stages it can lead to premature death through suicide. Because depression also acts as a stressor, it can cause harmful physiological effects as well, damaging the healing system and shortening your life span. Depression has been linked to such stress-related disorders as heart disease, diabetes, and cancer. Depression is more common in more intelligent people who, with their superior intellectual skills, tend to become prisoners of their own repeated negative thinking. For these people, learning how to relax, calm the mind, and get involved in activities that uplift the spirits is important. Even though depression is traditionally classified as a mental illness, physical factors often can contribute to this problem. In working with the healing system, a combined mind-body approach is usually the best strategy for reversing and overcoming depression, regardless of your age.

In most cases, you can avoid or reverse depression by staying involved and connected to family, friends, and loved ones; volunteering in meaningful activities; being around children, animals, and nature; developing a sense of gratitude; remembering to have fun and not take life too seriously; and focusing more on the spiritual aspects of life. Whether you are 22 or 82, the same strategies apply, and you will gain the same benefits.

Exercise and simply moving the body can be effective in lifting mild and moderate depression. A wholesome diet, combined with St. John's wort, a natural herbal medication commonly prescribed in Germany, may also be helpful. Learning to let go of unwanted mental and emotional baggage can lighten loads and lift spirits considerably. Practicing self-forgiveness and learning to release anger and hostility are also often helpful. A great book that deals with this subject is Dan

Millman's *The Way of the Peaceful Warrior*, based on the true story of an athlete who overcame depression and went on to win a gold medal in the Olympics. Remember that depression, like the vast majority of diseases, is not an age-related illness.

Diabetes is another disease commonly associated with the aging process, but recent research has shown that the causes of this disease have nothing to do with age. The most common type of diabetes has been linked to a lack of exercise, poor diet, stress, and emotional upheaval. Recent research has suggested that stress is a major contributor to diabetes. The medical community has known for quite some time that stress causes blood-sugar fluctuations that can be harmful. By working with your healing system in learning to manage stress, in addition to incorporating healthy eating and exercise, you can not only prevent but reverse this illness.

Heart disease was once thought to be a natural condition that accompanied the aging process. While it is true that heart disease is more common in the elderly, we have learned through the pioneering research of such noteworthy scientists as Dr. Dean Ornish that other factors in the genesis of heart disease are far more important than age. Factors such as poor diet, stress, lack of exercise, lack of love and intimacy, and repression of emotions have been shown to play a much greater role in the origin of this disorder. As noted earlier, in Dr. Ornish's studies, the oldest patients with the most severe heart disease generally showed the greatest reversal of disease and improvement in their heart health. Learning to work with your healing system, as Dr. Ornish's methods have proven, can both prevent and reverse heart disease, no matter how old you are.

High blood pressure, or *hypertension*, is a disease commonly associated with the elderly and is erroneously attributed to the aging process. Even though high blood pressure is markedly absent in younger people, the cumulative effects of stress and poor diets, along with a lack of exercise and the unhealthy suppression of such emotions as anger and resentment, cause the gradual narrowing and thickening of the arteries, which leads to this disease. Methods for reversing this condition center on diet and lifestyle factors, including learning how to relax, and releasing hostility and tension. More than 30 years ago, Dr. Herbert Benson, Director of the Hypertension Section at Beth Israel Hospital in Boston, in conjunction with

Harvard Medical School, proved that relaxation and meditation could substantially lower and reverse high blood pressure. Supporting your healing system by practicing stress management and incorporating other healthy dietary and lifestyle measures can help prevent and reverse this condition.

Parkinson's disease is another neurological condition associated with the elderly and believed to be caused by a specific biochemical deficiency in the brain. However, Parkinson's symptoms may occur in younger people, such as Michael J. Fox, whose challenges with this disease are well known. Many young Parkinson patients have suffered from trauma to the brain, are under stress, or have abused drugs. Parkinson's also flares up during periods of stress and emotional upheaval. If caught early, Parkinson's may be prevented and managed by proper diet, natural modalities that help improve blood flow to the brain, stress management, and other mind-body methods aimed at restoring balance to the nervous system and strengthening the healing system. Again, this disease is not reserved for the elderly, but can occur in anyone at any age, and it can be treated with the same methods.

Stroke can be a crippling and disabling condition that commonly affects the elderly. However, to associate stroke with the aging process alone is to overlook the key risk factors and underlying conditions that cause stroke, which in most cases are related to stress, diet, and lifestyle. In fact, stroke is an uncommon condition in most developing countries. Although several different mechanisms can result in stroke, the most common is an underlying condition of persistent, uncontrolled high blood pressure, not old age. Stroke is also commonly caused by constant irregular heartbeats, known as *arrhythmias*, which create blood-flow disturbances that can cause small blood clots to pass to the brain. Stroke, regardless of its underlying causes, is entirely preventable. Working with the healing system, a person with normal blood pressure who watches his or her weight, exercises regularly, drinks fluids, manages stress, and participates in the healthy release and expression of emotions will most certainly be successful in avoiding this condition. And even with strokes that already have occurred, successful rehabilitation is often possible thanks to the healing system, which is able to work with the nervous system to help transfer information from the damaged side of the brain to the other side, bringing life back to previously paralyzed limbs.

Remaining Flexible As You Age

Stretching to Support Your Healing System

The axiom "Move it or lose it" seems to be a fundamental principle in the universe, and it certainly applies to the health of our bodies. People tend to slow down and become more sedentary as they age, and so they tend to move less. This lack of movement can lead to stiffness, much like what happens when rust sets into an unused, neglected machine. The stiffness can lead to pain, which in turn discourages further movement. A vicious cycle perpetuates itself, leading to immobility and disability, not just of the joints and limbs, but also of the internal organs. When you stop moving, your healing system weakens, and life expectancy diminishes. To avoid these consequences, gently but persistently stretching the various muscles in your body is important.

Stretching keeps your joints mobile and ensures that your body will remain flexible as you age. For this reason, stretching is one of the most important things you can do to support your healing system and promote long-lasting health. Like a coconut tree in a hurricane, if your body is flexible, it can better endure adverse forces of stress and trauma as you age. If you were a dog or a cat, you would instinctively stretch every time you got up from sleep. All mammals and vertebrates instinctively stretch. Nothing else is as natural and beneficial for your healing system and body as stretching.

Chronic Disease

A Blessing in Disguise

One day while he was being interviewed, Sir William Osler, one of the most famous physicians of the twentieth century, was asked the secret to longevity. He gave an answer that surprised everyone: "Get a chronic disease, and learn to take good care of it!"

How could the secret of long-lasting health and longevity ever be found in having a chronic disease? To have a chronic disease and at the same time be able to extend your life span sounds like a total contradiction. What was on Sir William Osler's mind when he came up with this enigmatic statement?

In his greater wisdom and glory, Dr. Osler went on to clarify what he meant. He explained that having a chronic disease is really a blessing in disguise because it forces you to pay closer attention to your body than you would normally do. In so doing, you benefit all parts of your body, and so your overall health actually can be improved. He further went on to explain that when you have a chronic disease, your body becomes more sensitive, vulnerable, and demanding, and this makes you a better "listener." You become more aware of your body, and you can more effectively identify what causes flare-ups of your disease, whether toxins in the environment, unhealthy foods, irritating substances, stress or emotional upheaval, or other offensive factors. In the process, you have the opportunity to learn how to avoid these factors and lessen the intensity or frequency of the flare-ups. You also have the opportunity to discover how imbalances were created in your body to cause the disease in the first place. These imbalances may have been caused by unconscious, self-destructive habits and tendencies, as well as by unhealthy thoughts and attitudes. With chronic disease, you have the opportunity to learn how to undo the damage, reverse the disease process, and cooperate with your healing system to restore your body to its natural state of health. Doing this requires that you learn to nurture, and be kind and gentle to, your body, exploring ways to fulfill its needs and treat it better.

Having a chronic disease can teach you how to become your own best caregiver, your own full-time doctor, so to speak. And as you learn to cooperate with your healing system in your mission of returning to a natural state of health and wellness, your healing system can help you remain healthy, functional, and symptom free for the rest of your life. This is the hidden meaning behind Sir William Osler's statement that the key to longevity is to get a chronic disease and learn to take good care of it.

In contrast to this approach, as soon as they are diagnosed with a chronic disease, many people give in to fear, negative thinking, and despair. This response only reinforces the disease process and is a sure recipe for an early demise. Even well-meaning doctors often unknowingly support this pessimistic attitude. The following story illustrates the point.

A man I knew was suspected of having prostate cancer. His doctor ordered tests to confirm that he had cancer, and the tests came back positive. On his first doctor's visit after the diagnosis was established, this man asked his doctor whether he should quit smoking. To his astonishment, his doctor replied, "At this point, what's the use?" With his doctor's negative attitude, he left the office and immediately plunged into a deep depression. Even though the doctor didn't say it in exactly these words, what he heard was "It is too late to do anything at this stage. Face the facts. You are going to die." Six weeks later, the man died.

It is important not to deny the reality of an illness; at the same time, it is more important not to become passive or depressed, or to give in to the popular pessimistic notions about what will happen to you as you become more ill. As the late Norman Cousins used to say, "Don't deny the diagnosis, but defy the verdict!" Because of the connection between your mind and your healing system, remaining optimistic, even when the odds appear to be stacked against you, is crucial.

According to Dr. Osler's wisdom and experience, even if you have been diagnosed with diabetes, or heart disease, or any other chronic condition, it is possible for you to live to be 120 years old. If you watch your diet, regularly exercise, practice stress management, and use other methods and strategies that cooperate with your healing system, you can learn to positively influence your body's internal environment and improve your overall health. If you are currently taking medications, you may gradually be able to reduce your dependence on them and quite possibly get off them altogether. In my own practice, I have seen this happen quite frequently.

If you are sufficiently motivated, and you don't give in to pessimism and despair, a chronic disease can direct and guide you toward a much healthier lifestyle that supports your healing system and improves your overall health. In so doing, the disease can enable you to enjoy long-lasting health. Seen from this perspective, a chronic disease can actually be a blessing in disguise.

I'd like to make an additional point in support of Dr. Osler's wisdom. There is a saying, "You don't miss your water until your well runs dry." In my own experience, I have seen that many people do not honor or value their health unless they are at immediate risk of losing it. In this regard, contracting a chronic, life-threatening disease can serve as a much-needed wake-up call. When you realize your life is on the line and you are not here forever, it's amazing how quickly you can become motivated to improve the quality of your health and life. With this clarity and sense of urgency, it is often easier to make sweeping, constructive changes in your diet, lifestyle, and personal habits that strengthen and enhance the work of your healing system. When you live your life fully, with the awareness that being alive is truly a blessing, privilege, and unique opportunity, you begin to realize the critical importance of your health and your responsibility to take care of yourself. When you participate in healthful, wholesome activities that support your healing system, your overall health improves, and the prospects for greater longevity increase significantly.

As you learn to take better care of yourself, your illness can serve as your ticket to a longer and happier, more productive life. In fact, many people who have overcome chronic, life-threatening illnesses have looked back and declared that their illnesses were gifts, without which their lives would have never been transformed for the better.

And who is to say that once you have a chronic disease you are stuck with it? Since Dr. Osler's time, in addition to Dr. Dean Ornish's studies that proved heart disease can be reversed, many other studies are now showing similar possibilities for diabetes, arthritis, asthma, multiple sclerosis, cancer, and many other diseases. The same mechanisms that cause disease processes to occur in the first place can be reversed and eliminate the disease from your body. If you are currently plagued by a health problem, the sooner you adopt an active role in supporting and cooperating with your healing system, the faster you can heal and be back on the road to long-lasting health.

Memory Loss and Your Healing System As You Age

A simple fact of living is that, as people age, their brains accumulate more information than they need. Most people who age and have trouble with their memories suffer from a simple case of information overload, otherwise known as "brain clutter." There are just too many useless facts, memories, incidents, or other trivial pieces of information in their heads, stored up over a lifetime, and all these details slow down the quality of their brain's ability to process information and function efficiently. Although occasionally real organic or physical causes exist for memory loss or brain dysfunction, such as impaired blood flow to the brain or chemical imbalances in the blood, in my experience, the overwhelming majority of memory-loss and brain-dysfunction experiences are not the result of organic causes.

The dangers of memory loss and brain dysfunction are that they can cause disorientation and confusion, which lead to stress and anxiety, which can burden the healing system through the mind-body interactions that we have discussed earlier in this book. If a chronic physical disease is also already present, it can further jeopardize your health by interfering with the work of your healing system.

Many people who develop memory problems as they age contribute to their own difficulties by hanging on to memories and pieces of outdated information that no longer serve their best interests. For one reason or another, they are afraid to move forward with their lives, remaining stuck in the past and living their lives as if the best times were behind them. People who do this are closing the door to future experiences that may be wonderfully uplifting and enlightening. As their memory continues to fail them, they become more and more frightened, stressed, and anxious, and their brain function deteriorates further. This combination can become terribly unsettling and disorienting to their mental health and well-being.

Tips for Improving Memory and Brain Function

Taking an active role in preserving, maintaining, and restoring your very important mental health and well-being is essential. In fact, your survival depends on it. You can take definite actions to cooperate with your healing system in improving your memory and brain function as you age. The following key steps, while not all-inclusive, can serve as a starting point in this process:

■ Make sure you have investigated the possibility of underlying organic causes, including chemical imbalances in the blood or your body's internal environment that may be interfering with your brain function. Doing this may necessitate a visit to your family doctor for a checkup.

■ Clear your mind of unnecessary pieces of information, including phone numbers, facts, figures, memories, or experiences that do not serve your best interests.

■ If you cannot recall a piece of information that you feel is important, don't struggle, strain, or fight. Relax, breathe, calm your mind, and let go. If the information is really important, it will eventually come back to you. Your memory functions best when your mind is calm and relaxed, not when you are upset, tense, or anxious.

■ Make sure your diet is healthy and wholesome, and that you are drinking enough fluids. Avoid excess caffeine, alcohol, and other unhealthy substances that negatively affect your brain.

■ Avoid excess medications or medications that may interfere with your memory.

■ Make sure you are getting enough exercise. Exercise has been shown to improve blood flow to the brain, which improves brain function and memory.

■ Practice stress-management techniques to keep your brain and nervous system calm and relaxed. A naturally calm and relaxed mind is more alert and can concentrate better.

■ Avoid emotional upheaval, including anger and resentment, which compromises clarity and clouds thinking.

■ Experiment with natural supplements such as *gingko biloba* and *gotu cola,* which have been shown to improve blood flow to the brain; these herbs can improve memory and brain function. Make sure they will not conflict with other medications you already may be taking.

■ Consider trying other natural methods, including cranial-sacral therapy, acupuncture, yoga, tai chi, and other gentle, non-invasive, complementary therapies.

Advantages of Aging and Long-Lasting Health

As you advance in years, and whenever you begin to doubt your intrinsic worth, go to your local liquor store and ask to see its selection and price list of fine wines. You will notice that the older wines are the most expensive. Like a bottle of fine vintage wine, your net worth and value also increase as you age. Aging includes a number of advantages; proudly and nobly embrace them. Old age is a time to look forward to, and long-lasting health will ensure that you can enjoy it more fully.

For example, in the aboriginal culture of Australia, more than 40,000 years old, the elder members are regarded as the wisest and most powerful of all souls, and their people afford them the greatest respect. The culture relies upon their wisdom and experience to guide the aborigines through difficult times, to preside over disputes and to help settle differences, and to be available for consultation in all important matters, including those of a domestic, political, or spiritual nature.

In the Buddhist tradition, elder Buddhists are looked upon as the highest-ranking members of the society. In many other cultures throughout the world, the elder system is still intact. People are honored and valued for their advancing years, not banished, punished, and shamed, as they often are in the West.

As surprising as it may sound, getting older also confers many health advantages. For example, when you are older, you have more experience, more knowledge, and more wisdom about your health. You are more familiar with your body's strengths, weaknesses, and limitations, and you have probably discovered the virtues of moderation. Additionally, over the years that you have aged, you have learned how to feed and nourish your body; how to exercise it; how much water, sleep, and rest it requires; how it tolerates temperature changes; and what kind of clothes it requires to keep warm for each season. In the words of Plato, "It gives me great pleasure to converse with the aged. They have been over the road that all of us must travel and know where it is rough and difficult and where it is level and easy."

As you age, you possess a greater ability to avoid illness and injury. You learn to be more careful and safe in all activities, from walking and climbing stairs to driving. You become better at physical and mental energy conservation for your health and well-being. For example, when you were young, you may have thought that you were invincible, as if you were a superman or superwoman. As a consequence, you may have made some costly mistakes. When you are older, you tend not to be so foolish, to be more thoughtful and deliberate. When you are older, you are ruled not so much by your hormones or passions as by your common sense, tempered discipline, and your ability to listen to your body and act benevolently on its behalf. When you are older, you tend not to become so swept away or preoccupied with the affairs of the world, but, rather, to become more self-entertaining and self-contained. This process directs your mental energies inward, increasing your bodily awareness, and improving your ability to listen to and cooperate with your healing system.

As you age, you also tend to become more patient and tolerant of pain and physical discomfort, which increases your endurance. This is apparent in the Olympic games in which, in the endurance events such as the marathon race, the top athletes may be as much as 20 years older than athletes who compete in other events such as the sprints. In fact, many octogenarian marathon runners are active in the world today, and many senior athletes are still competing on the master's level in other sports such as golf, tennis, swimming, surfing, water skiing, and snow skiing. These elder athletes demonstrate that, regardless of their ages, they can keep their healing systems vibrant and youthful, stay competitive, and enjoy long-lasting health by remaining active.

With all of these advantages to aging, we should look upon old age as a time of maximum health and enjoyment. By understanding all of the factors that positively influence the performance of our healing systems, and then putting these factors into practice, we can successfully enjoy a superior state of health and a vibrant, active life for the rest of our days.

The Power of Laughter and a Sense of Humor

In previous chapters, we have talked about all of the factors that can improve the performance of your healing system. One of the most important of these factors, if not the most important, appears to be a sense of humor. I say this with good reason.

I have met many people who have lived well into old age and beyond, sometimes reaching 100 years or more, who defied the principles of what most experts would consider a healthy life. Many of these people had poor diets, drank alcohol or smoked excessively, did not exercise regularly, were overweight, and, strictly from a health standpoint, did just about everything else wrong. However, the persons among this group were rare who didn't also possess a keen sense of humor, an extraordinary ability to allow most difficulties, negative comments, and adverse situations to roll right off their backs. Most of these people understood that, to get the most out of life, they had to have fun.

Many good people miss the boat in this regard. They take their health and their life too seriously. One famous health expert even went so far as to say, "Seriousness is a disease more dangerous than cancer!" Being serious all the time creates tension in the body, which can drain the life force out of your healing system. We've all heard the saying, "All work and no play makes Jack a dull boy." What we haven't heard, and what is also true, is that "All work and no play can make Jack a sick puppy." Many research studies suggest that people who cannot take the time to relax, have fun, and laugh are at serious risk for developing a major illness. Dr. Bernie Siegel, a famous cancer surgeon, tells a story that helps illustrate this point.

A man ran six miles every day for 25 years. He never went to parties, never went to bed after 10:00 PM, never drank or smoked, and was a vegetarian. One day, he suddenly died. He was so upset by this sudden turn of events that when he got to the Pearly Gates he went straight up to God and demanded an immediate explanation for this apparent injustice.

"What the hell are you doing, God?" the man asked. "I've run every day for the past 25 years, never touched alcohol or tobacco, gone to bed early, and eaten only vegetables. I've worked hard my whole life just to remain healthy and live long, and you had to spoil everything by bringing me here. What's your point in doing this?" the man asked.

"My point is that you basically blew it!" God said. "You forgot to have fun and enjoy your life, which were the reasons why you were created!" He exclaimed. "And since you failed to learn your lessons this time, I'm sending you back to Hell for an attitude adjustment!" cried God.

"What will I do there?" queried the man.

"For starters, you'll have to run six miles every day, go to bed before 10:00 PM each night, and eat only vegetables," God declared. He continued, "Next time, try to enjoy your life, and come back when your attitude is a little better!"

Dr. Siegel goes on to make the point that it is important to do things not out of the fear of dying, but rather out of the desire to improve the overall quality of your life. Certainly there was nothing wrong with what the man was doing to improve his health, but his attitude and reason for doing these things were wrong. Again, the goal of long-lasting health is not just to live longer, but to improve the overall quality of your life in the process. If you are not having fun and enjoying your life, you are missing the boat. Just remember the French woman introduced earlier in the book, who lived to the age of 122 and who, when interviewed about the secrets of her longevity, replied that the only thing she knew was that "I only have one wrinkle on my entire body, and I'm sitting on it!"

Almost nothing in the world can keep your healing system as strong, vibrant, and healthy as cultivating and refining the ability to laugh . . . to laugh often, vigorously, and—what is even more powerful—to frequently share raucous belly laughter with your friends or family. Bob Hope passed away at the age of 100 years. I believe he was trying to beat George Burns' age when he died. It is not an accident that these two famous comedians, who earned their living with a sense of humor and making other people laugh, lived so long.

When you are laughing, having fun, and enjoying life, you are releasing tension and creating positive physiology within your body that strengthens and fortifies your healing system. Laughter kills pain by triggering the release of powerful neurochemicals from the brain, such as endorphins and enkephalins, which, as we noted earlier, are naturally occurring opiates much stronger than morphine. Laughter simultaneously stimulates the release of other powerful substances that boost the performance of your healing system. Some scientists have defined laughter as tantamount to "internal jogging," in that all the health benefits of jogging, such as improving the strength of your heart and circulatory system, can also be found in laughter.

Doing What You Love
Contributes to a Long and Healthy Life

Upon his retirement at the age of 89 years, an innovative artist and animator for Walt Disney Studios was recently recognized for his outstanding contribution to the field for more than 65 years. When asked how he managed to keep going all those years, and what motivated him, he replied, "You gotta love your work!"

When you love what you do, every day is a day of play and enjoyment. When you work at a job that you love, it doesn't feel like work. Loving your work is the healthiest tonic in the world for your body's healing system as it is injected with a continuous supply of dynamic, positive, mental and emotional energy every single day of your life. By the time you reach old age, this positive energy pays off in dividends. The following stories help illustrate this point.

Pop Proctor was a well-known surfer from California who fell in love with the sport when he picked it up at the rather late age of 50. He surfed for more than 40 years and retired from surfing at the age of 97. He died at the age of 99, and it was rumored that he died so young because he retired from surfing too soon.

Albert Schweitzer once told his hospital staff that "I have no intention of dying, so long as I can do things. And if I do things, I have no need to die, so I will live a long, long time." Dr. Schweitzer, who received the Nobel Prize in 1952, remained active until his final days; he lived until the age of 90.

Mrs. Minami was a Japanese-Hawaiian woman who was 101 years of age when I met her. She drank a cup of hot water after each meal and enjoyed perfect regularity. She worked in her garden, which she absolutely adored, every day, rain or shine. When she left me for another doctor because her insurance had changed, she was 103 and still going strong.

Harry Lieberman was an elderly, 78-year-old man who had been alone in a nursing home since the age of 75, silently awaiting his death. To help pass the time, every day at noon he would meet his partner for a game of chess. One day, unbeknownst to him, his partner died. When Harry showed up at the usual time the next day for his chess match, his partner didn't show. The staff, who was informed of his partner's passing and concerned about the effects on Harry, didn't want to break the news to him so suddenly. They told Harry his partner had become ill and had to go to the hospital. They asked Harry if he would like to attend an art class instead, just for the day.

Harry was shuttled off to the nursing home's art class, where he was seated at a table and handed a blank piece of paper, some colored paints, and a brush. He had never held a brush before in his life, and he felt totally awkward. The teacher announced that the class assignment was to paint anything the participants wanted.

While he was holding onto the brush, Harry's mind drifted back to the days when he was a boy growing up in a village in his country of birth, Poland. Slowly, he began to paint what his mind saw. At the end of class, the teacher looked at this painting, thanked him for his attendance, and encouraged him to return the following day.

The following day, however, Harry didn't want to paint another picture. Instead, he looked forward to resuming his chess game with his partner. At the appointed hour, however, when Harry sat down at the chess board and waited for his friend, one of the young volunteers came and informed Harry that his friend was still in the hospital. She encouraged him to please attend the art class one more time. Harry reluctantly agreed.

Now, for the second time in as many days, Harry found himself sitting down with a brush, a blank piece of paper, and some paints. Today's assignment: "Paint anything you want." Again, Harry drifted off to his childhood days and slowly began painting.

At the close of the class, the teacher again came by Harry's table, saw his painting, and made an encouraging comment. He told Harry he wanted him to attend the evening art class at the local junior college. The teacher told Harry that at the very least this would be a chance to get out and meet some new people, especially young, attractive college girls. Hesitant at first, Harry finally agreed.

In the evening of the next day, a van picked Harry up and took him several miles away to the art class at the junior college, where he was ushered inside with more than 40 students, most of them young enough to be his grandchildren. This setting was much different from the dull, sedate, and somber atmosphere of his nursing home.

For the third time in as many days, Harry found himself seated at a desk with a brush, a blank piece of paper, and paints. The assignment: "Paint anything you want." Once again, Harry's mind drifted off to his past as he dipped his brush into the paints and began applying strokes to the paper.

At the close of the class, the teacher walked around the room to critique each student's work. When he came to Harry's painting, he paused for a moment. Then he made a surprising comment.

"Would you be so kind as to autograph this painting for me?" he asked Harry.

Harry was dumbfounded. "Why?" he asked.

The teacher replied, "Because I have a feeling that someday you're going to be a famous artist."

Harry thought to himself, "Right, but first I'll be the next president of America!"

For the next 25 years, Harry Lieberman painted every day and eventually established himself as one of the preeminent artists in the world, painting village scenes from his childhood life in Poland, along with stories from the Old Testament. To this day, his works are displayed prominently in books, museums, and galleries all over the world. Doing what he loved to do, Harry Lieberman lived past the age of 103.

Do what you love, and love what you do. This is the essence of allowing the creative spirit within you to flourish and express itself, producing long-lasting health and a sense of well-being as byproducts. If you suppress or deny this spirit, it will wither up and die, and your health will surely follow. Suppressing or denying your inherent creative instincts, not doing what you love, or not loving what you do, will drain your life force and render your healing system powerless. When this happens, you will become sick.

Many people are allowed to pursue their dreams and are encouraged to follow their hearts from an early age. These are the lucky ones. Others, like Harry Lieberman, discover their true joy and passion when they are at an advanced age. However, regardless of your age, the health-enhancing benefits of putting your heart into what you are doing are undeniable. Organizing your life around doing what you love is one of the wisest and most effective ways to strengthen and fortify your healing system, allowing you the opportunity to enjoy long-lasting health.

Celebrate Your Years and Enhance Your Healing System

Old age is a time for celebration and enjoying the fruits of your labors. It is the time of your "second childhood," a chance to regain your innocence, to see beauty in simple, everyday things, and a time to play and enjoy yourself. Old age is a time to love, be loved, and to know that love is the fundamental underlying reality in all of life. With all of this to look forward to, it is critical that you keep your health as you age so you can maximize the enjoyment of your golden years. Strengthening and fortifying your healing system as you age is the best insurance policy I know to help you realize this goal.

Many people live healthy, pain-free, disease-free, active lives for a long, long time, and then they leave this world peacefully and gently without any pain or suffering. These people have found ways to cooperate with their body's healing systems, and they have learned to strengthen and fortify them as they have advanced in years. While I'm not denying that someday we all must depart this earth, there is no reason to buy into the false notion that you have to become sick and disabled before it is your time to leave. When you work with your healing system, you can enjoy long-lasting health, and stay healthy, until your final days.

From my own research and experience, I have found the following practical tips to be particularly helpful to strengthen and fortify the healing system as you age:

- Practice the principles, exercises, and techniques described in this book.
- Drink plenty of fluids.
- Eat plenty of fruits and vegetables.
- Get adequate fiber in your diet.
- Practice good bowel hygiene.
- Practice stress management.
- Relax regularly.
- Do breathing exercises.
- Think young. Remember that you are only as old as you think you are.
- Take the time to plan for a bright future.
- Learn to be spontaneous.
- Develop a flexible mindset. Avoid being too set in your ways.
- Do what you love to do.
- Stay active.

- Maintain a viable social support system.
- Stay involved with hobbies and creative activities.
- Be a nonconformist.
- Be adventuresome and try new things.
- Spend time in nature.
- If you get bored, learn to play a musical instrument or paint.
- Sing.
- Dance regularly and often, even if you are alone.
- Avoid getting angry.
- Cultivate and nourish loving relationships with your family and friends.
- Don't foster resentment.
- If you are single, date, or be active in social clubs.
- Spend time outdoors.
- Surround yourself with beauty.
- Have fun, and remember to smile and laugh genuinely from your heart.
- Enjoy comedy and keep a light-hearted attitude.
- Don't take life too seriously.
- Don't take yourself too seriously.
- Spend time with people who are busy and involved in doing something meaningful with their lives.
- Choose your friends and company wisely.
- Don't waste your time.
- Don't do things you don't want to do.
- Be true to your sense of purpose.
- Take the time to reflect on the meaning of life.
- Appreciate the fact that your life is a gift, no matter how difficult it has been.
- Acknowledge all the things in life for which you have to be grateful.
- Honor the dignity of your soul.
- Find a way to give back to the world.

- Perform some form of regular community service that makes you feel good inside.
- Spend time with children; let them teach you how to play and be in the present moment.
- Spend time with animals. If possible, have one or more pets.
- Vow to do at least one thing differently each day.
- Get up early every morning, and go to bed early every night.
- Listen to music that inspires and uplifts you.
- Travel if you can afford it and, if not, try to walk or go in a new direction every day.
- Write in a journal your most memorable experiences.
- Write poetry, even if you've never done it before.
- Wake up each morning and tell the world that it is a better place because you are here.
- Don't waste time being around people who don't inspire you or uplift your spirits.
- Read books and watch movies that inspire and uplift you.
- Read about people older than you who are more active than you.
- Keep connected to your family, friends, and loved ones.
- Remember that if you want to have a true friend, you have to be a true friend.
- Listen to music that stirs your heart and soothes your soul.
- Find a way to share your unique talents, gifts, and experiences with the world.
- Focus on how you can do your part to make this world a little better.
- Appreciate how age has mellowed you and made you a better person.
- Love yourself and your life, even if they aren't perfect.
- If you have faith in God or a higher power, pray for guidance and peace.
- Make peace with your soul. Forgive yourself for all you may have done wrong.
- Cry when you want to, and don't feel ashamed when you do.

> ■ Live from your heart.
>
> Remember that your body possesses an efficient and intelligent healing system that can keep you healthy through a multitude of life's challenges. Celebrate and honor your years on this earth, and enjoy your life!

Living Life to the Fullest Until Your Final Days

I hope I haven't given you the impression that you will live forever. Although I do expect you to live long, stay healthy, and enjoy your life, it would be irresponsible of me to try to deceive you into believing that you can remain on this planet indefinitely. Land is a limited commodity, and unfortunately, when it is our time to go, we have to leave to make room for the next person. Even if you reach the age of 100, 120, or beyond, some day you will experience the process of leaving your body as you depart this world. In many cultures around the world, this process, known as death, is regarded as a natural and sacred event, no less important than birth. In these cultures, death is seen as a release and a blessing, the final chapter of a person's earth-bound life in a story that would otherwise be incomplete. Further, in these cultures, death is seen to be not merely an end, but, rather, a new beginning. As a result, the anniversary of the day a person dies is usually remembered and celebrated even more than the person's birthday.

The benefit of accepting that you will not live on this earth forever is that you no longer have to live with the tension the fear of death creates. The acceptance creates a natural state of relaxation. As you know, your healing system works best when you are in a naturally relaxed state, and so overcoming your fear of death greatly improves your vitality and contributes to long-lasting health.

Death is certainly not an experience we should welcome, initiate prematurely, or glorify before its time; nonetheless, it need not be the difficult, painful, miserable experience it is commonly held to be in our society. Death can be a loving, special occasion, a profoundly healing experience for all those who've come to witness the sacred departure of a uniquely created soul. A good death can act as a powerful affirmation and a special blessing to those left behind.

Such deaths, rather than producing tension and prolonging the myth that death is a painful, horrible ordeal, contribute to overall healing by reinforcing the peacefulness, beauty, and serenity of this natural life experience. Such an attitude collectively strengthens and fortifies the healing systems of the individuals within the culture and society, and contributes to long-lasting health in those individuals.

A good death, which can be likened to childbirth, requires preparation. For example, it is well known that mothers who have not attended prenatal classes are usually poorly prepared for labor, and they often suffer far more complications, pain, and trauma than those who are well prepared. The same is true in death. In an ill-prepared-for death, far more complications, pain, and trauma often occur than is necessary. Such an experience reinforces the notion that death is a horrible event and creates fear in those who witness such a death. A vicious cycle perpetuates itself, influencing society's generally fearful perception of death, and creating unnecessary worry and negative outcomes in the process. Ironically, the best way to prepare for a good death is to have a good life.

It is possible to enjoy your final days on this earth and have a positive experience of death. How successful you are at doing this is strongly influenced by your ability to work with your healing system and remain healthy throughout your life, which is largely determined by the choices you make every day. Realize that your time on earth is limited, and then live your life as if it were a privilege, as if each moment counts. Focus on doing what you love to do. For example, a cowboy's dream is to die with his boots on and be buried with his horse. The probability of realizing this dream is increased with each day that he is can saddle up and ride off across the plains with his trusty steed. The same is true for you and any number of activities, hobbies, and vocations that you love to do and that are near and dear to your heart. The more you can organize your life around doing what you love to do, the better the chance that you'll depart this world in an uplifted state, without any sorrows or regrets.

In India, where I have traveled frequently, I have met many people in their eighties, nineties, and older who are active, healthy, respected members of their communities, and who enjoy their lives, totally free from the fear of death and unconcerned about their advancing age. Further, the Sanskrit literature, which dates back several thousand years, is full of historical accounts of accomplished souls who could accurately predict the time of their death and leave their bodies willfully, peacefully, and with courage.

Similarly, in Japan, Samurai warriors have traditionally greeted each new day with the thought, "Today is a good day to die!" Although this statement might initially appear to be fatalistic, the philosophy actually enriches the warriors' lives and improves their health. By facing their mortality this way, acknowledging that today could be their last day on this earth, they can live without fear and remain more relaxed. This relaxed attitude nourishes and supports their healing systems and helps them achieve long-lasting health. Because the Samurai creed permeates almost every aspect of Japanese society, it is not surprising to see that, on average, people in Japan live much longer than people in the West.

Understanding that you have tremendous control over your life circumstances and your health is the best way to prepare for a good death. It is also the best way to enjoy your life. Like the cowboy, yogi, or Samurai warrior, you can enjoy long-lasting health, and then, when it is your time, exit this world with peace and serenity, courage and conviction, grace and style. When you learn to work with your healing system, you can enjoy long-lasting health, and, when the time comes, experience a peaceful and pain-free death.

Closing Thoughts on Aging, Long-Lasting Health, and Your Healing System

The boundaries for what is considered to be old age are continually being expanded. A 70-year-old man, by today's standards, is now viewed as still young. You can prolong and maintain youthful vigor and health well into your eighties, nineties, and beyond if you work at supporting and nourishing your healing system. Your attitude about aging plays an important role in your longevity and influences physiological mechanisms that can either accelerate or slow down the aging process. If you develop poor health habits based on pessimistic, negative attitudes, you stand a greater chance of becoming ill and dying earlier. But if you are inspired to make the most of your life and your extraordinary healing system, and you are motivated to stay healthy, you can enjoy a long and fulfilling life. Maintain a positive mental attitude and develop sound personal health habits, and you will exude a spirit of youthfulness and improve your prospects of remaining healthy until your final days. Accept your mortality and understand that you are on the earth for a limited time, and you'll more easily overcome a fear of death. Cultivate a relaxed attitude. Your healing system will benefit significantly, and your attitude will facilitate your goal of achieving long-lasting health.

CHAPTER 8

The Healing System at Work
Personal Stories of Extraordinary Healing

Doctors deal with pain, suffering, and illness every day of their lives. Because of this, they tend to view life through a distorted lens that sees disease as normal and health as abnormal. Serving as society's appointed health experts, they are in reality disease experts. In this capacity, doctors exert a profound influence on our way of thinking, and so we have learned to be pessimistic, negative, and fearful when it comes to our bodies.

Going beyond this distorted lens and probing deeper into the miraculous workings of our bodies, however, we will discover a healing system that can overcome nearly every affliction known to man. We will discover that health and well-being are the rule, and illness and disease are exceptions to the rule.

Many people with advanced, serious medical conditions get better when they learn how to cooperate with their healing systems. And although these cases may seem extraordinary, in fact, they are quite ordinary. When you understand that you have a healing system, you should expect healing, regardless of how overwhelmingly the odds may be stacked against you. When you or a loved one is afflicted with an illness or injury, the real question is not "Will healing occur?" but rather "When will healing occur?" The answer is "When you decide to cooperate and work with your healing system, you will get better and heal; the sooner you do this, the faster you will heal!"

I offer the following stories to help you get to know your healing system better. Because your healing system is within you, it can be activated free of charge. It is ready to work for you "24/7," and it is your most powerful ally on life's journey. All your healing system asks is that you acknowledge its existence, listen to it, and make a concerted effort to cooperate and work with, not against, it.

Ronald's Story of Extraordinary Healing

Ronald Jenkins was 19 years of age and away at college. He was a strapping picture of health, on a full athletic and academic scholarship, and he had never missed a day of school due to illness since he was in kindergarten. Except for routine physical exams and immunizations, Ronald had never seen a doctor or been hospitalized. He was in the prime of his life, and it was all good. Soon, however, his life would change.

While he was a counselor at a youth camp during summer break, Ronald awoke one night with intense abdominal pain. He ran to the bathroom to relieve himself. Projectile diarrhea ensued, not just once, but so many times that Ronald had to spend half the night on the toilet. He began to feel feverish. He thought he might have contracted a case of food poisoning. He drank liquids and rested, thinking he would get better on his own. After one week, however, his symptoms continued without any letup in intensity. For the first time in his life, Ronald sought the help of a doctor.

The doctor diagnosed Ronald with gastroenteritis and treated him with rest, fluids, antibiotics, and anti-inflammatory medicines. After two weeks, however, there was still no improvement, so his doctor referred him to a specialist. The specialist ordered blood tests, X-rays, intestinal scans, and a *colonoscopy*, an exam in which a flexible tube is inserted up the entire length of the large intestines. After much deliberation and discussion, the doctors made the diagnosis of Crohn's disease, a severe inflammatory condition of the small and large intestines. Ronald was placed on a strict protocol of strong medications, including anti-inflammatories, antimicrobial agents and corticosteroids, and a highly restricted diet.

Ronald didn't do so well on this regimen. His pain and diarrhea continued, and he soon developed other symptoms, as well, such as stiff and painful swollen joints. A strange, blister-type rash appeared on his face. He was constantly nauseous and light-headed. The corners of his mouth began to crack and bleed. Day by day, he felt himself growing weaker, his vital life energy ebbing. He was forced to take a leave of absence from school and move back in with his parents. Fortunately, they were willing to do anything to help Ronald regain his health.

After six months, Ronald appeared to be on death's doorstep. His weight had fallen to an all-time low of 104 pounds, down from his normal weight of 180 pounds. His friends remarked that he looked like a concentration-camp victim. His diarrhea had increased to the point that he couldn't sleep for more than 45 minutes at a time before he would have to get out of bed and run to the toilet to relieve himself. He had no appetite, and his abdomen was bloated and full of gas. He forced himself to eat to stay alive, but he couldn't keep his food in—everything that came in the front door was immediately expelled through the back door.

In a desperate attempt to save Ronald's life, his doctor sent him to the nation's top specialists in gastrointestinal diseases. After reviewing his records and examining him, they all agreed Ronald's was one of the worst cases of Crohn's disease they had ever seen. If his life were to be spared, the consensus was that surgical removal of his colon and a lifetime of immunosuppressive medications was Ronald's only option.

Ronald returned home to contemplate his fate. He became extremely depressed, and even thought of suicide. Because he was malnourished, he had to be fed through a large, intravenous catheter inserted into a vein near his neck. This catheter, which could easily become infected, became Ronald's lifeline.

As Ronald lay in bed wasting away, one of his father's friends suggested something simple but radical. He suggested that if Ronald could regain the balance of natural flora in his intestines, he had a good chance of restoring his health. He based this idea on recent research that suggested that, in addition to the 500 good bacterial strains that reside in the human intestines, there may be many more types of beneficial bacteria, perhaps up to 10,000 strains. He asked Ronald to try several capsules a day of a special hygienic dirt cultivated for human consumption; this dirt contained many strains of these beneficial bacteria.

At first, Ronald was taken aback by the idea of eating dirt, but, because he was desperate, he was ready to try anything. After long hours of reading, research, and discussions with his father and his father's friend, he realized that what was being proposed was a return to the dietary habits of his ancestors. In those days, before pesticides and artificial fertilizers, people often ate vegetables right out of the fields, ingesting small amounts of beneficial soil organisms with each bite, and, in the process, replenishing their natural intestinal flora. When we think of cows' digestive systems, and how their multichambered stomachs are filled with many beneficial bacteria that help digest their food, this idea is not so radical.

The first day, Ronald took six capsules of hygienic dirt (two at a time, three times a day). The following morning, after his first sound night's sleep in a long time, Ronald felt his abdominal pain lessen in intensity. For the first time since his illness began, he didn't awaken with a fever. Throughout the course of the next several days, his diarrhea slowed in frequency and intensity. After several days, his stools began to firm up. After one week, his appetite began to return and he had his first normal bowel movement in almost a year.

Over the next several weeks, as he continued to swallow the capsules of beneficial dirt, Ronald's appetite and bowel movements continued to improve and normalize. His joint health, skin, mouth sores, energy level, and attitude all improved, as well. After six months, his weight was back up to 180 pounds, he was back in school, and he was completely well.

Eating dirt flies in the face of conventional medicine, which often views nature as the enemy and the cause of most diseases. When we work with our healing systems, however, natural solutions often work best. For Ronald, using beneficial organisms that are normally found in healthy, hygienic soil was the secret ingredient that ultimately cured his disease. Beneficial bacteria help in digestion, and they produce many valuable substances, such as vitamin K, thus restoring balance to the intestines; consequently, they are one of the most important ways to cooperate with your body's natural healing system.

Rani's Story of Extraordinary Healing

Rani was an elderly woman who lived in a community I regularly visited in India. She had suffered from asthma since she was a little child, and she took medicines regularly to control it. Whenever she caught a cold, breathed dusty air, or was under heavy stress, her asthma would flare up. At these time, sometimes even her medicines would fail her, and she would have to go to the hospital, where intravenous medications and special breathing treatments were administered.

Having been away for a long time, I returned to India one year to find Rani in a very precipitous condition. Not only was her asthma flaring up, but her feet, ankles, and abdomen were swollen. She had not eaten for days, she could not get out of bed without help, and she appeared to be on death's doorstep.

When I examined Rani, I discovered shallow respirations, a feeble, irregular heart rate and abnormal heart sounds, fluid in her lungs and belly, and an enlarged liver. She told me she hadn't urinated in several days. These were all ominous signs. I suggested she be hospitalized, even though her family couldn't afford it.

In the hospital, after many examinations and investigations, the doctors found that Rani was in congestive heart failure, her liver was failing, and her kidneys were shutting down. She was told that nothing could be done for her. Rani was discharged from the hospital with little hope of living more than a week or two. Her family prepared for her imminent death.

As a last-ditch effort to help Rani, I attempted to administer several very strong medicines I had brought with me from my hospital back home in the U.S. for patients with serious, life-threatening conditions. One of these was *lanoxin*, a derivative of *digitalis*, used for congestive heart failure. Another was *lasix*, a strong *diuretic* (water pill) used to remove fluid from the lungs, feet, and abdomen. I also hoped the lasix might flush her kidneys and restore their function. In addition, I brought the latest, strongest *bronchodilator* and *corticosteroid* inhalers to open up her airways in an attempt to treat her asthma. But several days on these medications only saw her condition worsen. She was going downhill fast.

One morning, when I was doing my usual rounds, I saw an Indian gentleman sitting down and talking with Rani as I approached her home. The family told me he was Dr. Vinod, a renowned doctor who practiced *Ayurveda*, India's ancient folk medicine. Ayurveda uses primarily natural medicines to help restore health to the body. Rani's family had called Dr. Vinod to see whether there was anything he could do to help her.

Dr. Vinod did something that I had never seen before, and which went completely against my medical training. He stopped all her medicines, went out back behind Rani's home, plucked a leaf from a particular tree, and placed it on her abdomen. He restricted her diet to three glasses a day of pure goat's milk. Every day a fresh leaf was applied. This treatment seemed primitive to me, and I was extremely skeptical that anything good would come of it.

However, within several days, Rani began sitting up in bed under her own power and eating full meals. Her breathing slowly returned to normal, the swelling in her feet and abdomen were gone, and, within a week, she was walking around the grounds outside of her home. Within three weeks, her breathing became normal, and she regained almost all of her previous strength. If I hadn't seen her recovery with my own eyes, I wouldn't have believed it.

Rani's case was more than a lesson in humility for me, a U.S.-trained physician who supposedly possessed the latest, most up-to-date education and high-tech medicines.

More importantly, it showed me how instituting the right treatment, even a ridiculously simple one, and even in the face of an apparently hopeless situation, can work with the healing system to help restore the body's natural state of health and vigor.

Pierre's Story of Extraordinary Healing

Pierre was an adventurous Frenchman I met during my earlier travels in India. The son of a royal French family, he had rebelled and run away from his homeland. Pierre had hitchhiked through Greece, Turkey, Iraq, Iran, and Afghanistan before he reached India.

Eventually, he built a hut on the beach in Goa, along the central western coast of India, and settled into a carefree life of an expatriate, international beach bum. His daily activities consisted of fishing, taking siestas, learning about the Indian culture, and panhandling for food. But the fun was soon to end.

One day Pierre awoke with a sharp pain on the right side of his abdomen, just beneath his rib cage. It was difficult for him to breathe. He noticed his urine was dark brown, almost tea-colored, while his stools were light yellow colored. He had a fever, no appetite, and was extremely nauseous. Food and water would not stay down—he frequently threw up. Several days later, while he was looking in a mirror in a public restroom, Pierre saw that his skin and the whites of his eyes had turned yellow. He was jaundiced. That's when he knew he had hepatitis. Being sick in your own country is scary enough, but when you are in a poor, developing country, far from home and without money, it can be even scarier.

Pierre went from hospital to hospital, hoping for a cure. He was told that there was no cure for his form of hepatitis, and that nothing could be done. Because he had a hard time keeping fluids down, and an even harder time keeping food down, he grew weaker and weaker and lost a lot of weight. Out of desperation, he was directed to the hospital and yoga research institute where I was studying and conducting research, about 400 miles northwest of Goa. In this hospital, all-natural treatments from the world of yoga are prescribed and administered to patients with diseases for which modern medicine has not been able to find a cure.

Pierre was prescribed things that made absolutely no sense to me whatsoever. For example, he was prescribed regular breathing practices, known as *pranayama*, that were supposed to calm his nervous system and improve oxygenation of the blood. He was also prescribed *kriyas*, specific intestinal water cleanses that flushed his intestines and were supposed to cleanse and purify his liver. Pierre was also prescribed certain *asanas*, or yoga poses, along with other gentle abdominal exercises to help massage his internal organs and promote blood flow to the liver. He also was instructed to drink lots of water and juices, and he was fed *kichari*, a traditional yogic food made up of cooked, split mung beans (dal) and basmati rice. I was told kichari was gentle and soothing, easy to digest, an excellent source of protein, and that it contained numerous vitamins, minerals, and trace elements that help restore liver health. Other foods, such as papaya, along with natural medicines that helped nourish and strengthen the liver, were also prescribed.

Following treatment with these unconventional methods, Pierre regained his health and in several months completely cured his hepatitis. His case demonstrates that even in the absence of modern medicines, healing can occur when treatment is aimed at cooperating with your body's healing system. In yoga, all attempts at restoration of health are designed to work with your healing system, not against it. For this reason, yoga remains one of the most promising areas of investigation if you're interested in working with your healing system to achieve optimal health and well-being.

Ned's Story of Extraordinary Healing

Ned Peterson was a professor emeritus in psychology at the University of Hawaii. He was 59 years of age when he was first diagnosed with heart disease. Before his diagnosis, Ned had been suffering from vague chest pain for several months, but he dismissed these pains as only a muscle strain. When he finally visited his doctor, he was referred to a cardiologist, who ordered a stress test and an angiogram, a test that measures the blood flow in the arteries that feed the heart.

Ned's cardiologist told him that the stress test showed heart disease. Results of his angiogram were also not good. The main artery was 100 percent blocked and two others were 80 percent to 85 percent blocked. A *thallium test*, which measures blood flow to the heart muscle, confirmed severe blockages to important areas of the heart. Because of the locations of the blockages, Ned had only one option: immediate coronary-artery bypass surgery. He was told that if he didn't have this operation, he would be dead within several months.

Ned was reluctant to accept surgery as his only alternative. He was not fond of the idea of having his chest cracked open and his heart stopped while the surgeon stitched tiny veins to his coronary arteries, bypassing the blockages. The significant potential complications associated with open-heart surgery caused him to seek another solution.

Ned told his cardiologist thanks, but no thanks; he would try another way. His cardiologist told him he was a fool and would probably be dead within the year.

By luck, Ned stumbled upon the work of Dr. Dean Ornish, the first person in the world to prove reversal of heart disease without drugs or surgery. Ned read Dr. Ornish's best-selling book, *Dr. Dean Ornish's Program for Reversing Heart Disease*, and he began a low-fat, plant-based diet. He also embarked on an exercise regimen of walking and bike riding three to six days a week, and daily gentle yoga stretching, relaxation, and meditation. And he learned how to get in touch with his feelings and express them.

After Ned had followed Dr. Ornish's program for two weeks, his chest pain diminished significantly. After one month, it had vanished completely. In three months, he could bike 12 miles while barely breaking a sweat. In one year, he went to another doctor who ordered a new angiogram and thallium test. Ned's repeat angiogram showed the blockages had dissolved significantly. The 100 percent-blocked vessel was now only 40 percent blocked, and the 80 percent to 85 percent blockages were reduced to 20 percent to 25 percent. The repeat thallium test showed 300 percent improvement of blood flow to the heart muscles. Ned was completely out of the danger zone.

Ned felt like a new man, and with laboratory proof to confirm his reversal of heart disease, he went back to the first cardiologist who had told him he'd be dead within a year if he didn't undergo open-heart surgery. Ned showed the doctor his angiogram and his thallium test results. The cardiologist stared at them in disbelief. He asked Ned how he had done it, how he had reversed his heart disease. Ned told him about the work of Dr. Ornish.

Today, Ned runs volunteer groups for newly diagnosed heart patients, and he receives regular referrals from the same cardiologist who originally told him he was a fool not to undergo open-heart surgery. He has written a best-selling book about caring for the heart, and he is completely free from heart disease. Because he was able to understand what contributed to the blockages in his heart, and he took corrective action that addressed the underlying causes of his problem, his healing system was able to repair the damages and reverse his disease. Today, Ned enjoys radiant health because he has learned to listen to and cooperate with his healing system.

Norman Cousins' Story
of Extraordinary Healing

Norman Cousins was the first person to tell me about the body's healing system. His own case is one of the most dramatic and vivid examples of the healing system in action.

A remarkable writer and international peacemaker, Cousins traveled to Hiroshima each year for 40 years to help heal people's wounds caused by the dropping of the atomic bomb on Japan in World War II. For many years, he also helped negotiate the release of important political and religious prisoners throughout the world. One day, after serving as a mediator during the famous SALT treaty talks between President John F. Kennedy and Nikita Krushchev, Cousins returned home from the Soviet Union completely exhausted, physically, mentally, and emotionally. He was extremely upset that the talks had not gone well and that the Soviets were defiantly moving forward on the buildup of nuclear weapons. It was a very stressful time for Cousins. Several days later, a mysterious fever surfaced.

In addition to his fever and exhaustion, Cousins' spine began to stiffen and become extremely painful. After many tests, he was diagnosed as having an advanced case of *ankylosing spondylitis*, a severe form of spinal arthritis that causes a progressive stiffening and fusion of all of the vertebrae of the spine. Cardiac involvement and death were a distinct possibility.

Cousins' family doctor checked him into one of the country's finest hospitals, and summoned and consulted the best specialists of the day. The expert medical opinions were unanimous: Nothing could be done; his was a hopelessly terminal case. Cousins was given six months to live.

The doctors monitored his *sedimentation rate*, which was a specific blood test that marked the severity of this disease. Already high, the rate continued to rise each day. Every day, the blood-drawing team would stick a needle in his arm to biochemically confirm his progressive, deteriorating condition. In his rare lighter moments, because the blood-drawing team wasn't really helping him, Cousins jokingly referred to them as "the vampire squad." During this time, Cousins realized that, because he had only six months to live, he might as well enjoy his final days. In his state of despair and hopelessness, he accidentally stumbled onto the secret healing power of humor and laughter as antidotes to pain and misery.

Cousins was a friend to many celebrities, from U.S. presidents to Hollywood movie stars. One of these friends was Allen Funt, the producer of the hit TV comedy series *Candid Camera*. Funt supplied Cousins with films of the show's most memorable episodes. Cousins also watched other funny movies, including Marx brothers' films. As he lay in his hospital room, lost in the gaiety and laughter of the movies, he began to notice his pain lessening. Specifically, he discovered that for every 15 minutes of solid belly laughter, he could get two hours of pain-free sleep. At the same time, Linus Pauling, Nobel Laureate chemist and a close friend of Cousins, insisted that he take vitamin C every day.

As Cousins continued on this program, he slowly noticed his symptoms improving. The "vampire squad" also reported that his sedimentation rate started to drop, indicating that his internal biochemistry was changing for the good. Within several months, he could get out of bed and walk without a cane or crutches. Within a year, he was completely pain free, his sedimentation rate was back to normal, and he was declared "cured," not only by his doctor, but also by the top specialists of the day, who had previously declared his case hopeless.

After writing his best-selling book *Anatomy of an Illness*, which describes the details of his miraculous healing journey and triumph over ankylosing spondylitis, Cousins went on to spearhead pioneering research in a new field of medicine known as *psychoneuroimmunology*, which, as noted earlier, studies how the mind and nervous system can affect the immune system and influence the course of illness and health. Many AIDS and cancer patients have benefited from these studies. As with all the systems in the body, the immune system depends on the healing system to do its best work. A strong healing system is necessary for the immune system to function optimally—as it did in Norman Cousins' case. After 10 years of work in this field, Cousins' next best-selling book was appropriately titled *Head First: The Biology of Hope and the Healing Power of the Human Spirit.*

Arthur's Story of Extraordinary Healing

Dr. Bernie Siegel is a well-known cancer surgeon, internationally acclaimed speaker, and best-selling author of numerous books, including the immensely inspirational, timeless classic, *Love, Medicine, and Miracles.* One of the earlier cases that helped inspire him involved a man named Arthur. Arthur was a patient of Dr. Siegel's who had been diagnosed with an advanced cancer. His condition was described as terminal, and he was given six months to live. Dr. Siegel did not expect to see or hear from him again.

One day five years later, however, Dr. Siegel ran into Arthur in the local grocery store, and he was astonished. He thought he'd seen a ghost. He told Arthur that he was supposed to be dead—what was he doing still alive?

Arthur replied, "Dr. Siegel, you probably don't remember what you told me, but you said I had only six months to live, and that it was important for me to make it the best six months of my life." Arthur went on, "I took your advice. I quit my job, which I never really liked. I went on a cruise, which was something I had always wanted to do, and I began taking piano lessons, which was something else I'd always wanted to do. After six months, I felt so good, I decided I didn't have to die. I've not been sick in the past five years, and I have never felt better in my whole life."

Dr. Siegel stood there scratching his head and thought, "I wonder how many more of my patients who I sent home to die are still alive, like Arthur."

The next morning, he had his medical-office staff call the families of hundreds of his patients who were assumed dead. To his surprise, he discovered that about 20 percent of these terminal cases were still living and were completely healthy.

He thought again and wondered why they hadn't come back to see him. Then it hit him: If you were a patient, your doctor said you'd be dead in six months, and after six months you felt better than you ever had in your whole life, the last place you'd go is your doctor's office.

Dr. Siegel then personally called all of these patients and asked them if they'd be willing to attend weekly group meetings. Over the course of the next 12 years, these patients, who were all survivors of cancer, met as a group. Dr. Siegel called them Exceptional Cancer Patients, and they served as his teachers. Their stories, and the many things they did to activate their healing systems while overcoming terminal cases of cancer, are described in *Love, Medicine, and Miracles.*

The beauty of Dr. Siegel's work is that it has given hope to millions afflicted with terminal, life-threatening illnesses. In his words: "There are no such things as incurable illnesses, only incurable people." He backs up these words by pointing to the scientific literature, which contains case reports of people from all walks of life beating every so-called incurable illness known to man. It is Dr. Siegel's opinion that if one person can beat an incurable disease, by definition, the disease can no longer be called incurable. Dr. Siegel's Exceptional Cancer Patients provide strong evidence that our healing systems can be accessed and activated through a variety of means and ways, and that, once activated, they can overcome even the most severe of life's afflictions.

Louise Hay's Story of Extraordinary Healing

Louise Hay was a young woman who barely finished high school. At a young age, she developed cervical cancer, and she was told that if she didn't undergo immediate surgery and chemotherapy, she would die.

Louise was reluctant to have an operation and put strange chemicals with potentially toxic side effects into her body. Instead, she decided to pursue alternative methods of healing. She researched the impact of nutritious foods on her health, and she changed her diet. She also explored the mind-body connection and discovered how her thoughts, emotions, and attitudes could be powerful influences on her physical health.

During this journey of self-exploration, Louise discovered that she had been sexually abused, and that, as a consequence, she had harbored shame and resentment for the part of her body where the cancer eventually developed. After she had discovered certain inner truths about herself, she realized that it was quite logical that cancer would show up there.

Slowly, as Louise's diet, lifestyle, and attitudes improved, and she learned how to care more for herself in thought, word, and action, her cancer went away, never again to return. She has since gone on to enjoy radiant health, and she has become an extraordinary teacher and healer.

In her healing work, Louise discovered that, in many instances, how we treat our bodies is a reflection of how we treat ourselves. This interaction has a powerful influence on our healing systems, and on our health. For example, when we think kind and loving thoughts about our selves and our bodies, we tend to treat them with love and kindness. This encourages us to eat right, and to exercise, rest, and sleep well, among other things. These behaviors help strengthen and fortify our healing systems and ensure our good health. When we are angry at life and resentful of ourselves and others, we tend to participate in self-destructive activities that are harmful to our bodies. These behaviors make extra work for our healing system and can ultimately contribute to illness.

Louise went on to write several international best-selling classics. Her first, and perhaps most famous, is *You Can Heal Your Life*, based on her own self-healing journey. She also has produced many other wonderful books and tapes to help others who are interested in healing. She even started her own successful publishing company, Hay House, which has grown rapidly since its inception.

Steve's Story of Extraordinary Healing

Steve was a carpenter doing framing work on a custom home. One day, while he was climbing a ladder and carrying his electric saw, he slipped and fell. In the commotion, somehow he accidentally hit the switch that turned the saw on. The powerful saw cut a clean track through his arm, completely severing it. He looked down and saw that his hand and wrist were no longer attached to his body. Blood was everywhere. He screamed for help, and his coworkers came running.

They called the ambulance, and someone had the presence of mind to apply a tourniquet to Steve's arm to help stop the bleeding. Another person grabbed his severed wrist and hand and put it in a bag.

The paramedics arrived on the scene within 20 minutes, and they took Steve and his severed hand to the UCLA Medical Center. He was immediately rushed to the operating room, where two teams of surgeons and nurses were already waiting to work on him. One team worked on the hand, dissecting the blood vessels, bones, tendons, muscles, and nerves, while the other team worked on his arm, preparing the severed end for reattachment. They were going to try to connect Steve's hand to his arm. This was in 1975, when these kinds of operations were not so common.

I was employed at the UCLA Medical Center as an operating-room assistant at the time. My shift started at 7:00 AM and ended at 3:30 PM. When I came back the next morning at 7:00 AM, the operation was still going on, and it continued for several more hours.

After the operation, Steve's arm was put in an immobilizing splint. After two months, the splint was removed, and he began physical therapy, during which he learned exercises to help stretch and strengthen his arm and hand. Thanks to Steve's healing system, the healing process was well under way by the time he reached physical therapy.

Within six months, Steve was able to gain full use of his arm, including his wrist, hand, and fingers. Within one year, most of the sensation had returned to his fingertips. Additionally, even though Steve had lost an enormous amount of blood from the accident (he had almost gone into shock), surprisingly, he didn't need any blood transfusions after the operation. By drinking lots of fluids and eating iron-rich fruits and vegetables, he was able to assist his healing system in making more blood for his body.

Because of Steve's healing system, circulation to his hand and fingers was restored. His severed bones knitted back together and were stronger than ever. The severed muscles and tendons were rejoined, mended, and healed. His nerves regenerated and registered almost fully intact sensation. Within one year, Steve was back on the job, healthy and strong, and cutting wood with his favorite saw. This time, however, whenever he moved around with it, he made sure the safety switch was on.

Rose's Story of Extraordinary Healing

Rose was an elderly woman who had been suffering from a rash on her arms and legs for several months. She went to see my good friend Dr. Elpern, who specializes in dermatology. Dr. Elpern had tried various remedies, and he had Rose come back several times for checkups. Each time, there was no improvement in her skin condition.

Becoming a little frustrated, Dr. Elpern decided to stop her medications and probe deeper into the possible causes of Rose's rash. He asked if she had been facing any unusual difficulties at home or had been under any kind of stress. Rose told Dr. Elpern that her husband had recently become very sick and that she was worried about his health. She went on to tell him that her husband's doctors had not been successful at making her husband better. Dr. Elpern discovered that her rash had first appeared about the time of the onset of her husband's illness.

Dr. Elpern asked to see Rose's husband. She brought him to Dr. Elpern on her next visit. He questioned her husband thoroughly, examined him, made a presumptive diagnosis, and treated him accordingly. In a week's time, Rose's husband was feeling much better. Oddly enough, Rose's rash also began to improve.

On Rose's next visit with Dr. Elpern two weeks later, her rash was completely gone. Dr. Elpern hadn't done anything other than treat her husband for an unrelated condition. Dr. Elpern knew that stress can affect a person's healing system, and he was wise enough to treat the source of Rose's rash, which was her husband's health. Once he regained his health, she regained hers, as well.

Sam's Story of Extraordinary Healing

Sam was an obese Hawaiian man who led a sedentary life and ate typical modern-day foods such as canned meats and high-fat Hawaiian foods such as pork lau lau. In addition to his obesity, Sam also suffered from several other chronic diseases, including insulin-dependent diabetes, which was poorly controlled. Sam's doctor wanted to send him to Dr. Shintani, a progressive young doctor who had a strong background in nutrition and preventive medicine. Dr.

Shintani had just launched a new preventive nutritional program for Hawaiians known as the Hawaiian Diet.

After taking his medical history and conducting a physical exam, Dr. Shintani recommended that Sam go on the Hawaiian Diet, which was formulated from a combination of modern science and traditional Hawaiian wisdom. According to historical accounts, the original Hawaiian people (before the arrival of the European explorers and missionaries) were quite healthy, athletic, and lean. Many diseases common among Western cultures were nonexistent among Hawaiian peoples when Captain James Cook first discovered them in the 1600s. The original Hawaiians ate mainly simple, wholesome, healthy foods such as fruits; complex carbohydrates, such as sweet potatoes and taro; vegetables; whole grains; nuts; seeds; and fish. This diet was in stark contrast to such high-fat foods as fried chicken, roasted pig, and fast foods, popular among present-day Hawaiians such as Sam. According to Dr. Shintani's research, it is because of their modern, perverted diet and unnatural lifestyles that Hawaiians suffer from high rates of obesity, diabetes, heart disease, high blood pressure, and stroke.

When he first met Dr. Shintani, Sam was more than 150 pounds overweight and required 100 units of insulin each day to control his diabetes. After one and one-half years on the Hawaiian Diet, Sam had lost 150 pounds. His blood-sugar levels had dropped to normal, and he was able to completely get off his insulin. He maintains normal blood sugar levels to this day by staying on the Hawaiian Diet.

The areas of nutrition and preventive medicine are sadly lacking in the practice of conventional modern medicine, and they are virtually absent from the curriculum of most medical schools in the West. But these two related fields of study, which most physicians rarely discuss with their patients, provide some of the most practical and important strategies to summon the support of the body's healing system in the healing and prevention of even the most devastating modern-day illnesses. This emphasis has been the main thrust of pioneering physicians such as Dr. Shintani. Sam's story provides a clear example of how cooperating with your body's natural healing system by applying these ideas about nutrition and prevention can reverse a deadly disease such as diabetes and effect true and permanent healing.

Jim's Story of Extraordinary Healing

Jim was a plumber in his early fifties. He led an active life, except when he became incapacitated with flare-ups of his psoriasis, a condition he had been suffering with for 30 years. Jim's psoriasis would flare up at the most inconvenient times. It caused him to cancel important scheduled events, such as family outings or fishing trips with his buddies.

Psoriasis can occur in patches on the skin, the knees, the feet and ankles, the elbows, the scalp, behind the ears, or just about any other place you can imagine. Although it is considered a skin disease, in severe cases psoriasis can also involve the joints, becoming a debilitating form of arthritis. Modern medicine does not understand what causes psoriasis. Unable to cure it, doctors treat it mainly with suppressive medications, which give temporary relief, at best. This approach is often referred to as *palliation*, or the process of easing discomfort without curing. Corticosteroid and immune-suppressing creams are usually administered daily to reduce the severity of the symptoms. These treatments are applied more frequently during flare-ups. Strong pills are often prescribed for more severe cases.

Jim had a drawer full of creams and pills that he had collected over the years during his many visits to doctors. However, as much as he used his medications religiously, his flare-ups were becoming more frequent and more severe. Each time his psoriasis erupted, his old patches grew larger and more angry, staying inflamed for longer periods. Additionally, new patches of inflamed skin were surfacing in areas that were previously normal. His condition was worsening, and, in addition to being painful and irritating, there seemed to be no rhyme or reason to the flare-ups or why his disease was spreading. His psoriasis was starting to drive him crazy. It was then that he began to understand the phrase "the heartbreak of psoriasis."

By luck, Jim came across the work of Dr. John Pagano, a chiropractor who had worked with many psoriasis patients over the years, and who had written an award-winning book entitled *Healing Psoriasis: The Natural Alternative*. This book contains many case descriptions and full-color plates of psoriasis patients (before and after) who have successfully cured their psoriasis by following Dr. Pagano's recommendations.

Dr. Pagano's approach to healing psoriasis is based on a broader understanding of the human body, the reality of a healing system, how all the other systems are interconnected, and how once balance is restored among these systems, healing can occur. In particular, Dr. Pagano's approach takes into consideration the unique relationship between the skin and the intestines. His work focuses on the eliminative properties of the skin, and how digestive disturbances such as constipation can lead to a buildup of toxins in the skin that contribute to psoriasis. His research has demonstrated that once intestinal health and hygiene are restored through proper diet, psoriasis is greatly improved or even completely eliminated.

When Dr. Pagano met Jim, he questioned him at length about his diet, something that no other doctor had done before. He then told Jim he had to give up his coffee habit, which was initially quite difficult for him to do, and to incorporate more fruits, vegetables, water, and fiber into his diet. He also told him to give up sodas and other junk foods that he had become habituated to over the years.

At first, Jim didn't think that all these sacrifices were worth it, especially when his condition didn't seem to change for the first six weeks. He asked Dr. Pagano if he really thought that the changes in his diet could heal his psoriasis. Dr. Pagano reaffirmed that Jim needed to stick with the program, that soon he'd start to see improvement.

After three months, Jim began to notice a reduction in the severity and frequency of his flare-ups, even during times of stress, which usually made his psoriasis worse. His patches looked less red and were more itchy than painful. After six months, his patches started to fade and look more like the color of his normal surrounding skin. After one year, his patches had receded and could only be discovered by persistent and deliberate probing. After two years, not a lesion could be found, and his psoriasis was gone. Five years have passed, and Jim has not had a recurrence. The "heartbreak of psoriasis" is now a distant memory. Jim hasn't missed a fishing trip or family outing in five years, and, instead of a drawer full of creams and medications, he now has a drawer full of shorts, which he never used to wear because of the embarrassment of his psoriasis patches.

Once again, the healing system went into action when Jim took measures to strengthen it through diet; and his psoriasis, which had been a major problem for years, was cured.

Hal's Story of Extraordinary Healing

Hal, a former athlete and now a medical student, had suffered chronic eczema on both of his hands for six years. When his eczema flared up, Hal couldn't even hold a football because of the cracking and bleeding on his hands, and, in particular, on the thumb on his throwing arm. This condition was especially debilitating and humiliating because Hal had been a star quarterback on his college football team.

Hal's eczema began when he was working as an orderly in a busy medical-center emergency room. During this period, he routinely used industrial-strength germicidal soaps, which seemed to irritate his hands, to clean the doctor's labs. The gloves he was supposed to use to protect his hands ripped and tore, and were more of a hindrance than a help. So Hal just did his scrubbing and cleaning without them. Other factors, such as stress, could have contributed to Hal's eczema, as well. After six months, his hands became extremely itchy, and they started to crack and bleed.

Doctor after doctor saw Hal's hands and prescribed treatments, but there was no improvement. He took a truckload of various creams and pills, and he was eventually referred to an allergist, who did some skin tests on Hal. The skin tests indicated positive for more than 20 allergens. Based on these tests, Hal underwent a series of allergy injections, all to no avail. After several years, he gave up all hope that his condition would ever be healed.

Six years to the day after he began, Hal had just finished the academic and clinical work for his senior year in medical school. He had a few weeks off before beginning his internship, usually the most difficult year in a young doctor's training. He was awaiting the results of the national match program, to find out which hospital he would be assigned to for his postgraduate residency training.

Every day for four years, on his way to medical school in Philadelphia, Hal had passed a pottery studio that offered beginning classes in making pottery. He had remarked to himself that someday, when he had a little extra time, he would like to take one of those beginning classes. Now was his chance.

Hal walked into the pottery studio and signed up for a beginning class that lasted six weeks. He informed the teacher that his goal was to make a complete dinnerware setting for six, including plates, soup bowls, and coffee mugs, before the six-week class was finished. The teacher thought this was a bit too much, not realizing that she was dealing with a typical type A-personality medical student.

Hal came to class the first day and was given a lump of wet clay to mold and form between his hands. He was told how to care for the clay, how to add more moisture when it became too dry, how to dry it if it became too wet, and how to roll and knead it, just like bread dough. That first day, Hal thoroughly immersed his hands in the clay. He followed the teacher's instructions earnestly and sincerely.

After several classes, the students were introduced to the potter's wheel, on which pots are "thrown" or spun into shape by the skillful hands of the potter. Hal absolutely loved the potter's wheel, and he came in during his free time after class, working long hours with the clay. Even though he was only a beginner, Hal again reminded the teacher of his goal to create a complete dinner setting for six.

Six weeks later, at the end of the last class, Hal had completed his dinnerware set for six, which he removed with joy from the kiln and proudly displayed in front of the other students in the class. After he did this, he happened to glance down at his hands. They were no longer cracked or bleeding, and they had no signs of eczema.

Now, 20 years later, the eczema has never returned. We don't know exactly how Hal was cured. Perhaps doing something relaxing that he loved was enough to stimulate his healing system into action. Perhaps working with the clay itself had a healing effect on Hal's hands. Perhaps the cure involved a combination of the two; we'll never really know. What we do know for sure is that Hal's healing system was ready to do its work, and all it needed was the right catalyst for it to spring into action.

Sister Esther's Story of Extraordinary Healing

Sister Esther was senior nun at the Good Counsel Hill convent in Minnesota, the site of a groundbreaking 15-year study of Alzheimer's disease. The study was conducted by Dr. David Snowden, a researcher at the University of Minnesota, and it was important enough to appear on the cover of *Time* magazine. Sister Esther, who was 106 years of age, and many of her fellow nuns, who were in their eighties and nineties, showed no signs of Alzheimer's disease, despite significantly advanced ages. This fact was in sharp contrast to what conventional science would have predicted.

Dr. Snowden was particularly interested in Esther's life story, as well as those of her sister nuns who were free from Alzheimer's disease. Because Esther was fully functional and mentally sharp as a whip despite her advanced age, Dr. Snowden decided to look deeper and try to discover other causes than merely age or genetics that might explain the riddle of Alzheimer's disease, which annually affects about 4 million Americans.

Dr. Snowden's research revealed a completely different scenario for Alzheimer's disease than is currently theorized by most researchers. Because of the length and thoroughness of his study, Dr. Snowden's findings are not only credible, but they also offer tremendous hope and insights about how the healing system works and how we can stay healthy as we age. In Dr. Snowden's scientific opinion, Alzheimer's disease is strongly linked to lifestyle, environment, and social and emotional factors, all of which can affect the anatomy and physiology of the brain.

Likening the brain to a muscle, and applying the familiar axiom "Use it or lose it," Dr. Snowden found that the nuns who kept mentally stimulated and socially connected showed the fewest symptoms and were able to avoid the disease altogether. Age didn't seem to be a critical factor. The older nuns who continued to exercise their brains by thoughtful writing and speaking while remaining engaged in other meaningful work and activities continued free of the symptoms of Alzheimer's disease, while younger nuns who were socially withdrawn and not mentally stimulated developed symptoms of the disease.

Sister Esther enjoys working on various craft projects, and she rides a stationary exercise bike for 10 minutes every day. She stays actively involved with other nuns and with the affairs of her convent. In our attempts to understand how the mind affects the body, and vice versa, Sister Esther's example and Dr. Snowden's research remind us of how important it is to keep using our brains, remain socially connected with our friends and family, and find ways to keep ourselves stimulated and actively involved in life. A well-rounded, healthy lifestyle that involves mental challenges as well as strong emotional and social connections helps support our healing systems, which can keep us healthy, even when we reach ages approaching Sister Esther's.

Gerry's Story of Extraordinary Healing

Gerry was an elderly patient of a doctor whose practice I was covering while he was away. Gerry had a long-standing history of diabetes, and she had suffered from hip pain for many years, pain that caused her to walk with a cane. Her medical chart was thicker than a phone book, and every time she came in to complain about her hip pain, she was told it was from her diabetes, which is known to cause nerve problems that can result in pain in the legs and lower extremities.

One day while I was examining her, Gerry asked me if I thought a visit to a chiropractor might help her hip pain. Not wanting to discourage her, but not wanting to build up false hopes either, I told her it might be worth a try and probably wouldn't hurt her. Because her regular doctor was adamantly opposed to chiropractors, he never approved of her doing this. She had never seen a chiropractor before, and she was somewhat apprehensive. She seemed relieved that I wasn't so against them, and perhaps my reaction helped her get up the courage to visit one.

Two weeks later, on her next visit with me, Gerry walked into the exam room smiling. I saw that she didn't have her cane.

"Gerry, you forgot your cane. What's up with you? " I asked.

"Doctor, I don't need my cane anymore," she replied. She added, "Last night, I went dancing for the first time in 30 years! My hip pain is completely gone!"

She then burst into tears and thanked me for healing her hip pain. All I did was give her permission to go to the chiropractor, who, after one simple adjustment, was able to relieve 30 years of pain and misery.

Even though Gerry's is a rather straightforward case, I learned something important from her. Sometimes, an open mind, a new way of thinking, and a simple adjustment are all that are necessary to assist your healing system in restoring health to your body.

Merry's Story of Extraordinary Healing

Merry was a young nurse I worked with who used to be a dancer. As Merry began to attend to her patients and concentrate more on her professional career, however, her time for dancing became less and less. Trying to maintain an active lifestyle, instead of dancing she took to a program of regular exercise, including jogging. Soon, however, Merry began to notice pains in her hips. At first the pain occurred only when she tried to exercise. Then, she experienced pain when she was getting in and out of her car, walking up stairs, and performing other simple movements. Over a several-year period, the hip pain became worse and worse, and although she was not yet 30 years old, she began to exhibit a noticeable limp. Merry had to curtail all exercises other than slow walking, and even that caused her considerable discomfort.

Merry eventually could ignore the problem no longer, and she had to go to see several doctors. The doctors did X-rays and blood tests, and after extensive investigations made the diagnosis of severe, progressive osteoarthritis. They placed Merry on strong anti-inflammatory medications, including corticosteroids, but they told her that eventually she would need a double hip replacement.

Because I was working with Merry, I had only a professional relationship with her and was not familiar with her medical history. When I went for a walk with her one day after work, however, I noticed her limp. I asked her why she was limping. It was then that I found out about her diagnosis of osteoarthritis. She shared her pain with me, and told me that she was not looking forward to having her hips replaced at such a young age.

As an alternative to surgery, even though there weren't a lot of scientific studies to support my work, I had had some previous clinical successes with yoga and gentle physical therapy for my patients with various types of arthritis and joint deformities. By having an open mind, self-discipline, and a genuine will to improve, many of these patients were able to avoid surgery and improve the health of their joints.

I spoke of this work with Merry and suggested several specific yoga stretches and other gentle therapeutic activities that might help open up the joint spaces in her hips and reverse her arthritis. She was looking for a more permanent solution to her problem and wanted to avoid surgery, and so she was very open to this more conservative approach. She applied the stretching and other activities diligently and persistently.

Soon, however, my military duty and clinical training took me far away from Merry's world. It wasn't until nine years later that our paths crossed again, when we met at a medical conference. We walked as we talked, catching up on old times. It was then that I noticed that her limp was gone, which reminded me to ask her about the arthritis in her hips.

Merry told me that her hips were now disease free. She was dancing again, and it felt wonderful. She told me that she had followed my regimen faithfully during the first several months, and, after feeling great improvement, decided to stick with it. She has stuck with it to this day and continues to enjoy excellent health in both her hips. Merry's healing system was willing and able to go into action, but it needed her cooperation. By working with her healing system using natural, noninvasive techniques, Merry was able to reverse her arthritis and live her life to the fullest once again without resorting to the extreme solution of surgery, which also might not have been a long-term solution.

Clyde's Story of Extraordinary Healing

Clyde was a physics professor who had suffered from back pain for many years. One day, while he was lifting luggage from the trunk of his car, his back locked up on him and dropped him to his knees. The pain in his back was excruciating, and it shot down his right leg like a bolt of lightening. He couldn't move, not even with his wife's help. Luckily, she had their cell phone and called 911. The ambulance crew arrived shortly after.

In the emergency room, Clyde was given strong narcotic injections to relieve his pain, relax his muscles, and help break the intense muscle spasms. His spine was X-rayed, and the orthopedic surgeon was called in. Clyde was admitted to the hospital and underwent an MRI the next day. The MRI showed a severely herniated disc in the lower lumbar spine and a synovial cyst in the joint space between the adjacent vertebrae. Other specialists were called in, including the neurosurgeon, and it was determined that spine surgery to repair the disc and remove the cyst would be necessary.

Clyde, however, was not ready to undergo spine surgery, and he asked if there was any urgency to the surgery. Clyde was hesitating because one of his friends had had a poor outcome with a recent spine operation. His friend had ended up with an infection that almost killed him, and that had kept him hospitalized for than six months after his surgery. Clyde was told that if he wanted to go home and rest, the surgery could be scheduled within the next couple of weeks.

When Clyde went home, he decided to find out whether there were other options that didn't involve surgery to correct his spine problem. He researched on the Internet and found a book about a doctor's own journey through back pain and an ultimate cure that involved holistic methods, including nutrition, exercise, stretching, and stress-management techniques, such as relaxation, meditation, and guided imagery.

Clyde thought he would give this alternative approach a three-month trial, and if it didn't work, he would then consent to the surgery. He contacted the doctor who wrote the book, and the doctor concurred that this might be a wise approach.

After three months of diligently applying this doctor's program, Clyde's back pain and the pain down his leg were completely gone. His herniated disc had shrunk significantly, and there was no evidence of his synovial cyst.

More than 300,000 people undergo back surgery each year in the U.S. Many of these people will undergo a second operation. It is not uncommon to meet people who have had 20 or more operations, and many of these people end up with chronic pain.

Fortunately for Clyde, he is not one of these people. Nor is he ever likely to be. Because he learned to work with his healing system, Clyde was able to heal his back pain naturally and restore health to his spine through the regular practice of simple, effective methods that work with his healing system.

The people you have just met are only a handful of the thousands I've either known myself or heard about who have learned to cooperate with their healing systems to eliminate a variety of health problems. From serious, life-threatening illnesses such as cancer or heart disease to more benign conditions that, while not necessarily life-threatening, significantly compromise the quality of your life, your healing system can perform remarkable feats if you just learn how to work with it. You have the power to strengthen and fortify your healing system, just as Rani, Steve, Rose, and the other people in this section did, and, with extraordinary healing, overcome any health challenges you face.

PART TWO

Activating Your Healing System When You're Sick

Before You Begin

Now that you understand how your body's healing system works and how you can strengthen and fortify it, you can apply this knowledge to the treatment of specific health problems. Before you begin, however, there are seven key points to keep in mind while you are working with your healing system:

1. Remember that you are not a machine.

   Keep in mind that you are not a machine, but a complete human being with a body, mind, and spirit, and that all are interconnected. You need to take all three aspects into consideration if any physical disease is to be truly eradicated from your body. This is particularly true for chronic problems.

   When serious illness strikes, it is easy to become overwhelmed, not just physically, but mentally, emotionally, and spiritually, as well. You can become depressed and give up any hope that you will ever live a normal life again. At times like these, when you are in a weakened physical and emotional state, the task of getting better may seem daunting. Because your mind is connected to your body, when you are in this hopeless state of mind, it is difficult for your health to improve. As you recall, your mind is connected to your healing system and exerts a tremendous influence over your internal mechanisms of repair and recovery. To enlist the services of your mind while you are working with your healing system, refer to the strategies, methods, and techniques given specifically for this purpose in Chapter 6.

2. Focus on your healing system, not on your illness.

Be careful not to pay more attention to your disease and the external agents that may be causing it than to your own healing system and the steps you need to take to bring it up to speed. The most common strategic mistake most people make when illness strikes is that they invest more time, energy, and fear into what has invaded their bodies, or what is wrong with their bodies, than they do focusing on their natural internal healing resources. This emphasis sabotages the healing process. When your are sick, you can easily lose sight of your body's intrinsic state of health and instead erroneously succumb to the belief that the illness is more powerful. When you do this, you waste precious energy that could be used for healing.

Focus your attention on your healing system and not on your disease, pain, and discomfort. When you do this, your mind will join forces with your body to more effectively overcome your illness. This powerful healing partnership can maximize the flow of your healing energies, mobilize the forces of healing that exist within you, and produce a more rapid, effective, and thorough healing response.

If you are motivated to get better, you can even use your illness as an opportunity to learn more about the factors that contributed to your loss of health in the first place. Your illness can show you not only the way to remedy your current situation, but how to stay healthy and remain balanced in all areas of your life, so you can avoid getting sick again in the future. In this respect, illness can be a blessing in disguise, a valuable learning experience, and a time of transformation, renewal, and healing.

3. Practice prevention.

We all remember the saying "An ounce of prevention is worth a pound of cure." Anything, including your body, is easier to fix when problems first begin and damage is minor, than it is if you wait until the problem has escalated to the point at which extensive damage has occurred. More time, energy, and expense is required to repair the damage when you wait to address a problem than if you can prevent it from happening in the first place. Investing in your health by supporting your healing system when you are well, so that you can avoid illness, is more cost effective, in both time and money. Additionally, when you have the momentum of good health on your side, any illness or disease has far more difficulty invading your body.

If you can't prevent a health problem, at least intervene early to nip it in the bud. Institute corrective measures as soon as possible. Illnesses and diseases that are caught in their early stages are much more easily treated than those that have been allowed to progress, spread, and establish themselves in your body.

4. Pay attention to your body.

Remember to listen to your body whether you're sick or well because it can provide valuable information concerning your health. Although there are a few exceptions, do your best to avoid any activity or treatment that drains your energy, makes you irritable, interferes with sleep or other vital functions, increases your symptoms, or makes you feel worse. With a few exceptions, continue and pursue any activity or treatment that makes your mind and body feel stronger, clearer, lighter, more energetic, and more at ease. It is important to use common sense here, and to avoid artificial substances, such as anabolic steroids, opiates, stimulants, or other drugs that may provide temporary, short-term relief, but that in the long run often prove harmful. To help you access invaluable support for your healing during times of illness, review and regularly practice the exercise for listening to your body described in Chapter 4.

Remember that distinguishing between a symptom of disease and a healthy physiological response from your healing system is vitally important. For example, as discussed in Chapter 2, many symptoms of illness, such as coughing, sneezing, or fever, are commonly attributed to the actual disease process when, in fact, they more accurately reflect activation of your body's healing system. Recognize these symptoms for what they really are, learn to cooperate and work with them, and don't panic when they occur.

5. Use natural medicines and treatments responsibly.

Natural medicines and treatments, when used responsibly, can be highly effective. They are particularly effective when they are used early on in the course of an illness, or for an illness that is chronic. And even though many natural medicines and treatments are safe, it is important that someone knowledgeable administers them, their use doesn't cause you to delay conventional treatment that may be more effective, they don't interact with conventional medicine you may be currently taking, and they don't cause any untoward reaction in your body. Natural medicine or treatment is best administered by a trained health professional who also has worked and trained in conventional medicine and is open-minded enough to understand the practical contribution and benefits of a variety of treatments that can support your healing system.

6. Use conventional medicines and treatments when necessary.

There are times when it is appropriate, particularly in acute situations, to use conventional treatments such as modern pharmaceutical agents and surgical procedures, even those that may be extremely invasive. These treatments can often be life saving, particularly in emergencies. When you are in a car accident and have sustained critical injuries is not the time to eat brown rice, meditate, and do acupuncture. You need to go by ambulance with the help of trained paramedics to the finest hospital emergency room. There, skilled surgeons and critical-care nurses will give you the treatment you need. In addition, conventional diagnostic methods, such as laboratory and imaging techniques, can provide key detailed information about your illness and serve as invaluable aids in monitoring your healing progress. While the least invasive methods usually should be attempted first, conventional medicine used appropriately has much to offer for supporting your healing system and facilitating the healing process.

7. Understand your pain, and learn how to work with it.

Pain is one of the most potent messages your healing system sends to you. Pain gets your attention and is an urgent wake-up call from your healing system's communication center that something is out of balance and wrong with your body. Pain tells you that, if you don't take immediate action, things could get worse. (There are exceptions to this, such as the pain of childbirth.) Don't be frightened or intimidated by your pain; rather, try to understand it. Pain is a valuable message from your healing system and in the long run is intended for your benefit.

The purpose of pain is to help you direct your healing energies to a particular area of your body where the normal flow of energy has become blocked. Pain conveys a sense of urgency, and, if you don't respond, its intensity increases. When pain escalates but is ignored or suppressed, it evolves into numbness. When this lack of feeling or sensation sets in, it is accompanied by a loss of function. Numbness is an ominous sign: It is difficult to heal that which you cannot feel.

Always remember that where there is pain, there is life. Your pain tells you that your nerves and your body's tissues are alive and well and are trying to communicate with you. It is telling you to take corrective action to restore normal function to your body. Where there is pain, there is always the opportunity for healing. Pain is not negative or punitive, but rather a positive, instructive, helpful message from your body's healing system. Pain is a consummate teacher, and you should consider it your friend, not your enemy.

Pain is always temporary and needs to be understood, not ignored or suppressed. When you suppress pain through artificial means, you are turning a deaf ear to valuable information your body is trying to share with you. A smoke alarm is installed for your protection, and if you were to snip its wires because you didn't like the irritating sound it made every time it was activated, your house might burn down. Snipping the wires to your internal alarm system is what you do when you suppress your pain. Unfortunately, through the widespread use of pain-suppressing medications, people in our society are learning how to successfully ignore their bodies. Doing this is often very harmful because most conditions get worse when the underlying causes have not been addressed.

Sometimes, chronic pain doesn't have a physical cause but has its roots in deeper emotional pain. This emotional pain seeks bodily expression, which can come in the form of unbearable physical pain. This type of pain is often described as functional, which means that nothing structural can be found as the source, as opposed to organic, which means that there is a definite physical cause for the pain. You must address functional pain just as seriously as you do organic pain, and you must listen to these important messages from your body to activate your healing system and begin the healing process.

Learning to Work with Your Pain

Pain is a potent message from your healing system that something is out of order. Underlying causes always need to be addressed, but if no serious or life-threatening cause has been found, and your pain still persists, you can take the following steps to work with your pain, no matter how long it has been with you:

- *Listen to your body.* Regularly practice the "How to Listen to Your Body" exercise according to the instructions given in Chapter 4. If your pain is severe and longstanding, you initially might need to practice this exercise up to four times a day, for a minimum of 30 to 45 minutes for each session. Allow several months for improvement if your pain has lasted for six months to a year. Allow more time if your pain has been present longer.

  If you are taking strong pain suppressants, practicing this exercise and gaining full benefits may be difficult. To gain full benefits and for maximum healing, reduce or defer taking these medications while you are practicing the exercise of learning to listen to your body. As the pain eventually begins to lessen in intensity and your body heals, you will come to appreciate this discipline and see that it was well worth the effort.

- *Dialogue with your pain.* Through the guided-imagery and visualization techniques presented in Part One, you can learn to have a conversation with your pain and gain valuable insights about its specific purpose and function. You can gain much healing information in this way. Your healing system is intelligent and knows more about your illness than you do, and by practicing these techniques you can access information that may be completely unavailable through other means. This information can guide and direct your healing efforts and help you decide what other treatments may be of benefit. It is critical, however, that you make a commitment to implement into your life whatever insights you gain from these techniques. (For more information about these valuable techniques, consult the "Resources" section in the back of this book.)

- *Breathe with your pain.* In yoga, breath and energy are nearly equivalent. By working with your breathing, you can increase your energy and gain tremendous control over your pain. When you learn to slowly and gently lengthen your breathing, not only do you bring more oxygen and healing energy into your body, but you also help relax your nervous system, the master system in your body.

  Your nerves control all of your muscle tissues, which contain the largest number of pain receptors in your body. So when your nerves are calm and relaxed because of your breathing, your muscles relax. When your muscles relax, tension and pain automatically diminish throughout your entire body. Breathing is one of the most powerful modalities known to help diminish pain and strengthen your healing system. Breathing is simple, easy to practice, and always available to you. (For more information on breathing, please refer to the breathing exercises in the stress-management section in Chapter 6.)

- *Stretch with your pain.* Stretching lengthens muscles in your body, decompresses nerves, helps to restore vital movement of important structures and fluids, improves lymphatic circulation (which aids immune function), and creates space within which more blood flow and healing energy can enter problem areas of your body. Stretching, when done gently and correctly, and when combined with slow, gentle, deep breathing, is a powerful modality for eliminating pain. When you are stretching, keep these basic tips in mind:

1. Follow the guidelines for stretching described earlier, and remember not to stretch too far.

2. Remember to avoid any movement that increases your pain.

3. Remember never to force or strain while stretching. (For a guide to

specific stretches that may apply directly to your condition, an excellent book to start with is *Yoga for Dummies* by Drs. Larry Payne and Georg Feurstein. Other books are listed in the "Resources" section at the back of this book.)

■ *Grow from your pain.* Most machines, when they exceed their capacities and shut down, have reset buttons that you can push to resume their normal functioning. Pain serves a similar function for us. Because our own poor personal health habits, attitudes, and thoughts create much of our pain and disease, pain forces us to take a deeper look at ourselves, reevaluate our lives, and change. Without pain, we cannot grow. In the words of well-known cancer surgeon and author Dr. Bernie Siegel, "Pain is nature's reset button."

Pain, particularly of a chronic nature, often carries with it deeper messages than merely indicating that something is wrong in your body. Although pain can be a living hell, it can also be a great teacher and a blessing in disguise. Pain opens us up, broadens our horizons, enlarges our perspectives, expands our minds, makes us more tolerant, teaches us patience and endurance, and toughens our spirit and moral fiber. Pain teaches us compassion and understanding, and helps us to become better people. After you've been through pain and you've survived the sheer brutality of its force and power, you'll never take anything in life for granted again. As gold is purified by superheating, so too the hell fires of pain can purify your soul and make you a better, stronger, more caring person.

No matter how long it has lasted, pain is always temporary. Once you have learned its deeper lesson, the pain will be released from your body and you will be free from its tyranny.

There's No Such Thing as an Incurable Disease

Diseases that are difficult to treat have always been with us, and they are challenging for both doctors and patients alike. But because you have a powerful healing system, there is another way to understand what the word *incurable* really means.

A number of years ago, Dr. Bernie Siegel spoke the following words that forever changed the way I viewed the word *incurable*: "There are no such things as incurable diseases, only incurable people."

The reasoning behind this statement is that, if you search the medical literature, you will find individual cases of people who have beaten every single supposedly incurable disease in the world. In Dr. Siegel's opinion, if only one person has found a way to cure himself or herself of a supposedly incurable disease, then, by definition, the disease is no longer incurable.

Just as human flight was once considered impossible in the days before the Wright Brothers, and it is now a routine experience, the incurable diseases of today will most likely be declared curable tomorrow. In the fields of health and healing, in which sorrow and suffering are our greatest enemies, it is important to think optimistically, as the Wright Brothers did when they ventured into previously uncharted territory on only a wing and a prayer, with no prior studies documenting that human flight was possible!

New cures are being discovered every day. One by one, diseases we previously thought of as incurable are being contained and overcome. The more we understand how our bodies work, the more we can acknowledge the incredible service our healing systems perform. The more we know about our healing systems, the better we will be able to understand the factors that contribute to disease, and the more effectively we can demystify, defuse, and defeat these afflictions.

The list of illnesses for which we have proven cures and preventions has grown considerably, and it continues to grow. Leprosy, the historical scourge of all societies and once thought to be incurable, is now easily treated and quite rare. The deadly plague that wiped out millions in the Middle Ages is now extremely rare, and if someone contracts it, he or she can be cured in fewer than 10 days with modern antibiotics. Cholera can now be easily cured in less than 72 hours. Smallpox, once a deadly killer, has been eradicated. Scurvy and rickets are almost unheard of. Gangrene is rare. Ptomaine poisoning and botulism almost never occur. Tuberculosis is also disappearing rapidly on a global level. Syphilis, comparable to HIV and AIDS, is now easily treated with penicillin, entirely preventable, and quite rare. Heart disease, once thought to be incurable, has been shown by Dr. Dean Ornish and others to not only be reversible even in its severe forms, but completely preventable. The same is proving true for arthritis, diabetes, asthma, and other chronic conditions. Many forms of cancer are also being defeated, and the number of cancer survivors in the U.S. alone has reached more than 8 million. The more we are able to focus on preventive efforts and our healing systems, the sooner this condition also will become rare, as will many other afflictions that we currently fear.

When we go to a doctor and are told we have an inoperable brain tumor, terminal heart disease, multiple sclerosis, HIV, or some other horrible affliction, most of us have a tendency to go into a state of shock, followed by depression, because we assume that nothing can be done for us. Most of us have an unhealthy tendency to give all our power over to our fears, abandon all hope, and give up in the face of such a difficult challenge. But studies have shown that this response only accelerates our early demise.

Many people, however, have healed themselves of afflictions labeled as *terminal conditions* by their doctors. Even though doing so may not have been easy, most of these individuals reported a refusal to give up and an unwillingness to give in to a spirit of hopelessness. With this commitment and resolute attitude, a shift in their preconditioned beliefs and a subsequent improvement in the physiology of their body's internal environment occurred, which activated their healing system and reversed the tide of disease and debility. This process allowed the pendulum to swing back in the direction of a more positive state of health. A clear example of this is evident with HIV and AIDS. When HIV and AIDS first went public, there was mass fear and hysteria. People lost all hope, gave up, and succumbed quickly when a doctor rendered the diagnosis official. A positive HIV test was tantamount to a death sentence. Now, however, people with HIV are living 15 years, some longer, after the original diagnosis, and many of them are symptom free. Cases also are now being reported in which people who had HIV-positive blood tests are now being tested as HIV-negative. Those who take the time to tune into the wisdom and energy of their bodies, and learn to work with their healing systems, discover the body's ability to heal and recover its natural health, even from HIV and AIDS.

It is important to understand that these optimistic ideas are not based on theoretical conjecture. An increasing number of studies in the medical literature have demonstrated that positive attitudes and beliefs contribute in large measure to your health, and that, once mobilized, they can help activate internal healing forces and reverse serious, life-threatening situations. As I continue to repeat, your mind and body are connected, and hope and the "will to live" have been recognized to produce biological consequences that can improve your state of health, strengthen your defenses, and stimulate your body's intrinsic healing mechanisms.

In her courageous book *Who Said So? A Woman's Fascinating Journey of Self Discovery and Triumph over Multiple Sclerosis*, Rachelle Breslow documented her successful 12-year struggle and epic victory over multiple sclerosis, and she came to similar conclusions as Dr. Siegel regarding the label of "incurable disease." In Ms. Breslow's words, "I learned that there is no such thing as incurable, that when a doctor says something is incurable, he really (and more accurately) is saying that the medical community has not yet found a cure. Who can accurately predict anything? The facts are never in. Saying that a disease is incurable and saying that a cure has not been found are two entirely different statements."

When you are confronted with the challenge of a serious disease, don't focus on the dynamics of the disease process and give your power over to the fear that is generated and reinforced by the disease. Try to understand the circumstances that might have led to the affliction in the first place. Try to recall that, before the affliction, your natural state was health. Do all you can to cooperate with your healing system so it can do its job properly for you. Remember that, as long as you are alive, you have a healing system with the capability to restore your body to its natural state of health.

Obstacles to Healing
Factors That Interfere with Your Healing System

I frequently meet people who tell me that they have tried every conceivable form of treatment and method for healing, and they still are not getting better. Upon further questioning, I often find that these people have not given these methods sufficient time to work. For this reason, I strongly recommend that you give each healing method you select at least a six- to eight-week minimum trial period to notice improvement before you dismiss it as ineffective for you.

It is also important to remember that although external agents of healing can be important, your greatest resource for healing is the activation and stimulation of your body's own healing system. This is an internal job that requires commitment, courage, persistence, patience, and a willingness to acknowledge that, together with your body, you also have a powerful mind and a spirit. Solutions to difficult physical problems usually require that you utilize all aspects of who you are for healing.

If you are currently afflicted with a disease or illness, and you have been trying hard but still are not getting better, consider the physical, mental, emotional, and spiritual obstacles that could be keeping you from achieving your goal. Some of the physical obstacles to healing are

- An unhealthy, unwholesome physical environment, including poor air, poor water, irritating noise, overcrowded surroundings, and pollution, such as chemical pollution, microwave ovens, X-rays, and toxic waste
- A poor diet
- Not enough water in your diet
- Poor hygiene
- Not enough exercise and movement, including stretching
- A lack of space, privacy, or solitude
- Inadequate relaxation or rest
- Poor breathing
- Not enough contact with nature
- An absence of touching in a loving way (no hugging, physical intimacy, or warmth)

There are many potential mental obstacles to your healing, as well. Some of the more significant are

- Chronic mental tension, anxiety, fear, or worry
- Lack of focus

- No time spent in reflection, contemplation, or meditation
- Lack of gratitude for one's life and good fortune, whether big or small
- Poor mental attitude, including harboring a grudge ("chip on the shoulder"), being cynical, and having a pessimistic outlook
- Unresolved anger, hostility, or resentment
- No sense of humor
- Excess attachment to people or things
- Too much focus on goals and not enough focus on the process of getting there
- Worrying about the future, lamenting the past, or not being in the present

The potential emotional and spiritual obstacles to your healing are numerous. They include

- Self-punishment, self-blame, guilt, shame
- Self-destructive thoughts
- No love or joy in your life
- No sense of freedom in your life
- No support system, including family, friends, confidants, community
- No sense of purpose
- Lack of spirituality, universal wisdom, and prayer
- Lack of meaning and fulfillment in life
- A broken spirit

You can see that many elements in life can either contribute to your healing or interfere with your healing, in addition to the specific treatment you're undergoing. The first step in overcoming any obstacle is recognizing it. If you recognize any of these obstacles as ones that might be standing in your way, use this knowledge and the condition-specific guidelines that follow in this section of the book as an opportunity to activate your healing system and regain your natural state of health.

A Word About Hereditary Conditions, Familial Diseases, Genetic Disorders, and Congenital Problems

Many diseases and conditions appear over and over again in families and therefore are thought to be genetic in origin. However, there is a difference between *familial* and *genetic* conditions. Although defective genes and inherited disorders do exist, it is important not to lump all diseases that turn up again and again in families into these genetic categories.

Identifying genetic disorders can help prevent the possibility of their occurrence, but to over-generalize and label all serious diseases that run in families as genetic is dangerous. This label causes people unnecessary helplessness and hopelessness. Many diseases that run in families are not the result of genetic factors but rather are based on deep-seated, maladaptive behaviors, attitudes, and emotions, and on psychological coping mechanisms that express themselves in poor personal health habits and self-destructive tendencies. Family members and subsequent generations can avoid and overcome these conditions. Do not feel bound to inherit your parents' or families' disease-oriented, maladaptive legacies; rather, realize the full potential of your body's natural state of health and the incredible healing system that you have to help you.

Congenital conditions, such as cerebral palsy, often can be traced back to unfortunate events or trauma sustained at birth or while a child was still in the womb. And even though the management of these difficult conditions can often be trying, many such problems can be prevented with proper prenatal education, care, and preparation for childbirth.

Getting Started

A Daily Program for
Enhancing Your Healing System

It is said that a journey of a thousand miles begins with one step. Even though the first step and each subsequent step along the way may seem small and insignificant, when they are added together, they eventually take you to your final destination. In the same way, the following daily program to strengthen and fortify your healing system provides a starting point on your journey toward improved health. At first, the activities that make up this program may seem quite ordinary and not very significant or life-changing. When combined and continued over time, however, they can make a huge difference in your health. In short, they can create extraordinary healing. After just 10 days of following this program, you will notice a marked improvement in your health, and you should experience a much greater sense of well-being.

A word before you start: Because your healing system is vast and complex, you should not consider this program all-inclusive. As you apply the activities in this program to the rhythms of your own life, you will want to use the methods, techniques, and information described in earlier chapters to suit your own particular health needs. Be flexible and practical when you use this program. You need to arrange the order of daily activities, and the types of activities, to fit into your daily schedule. For example, with breathing, relaxation, guided imagery, meditation, or prayer, you might be starting out with 5 to15 minutes a day that you can do in the morning before work. But you can gradually build up to at least 30 minutes, once or twice a day; when you do that, you might then have to do these activities in the evening. If you are suffering from a serious illness, it will be most beneficial for you to do these activities whenever you have the time to do them for at least 30 minutes.

In terms of the dietary suggestions, experience has shown me that each person has his or her own specific nutritional needs. For this reason, I don't advocate only one type of diet for all people. I honor the ancient axiom, "One man's meat is another man's poison." Although I do make some general dietary suggestions, do not adhere to them so strictly that you ignore common sense. For instance, if you have a fever, you need to drink lots of fluids and abstain from eating solid foods until the fever passes. If you suffer from a specific digestive disorder, follow the dietary guidelines in the sections in the earlier chapters that describe in more detail what and how you should be eating. When it comes to diet and nutrition, listen to the voice of your body's inner intelligence; that voice is closely connected to your healing system.

If you have a question about any activity in the daily program, refer to the earlier chapters in the book. They describe in more detail how each activity benefits your healing system.

Strengthening and Fortifying
Your Healing System in 10 Days

In the Morning

Personal Hygiene for Your Healing System

Personal hygiene consists of the daily cleansing that strengthens and fortifies your healing system. Over a lifetime, your personal hygiene accumulates to wield a powerful influence on your health. In addition to brushing your teeth and other related activities, take a bath or shower each morning. Bathing supports your healing system by cleansing and protecting your body; keeping your skin healthy and free from dirt, germs, and other potentially harmful microorganisms; and aiding in the elimination of toxins.

Elimination (Moving Your Bowels) for Your Healing System

In addition to urinating, it is important to move your bowels each morning. Doing this prevents unwanted waste and toxins from building up and helps keep your internal environment clean and healthy. Regular daily bowel movements reduce the burden on your healing system and make it easier for it to perform its duties of repair, reconstruction, and regeneration more efficiently for you. Here are a few tips to aid the process of elimination:

- Drink a cup of warm liquid (water, tea, decaffeinated coffee) to help move your bowels. You may need to drink several cups until you get a result. Warm beverages are better than cold because heat relaxes the smooth muscles in your intestines, enabling them to expand and dilate. As the warm fluids help flush the fecal material through the more relaxed and expanded bowels, unwanted waste products can be eliminated faster and more easily. Cold liquids, in contrast, constrict the muscles in the intestines, which narrows the opening of the bowels, and so they are usually not as effective in aiding the processes of elimination.

- If you are frequently constipated or suffer from irregularity, and you need more than several cups of warm liquids each morning to move your bowels, stir one or two heaping teaspoons of psyllium seed husks, or any other gentle natural fiber supplement, into a glass of warm water and drink it each night before you retire.

- If you want to prevent constipation, eat a healthy diet with lots of fluids and fiber, which you can find in fruits, vegetables, and whole grains and legumes. Soups at lunch or in the evening, along with herbal teas, are also ideal for this purpose.

- Although it is sometimes unpopular, okra, eaten either at lunch or dinner, is one of the best vegetables to help ensure healthy elimination in the morning. Lightly steamed or cooked, okra is one of the gentlest and most effective of all natural food fibers in the world.

Gentle Stretching for Your Healing System

Stretching helps to loosen up and tone your muscles and joints, and to improve circulation. By increasing flexibility in your joints and limbs, stretching can also improve lymphatic drainage in your body and stimulate your glands. When your muscles are lengthened and their flexibility is increased, space for the passage of nerves increases. Gentle, regular, systematic stretching often relieves pinched nerves. Stretching can keep your body lithe, young, and free from disease, and it is one of the best methods I know for strengthening and fortifying your healing system.

- Stretch for 5 to15 minutes each morning, following the guidelines provided in the section on stretching in this book. You may also find it beneficial to stretch in the evenings. Stretch on an empty or light stomach, not right after eating.

- You can start stretching with the help of a yoga book or video for beginners, or you may want to sign up for a beginner's yoga class. If you've never done yoga before, or you have specific health issues, make sure you tell the instructor so he or she can accommodate your needs. (If you have back problems or are stiff, try my comprehensive yet gentle stretching routine called the Back to Life Stretching Program, which you will find in my previous book, *Healing Back Pain Naturally.*)

Breathing, Relaxation, Guided Imagery, Meditation, Quiet Reflection, or Prayer

All of these activities help to relax your body, calm your mind and nervous system, relieve stress, and strengthen and fortify your healing system. They can also help you discover a higher power that organizes and directs the flow of energy in the universe and in your body. Attuning your awareness to this force can be extremely empowering for your healing system. A great time to do these activities is right after stretching, when your body and mind are already in a naturally relaxed condition.

- Take 5 to15 minutes each day to sit in a quiet place, relax your shoulders and entire body, and close your eyes. Begin by watching your breath flow in and out of your nose. You can practice one or more of the breathing techniques described in the section on breathing. These techniques will help to calm and focus your mind and nervous system, bringing them into harmony with your healing system.

■ Once you feel calm and relaxed, try one of the guided imagery/visualization techniques described in this book. Allow your awareness to go into the interior of your body. As you focus your mental energies on your body's internal structures, imagine your healing system springing into action to help repair any damaged tissues as it restores your health and vitality.

Exercise for Your Healing System

Exercise helps your healing system by toning the heart, strengthening circulation, and improving mental health. Morning exercise is a great way to start the day. If you are not already doing so, try to find a way to fit morning exercise into your schedule.

■ Each day, do 15 minutes of simple walking, swimming, bicycling, jogging, aerobics, calisthenics, or any other exercise. If you feel like doing more, or are used to doing more, do so. However, if you are new to exercise, or you haven't exercised lately, it is better to start out gradually. Do not to force or strain when you exercise. Observe your breathing to see whether you are overdoing it. When you exercise, you should be comfortable with your breathing. Remember, slow and steady wins the race. For maximum benefit to your healing system, gradually build up to 30 to 60 minutes a day, three to six days a week.

Breakfast for Your Healing System

Eat a light, healthy breakfast each day. If your job requires a lot of physical activity and greater caloric intake, use your common sense and eat more. If you have a sedentary job, such as a computer operator or office worker, eat a lighter breakfast. If you are overweight or normally eat a larger lunch, you may want to skip breakfast and just drink water or juices. Here are other suggestions for breakfast:

- If you are on a carbohydrate or starch-restricted diet, eat lean protein and vegetables, and drink warm fluids such as herbal teas, decaffeinated beverages, and soups.

- If you are not a diabetic or not on a carbohydrate-restricted diet, eat fresh fruits, whole grains, and organic cereals, which can help reduce sugar cravings later in the day. These foods also provide key caloric energy and contain a host of vitamins, minerals, and trace elements, as well as essential fiber and fluids to aid your healing system. If you're allowed to have natural sugars in your diet, try dried fruits, including raisins, figs, dates, and apricots, and organic, naturally sweetened jams and jellies in limited quantities. These foods can be nourishing and healthful.

- You can also add small quantities of nut butters, such as peanut, cashew, almond, or sesame tahini, or other protein sources for breakfast.

- You can also eat dairy products, such as yogurt and low-fat cottage cheese, in limited quantities if you are not lactose intolerant or do not have other dietary restrictions.

- If you are diabetic, eat more protein and whole grains for breakfast, and avoid sweets of all kinds. Breakfast proteins and grains could include a whole-wheat bagel, or rice crackers with cottage cheese. You can also eat other proteins, such as nut butters. These foods will provide long-lasting fuel throughout the day without drastic increases in blood sugar. Natural sweeteners, such as *stevia,* also are available that can satisfy your sweet cravings while not increasing your blood-sugar levels.

- Avoid sweet, starchy, oily breakfast items such as donuts or pastries.

- Taking a natural supplement or daily vitamins may be appropriate, especially if you're not getting all the nutrients you need from your regular diet. (Review the section on vitamins and natural supplements earlier in this book for more information.)

Remainder of Morning and Afternoon

If your work takes you away from home, you can still find simple, easy ways to strengthen and fortify your healing system, even though your schedule may be hectic. Even if you stay at home, try to incorporate the following activities into your morning routine.

Breathing, Relaxation, Guided Imagery, Meditation, Quiet Reflection, or Prayer

Throughout the day, because of your mind's influence on your healing system, which operates best in a calm, quiet, and relaxed internal environment, it is important to keep your mind calm, cool, and collected. Breathing, relaxation, guided imagery, meditation, quiet reflection, and prayer are ideal methods for helping to keep your mind tranquil. The more you practice these methods, the easier it will be for you to retain your composure and keep your healing system strong and vibrant.

- Take short, 30-second to one-minute breaks at least once an hour to calm your mind by practicing one or more of the methods for breathing, relaxation, guided imagery, meditation, quiet reflection, or prayer that are described in this book. In the beginning, you may need to experiment with several of these options to find out what works best for you. After you have found one that works for you, learn one or more of the other techniques, as well. I usually recommend giving each technique at least a one-week trial, until you are comfortable with it and have noted its positive benefits.

- During stressful times, or when you feel yourself becoming upset or losing your composure (especially in the presence of another person), momentarily excuse yourself and retreat to a safe, peaceful place. Once you are out of harm's way, practice one or more of these peaceful, calming techniques. After you have calmed down, you will be in a much better position to deal with your situation.

    One of the tricks to this strategy is learning how to recognize when you are first beginning to lose your composure. When you lose your composure, in addition to your mental agitation, you will most likely experience one or more of the following symptoms:

    - Rapid, fearful, or angry thoughts

- Shallow, rapid breathing
- Rapid heartbeat
- Increased perspiration
- Queasy stomach ("butterflies in your stomach")
- Weak knees

From your earlier reading, you might recognize these symptoms as part of the fight-or-flight response, which, if allowed to continue or escalate, can interfere with your healing system and cause harm to your body, especially if they are sustained over a long period of time.

In my work as a doctor, these strategies are particularly helpful. For example, I sometimes meet new patients who have a lot of anger and are quite upset at "the medical system" in general and doctors in particular. They may be upset for other reasons, too, of which I may not be aware. In these situations, I am a prime target for their anger. Sometimes, the slightest thing I say can trigger a huge explosion of angry emotions. Naturally, this reaction from a patient will cause a wave of fear and anger to well up inside of me, too. In this state, I could easily retaliate with fear and anger of my own, but I try to stay composed. When I notice my heart rate speeding up, my breathing getting shallower and rapid, and my mind becoming agitated, I excuse myself and quickly retreat to the safety of another room. There, I close my eyes and do one or more of the following: breathing, meditation, relaxation, imagery, or prayer. I do this until I feel my breathing and heart rate slow down, and I am able to regain my composure. Usually, a maximum of five minutes is all that I need. Afterward, when I go back to see the patient who has provoked me, I am more relaxed and comfortable, and better able to help the patient.

Water for Your Healing System

Your body is 70 percent water, and because water constantly circulates throughout every cell, tissue, and organ in your body, the more water you introduce into your system, the faster it can distribute nutrients and eliminate toxins. Drinking water and fluids is one of the best ways to strengthen and fortify your healing system.

- Throughout the day, sip water or other fluids, such as juices or herbal teas.

- Drink six to eight glasses of water, or the equivalent, over the course of each day.

A Mid-Morning Snack for Your Healing System

You might need a light, mid-morning snack if your work requires you to take a late lunch, or if you have a fast metabolism and are prone to blood-sugar swings. It is important to listen to your body when it comes to getting the nutrition you need to function at your best. Here's some advice about mid morning snacks:

- Don't eat if you're not hungry.

- You can eat fresh fruits, carrots, wholesome crackers, or an herbal tea or other beverage if you feel you need to eat something before lunch.

Lunch for Your Healing System

For most people, eating a healthful, wholesome lunch is important. In many cultures around the world, lunch is the main meal of the day. To ensure a steady flow of nutrients and optimum fuel for your healing system, take the time out of your busy schedule each day to eat lunch. Skipping lunch is generally not recommended. And just as proper food is essential fuel for your healing system, eating that food in a way that optimizes its digestion is equally important. The following suggestions should be helpful:

- Avoid fats and oils, as well as processed snack foods, which are heavy and often difficult to digest.

- Try a cup or bowl of soup.

- Try a hearty salad, but avoid rich, oily dressings or toppings.

- If you eat carbohydrates, a healthful sandwich with fresh lettuce, tomatoes, sprouts, cheese, tofu, tempeh, or any other lean protein can often be a complete meal in itself. Eat breads made from whole grains, such as wheat, barley, rye, and oats.

- If you are not diabetic or on a sugar-restricted diet, a fruit dessert will provide an adequate balance of essential nutrients, including vitamins, minerals, trace elements, fluids, and fiber.

■ You can take water or another liquid with or immediately following your meal.

Here are a few more tips for eating lunch:

■ If you are at the workplace or at home, take a break and focus solely on eating and digesting your food. Turn off your computer, TV, or radio, and make sure you aren't talking on the phone or reading a magazine or newspaper when you eat.

■ When you are eating, your body needs to concentrate on the process of digestion. It should be a time of rest and relaxation, and you should devote all your attention to the process of eating. If you continue to talk on the phone, drive, or work on the computer while you are eating, you won't be able to feel your body's response to the food you are consuming. When your mind is in more than one place at a time, it is hard to fully taste your food. It also is easy to overeat and experience indigestion under these circumstances.

■ If you eat with coworkers, family, or friends, lunch can be a pleasant social occasion. Avoid arguments, conflicts, or talk of business or finances. The mood and atmosphere should be pleasant and uplifting. Your emotional state at the time of your eating affects your digestion.

Consider an Afternoon Nap for Your Healing System

Studies show that most Americans are sleep deprived. Sleep deprivation has been linked to numerous chronic diseases, including heart disease. It has also been linked to accident-prone behaviors. Your healing system performs most efficiently when you are sleeping or resting, and an afternoon nap can be an effective way to help strengthen and fortify it. Most cultures around the world eat their largest meal at lunch time, followed by a nap, or siesta. This is a time-tested method to help optimize digestion. If you can, take a light nap after lunch.

In the Afternoon

Play, Fun, and Hobbies for Your Healing System

Not enough can be said about the health-promoting effects of a playful attitude, a sense of humor, and the ability to have fun. Bob Hope and George Burns, both famous comedians, each lived for 100 years by cultivating light-hearted attitudes. They pursued lives of fun and laughter while they tried to make others laugh. And as we discussed earlier, well-known doctor and author Norman Cousins cured himself of a painful, life-threatening disease with laughter and a little vitamin C. Humor and a light-hearted attitude can add years to your life, and they are powerful stimulants for your healing system.

Keeping your spirits light throughout the day is important. If you are working long, hard hours or are having an extremely difficult time in your life, you don't have to be serious all the time. Seriousness creates tension, which can drain vital energies away from your healing system and lead not only to disease, but also to pain. Keeping your spirits light will have a powerful strengthening and fortifying effect on your healing system. Here are a few tips for keeping your spirits high:

- Do at least one fun activity each day, for at least 30 minutes, preferably longer. Here are some suggestions:

  - Find something funny to laugh at. Share a joke with your family or coworkers.

- Watch a comedy movie, or engross yourself in a favorite personal hobby, such as painting, sewing, quilting, jewelry, or model-airplane building.

  - Play or listen to uplifting music.

  - Dance to your favorite music.

  - Play with children.

  - Go to a musical production, a movie, a play, or a sporting event.

  - Participate in your favorite sport.

  - Read a favorite book.

  - Write in a journal.

Social Activities for Your Healing System

Man is a social creature, and for this reason, it is important to stay connected to other people. Conversely, social isolation creates stress, which can lead to disease, both mental and physical. For example, heart disease, the number-one killer in the Western world, has been linked to feelings of social isolation. Studies have shown that heart patients who live alone fare much worse than heart patients who have connections with family, friends, or pets. To further illustrate this point, consider that, even among hardened criminals, solitary confinement, which is nothing more than social isolation, is one of the most dreaded of all forms of punishment.

Social support is important to help strengthen and fortify your healing system. Plan to spend time each day in an activity that supports your feelings of being connected to others. Try one or more of the following:

- Make a special effort to call or write a close, trusted friend or family member.

- Tell a loved one or a family member that you love them, even if doing so at first feels awkward or phony. The more you do it, the more real it will feel, and you will soon become comfortable saying it. What you give comes back to you, so you are really only telling yourself that you love yourself. The same principle applies to any other loving act of kindness.

- Give hugs to your family members, friends, and coworkers. Don't do it for their benefit, even though they will like it, but for yours. Nothing heals like love, and nothing stimulates your healing system more powerfully than love. Love starts with you.

- If you have the time, you can volunteer at least once a week at a senior citizens' center, hospital, library, school, local day-care center, or one of hundreds of other charitable and community organizations. You could also lend your special talents and energies to any of a number of state, national, and international organizations. Make a commitment to take the time to get involved in one or more of these types of activities. Your healing system will benefit from these activities, so do them first for yourself, knowing also that others will later benefit from your generosity.

Rest and Alone Time for Your Healing System

In sharp contrast to what I recommend for social connectedness, I also feel it is important to learn how to socially withdraw, to rest and be alone. Many people spend practically every waking moment taking care of others, or they are involved in too many activities that leave them emotionally, mentally, and physically drained. This pattern can result in chronic fatigue, "burnout," and even serious illness. If you are one of these people, it is imperative to learn how to say "No" to others and carve out a chunk of daily time for yourself. To rejuvenate your health, recharge your batteries, and strengthen and fortify your healing system, doing this is a basic necessity of life. Here are a few tips:

- Each day, take 10 to 15 minutes to be alone, shutting yourself off from the world and the constant onslaught of others. Make arrangements to have trusted family or friends perform your duties and take on your responsibilities during this period. Find a safe, quiet, uplifting place, either outdoors in nature, or in a room in your house or apartment.

- You may wish to use this time to meditate, breathe, pray, paint, listen to music, or do absolutely nothing.

- Honoring your special time alone, which your healing system requires to maintain its strength and vigor, is important. If you don't insist on the right to be alone to rest and rejuvenate, your healing system will have difficulty functioning optimally.

In the Evening

Dinner for Your Healing System

Try not to eat too heavy, or too late. Eating heavy or late will cause indigestion and disturb sleep, causing you to wake up tired and low on energy in the morning. In addition, eat peacefully, without the TV or stereo blaring, and without discussing business or other potentially stressful topics. Keep the family dinnertime conversations light and harmonious, which will improve digestion while it strengthens and fortifies your healing system.

Here are a few suggestions for dinnertime meals:

- Try a vegetable soup, such as squash, split pea, or carrot, which can be hearty, nourishing, and soothing.

- Try a dinner salad, with leafy greens such as lettuce, spinach, and one or more vegetables, including tomatoes, cucumbers, olives, mushrooms, artichoke hearts, or garbanzo beans (chick-peas).

- You can eat cooked whole grains, such as fluffy brown rice or barley, or organic pasta, separately or mixed together with a vegetable or protein side dish.

- A vegetable casserole or mixed-vegetable stir fry can be tasty and nourishing. You can add tofu, a touch of light cheese, or another lean protein. Minimize the use of heavy oils and butter when you cook these dishes.

- You may also have a light dessert such as yogurt, sherbet, or fresh fruit. (If you are diabetic, you can have a light dessert with a sugar substitute.)

- Drink water either before or after dessert.

Emotional Well-Being for Your Healing System

As we discussed earlier, emotions are powerful sensations of energy felt in the body. For healthy living, most emotions need to be released and expressed in your life. If they are suppressed and allowed to remain in your body longer than is necessary, or dragged around as energy-draining emotional baggage, emotions can severely hinder the work of your healing system and can contribute to illness. To know how you are feeling at any given moment, and then have the courage to share these feelings with others, is one of the most powerful ways to strengthen and fortify your healing system. Here are some suggestions for expressing your emotions in a beneficial way:

- To learn to express your emotions in a healthy way, it is often helpful to join a group and learn to participate in group activities. Join a group that meets at least once a week, or, if you have the time, more often. The group could be a support group or a therapeutic group. It should be a group that you feel comfortable and safe with, a group that you feel will not sit in judgment of you should you choose to air your "dirty laundry" in public. Many non-alcoholics join AA (Alcoholics Anonymous), which has groups in nearly every major U.S. city, just for the sake of being in a group and learning to share their feelings. Take the time to find out about groups in your area, and make a commitment to participate in one.

- If you are not comfortable in a group, or you cannot find one in your area, professional counseling is available and might be offered through your house of worship, local YMCA or YWCA, or other community organizations. One-on-one counseling, especially with an effective counselor, is also a valuable way to express your feelings. Find out about counselors in your area, and make a determined effort to participate in this activity.

- Get a small notebook and pen, and start writing about your feelings. Writing in a journal, expressing all that is inside of you and all that you are feeling, can often be an effective way to release your emotions, your thoughts, and deepest feelings, even if you write for only 5 to 10 minutes each day.

- Each day, in a conversation with your family, friends, or loved ones, speak from your heart and share your deepest feelings. If you are not comfortable doing this, write a letter to someone with whom you wish to share your deepest feelings.

Spiritual Well-Being for Your Healing System

Your healing system functions best when you are spiritually healthy. Many physical diseases have their origins in the spiritual realm. For example, when your spirits are continually down, you can become depressed, which is a form of mental disease. As noted earlier, depression has been shown to contribute to heart disease, diabetes, cancer, and many other serious ailments.

If you are an atheist, you can still enjoy spiritual health and well-being. Try to connect to a higher cause, purpose, or force other than yourself. Ponder the fact that some intelligent, powerful, creative energy has put you on this planet. Doing this will take a huge burden of stress off your shoulders and allow your healing system to work more effectively. Thinking that everything in the world and your life depends solely on your constant mental vigilance and surveillance creates tension and stress, drains vital energies, and can be emotionally and physically exhausting. These factors conspire against your healing system and can eventually lead to physical illness.

If you believe in God or a higher power, your plight is not much different from that of the atheist. Doubts about God and the Divine still might bombard you when you encounter rough waters or come up against a brick wall, and so it is necessary to continually renew your faith many times throughout each day, and ponder the meaning and purpose of your existence.

- This week, take a brief respite from your work and hectic schedule, and think about your life and its significance. Think about a higher power, a divine, creative, intelligent energy at work in the universe and your life. Do this for at least 5 to 10 minutes each day.

- If you are comfortable doing so, pray for 5 to 10 minutes each day.

- Before going to bed, take 5 to 10 minutes each night to read scriptures or other related books that can uplift your spirits.

Sleep for Your Healing System

Sleep is fundamental to all living things and is an intrinsic part of the natural rhythms and cycles of life. Sleep is a required physiological activity in all living species, a basic biological principle of life. Some animals hibernate and go into a cave to sleep for months at a time to restore their bodies' health and energies; humans generally require between 8 and10 hours of sleep each day.

Your body requires regular sleep to restore vital energies and to heal. As you may recall, your healing system does its best work when your body is resting. Regular, restful sleep is one the most potent things you can do to strengthen and fortify your healing system. When sleep is disrupted, healing system function is compromised, and ill health can develop. It is not surprising that as sleep deprivation and insomnia increase in epidemic proportions in America, the number of chronic, stress-related diseases, including heart disease, high blood pressure, cancer, and autoimmune disorders, is also increasing.

To ensure proper sleep, try the following:

- Get up early each morning.

   Sleeping late disturbs the natural rhythms of your body and will cause you to go to bed late. This pattern will perpetuate an unnatural cycle that can be harmful to your healing system.

   Getting up early improves your chances of having an active, full day. Having a long, full day will improve your chances of going to sleep at night at a decent hour. A restful, good night's sleep will allow you to awaken early each day feeling refreshed and renewed, with abundant energy.

- Don't engage in agitating or disturbing activities before you go to sleep. (Such activities include watching the news or violent movies.)
- Avoid late-night arguments or conflicts with your partner or family members.
- Make sure your bed is comfortable.
- Make sure your bedroom or the place where you sleep is clean, neat, and peaceful. A clean, orderly environment reduces confused, chaotic mental stimuli and allows the brain, mind, and nervous system to relax more effectively. All this brings about a much deeper, more restful quality of sleep.
- If you live in a noisy place, where traffic or other noise is likely, consider using comfortable ear plugs to ensure a good night's sleep.

   Whenever I travel to large, congested, bustling cities, and I'm disturbed by the constant noise of the city at night, I use a simple pair of earplugs while I sleep. Instead of waking up fatigued, foggy-headed, grumpy, irritable, and low on energy, thanks to the earplugs, I can wake up feeling refreshed, renewed, and ready to greet the new day with enthusiasm.

- Make sure the air you breathe when you sleep is fresh and clean. Avoid dusty, foul-smelling, stale air. A good, fresh breeze can do wonders to improve the quality of your sleep.
- Don't eat a late dinner just before you go to sleep. A full stomach and heavily laden digestive system will put pressure on the

diaphragm and lungs and interfere with normal, natural breathing. Many people with sleep disturbances and other illnesses are overweight and have poor, late-night eating habits that cause indigestion and interfere with the quality of their sleep.

■ Try a warm beverage before you go to sleep. A warm beverage can be soothing and relaxing, improving digestion, and helping to settle down the nerves. Herbal teas, such as chamomile or peppermint, can be particularly comforting.

■ Relaxation, gentle breathing, meditation, imagery, or prayer can help calm and relax the mind and nervous system. When they are performed before bedtime, these methods can be a gentle and soothing way to induce deep, restful sleep.

■ Listen to soft, soothing music. Doing this can be relaxing and restful, and can help induce gentle, effective sleep.

■ Before bed, read an inspirational novel, book, or scripture, or some other uplifting material. This activity can be comforting and reassuring, and a pleasant way to wind down and relax before sleep. Some people I know read the *Yellow Pages* or *Webster's Dictionary* to help them get to sleep. This method works, I am told, because these books are so boring!

The suggestions included in this "Getting Started" section may seem simple and insignificant, but, when taken together, they will make an enormous difference in your life and the functioning of your healing system. Just five minutes a day of meditation, an uplifting phone conversation with a friend, a cup of delicious soup for lunch, and a good night's sleep can have a great impact on your healing system and your physical, mental, and emotional health.

Conquering Common
Health Conditions

In this section, you'll find strategies and approaches for tapping into, enhancing, and strengthening your healing system to heal a variety of specific health problems. Keep in mind, however, that these recommendations are only guidelines and are not intended to replace responsible, intelligent, personalized professional healthcare. Additionally, because every person is a unique individual, not every one of these recommendations may be effective for you. I have purposely avoided prescribing exact amounts, dosages, or schedules for treatments, because, when you are working with your healing system, no simple formulas or recipes will work equally well for everybody. In the art and science of medicine and healing, every treatment and therapy needs to be adjusted to meet the unique needs of each person. However, by following the recommendations that follow and incorporating those presented in previous chapters, your chances for success will be greatly increased. Remember that with each malady listed, what is recommended is not intended to be all-inclusive; additional options might be available for your problem.

For your convenience, the following list of health problems is organized in the simplest way I know—according to the various systems and anatomical regions in the body. This list, while not all-inclusive, represents the most common maladies presented to me as a primary-care physician. If I have omitted a health problem that you may be currently suffering with or are interested in, just follow the general recommendations given throughout the book, and see the "Resources" section at the end. If you learn to work with your healing system to overcome your health problems, you will achieve success in your quest for greater health.

Skin Problems

Your skin is a reflection of your general state of health. People who are generally healthy exhibit healthy skin tone and color. Conversely, in diseased or weakened states, the skin is often pale or mottled and lacks a healthy sheen. When you have liver disease, for example, your skin becomes jaundiced and takes on a yellowish appearance. Skin rashes are also often signs of deeper problems. For this reason, doctors have traditionally relied upon the skin for diagnostic clues to deeper internal problems.

Abrasions, Contusions, Lacerations, and Punctures

These four types of injuries are among the most common that the skin sustains, and they are usually present whenever physical trauma of any kind occurs.

Abrasions occur where the skin is scraped, revealing the raw under-surfaces of the skin. Abrasions most commonly occur from falls on pavement or asphalt, and, although painful, they usually heal up uneventfully if they are kept clean and dry. Topical aloe vera, turmeric, and other herbal and natural plant and mineral salves may also be helpful to prevent infection and speed the work of your healing system with abrasions.

Contusions are bruises that appear in the form of "black and blue" marks on the skin, which reflect broken blood vessels underneath the surface. Contusions may be accompanied by swelling and pain, but they usually do not result in a break of the skin. Unless there is damage to underlying tissues, your healing system can repair the damages caused by contusions in a relatively short time. Ice applied for the first

24 hours to minimize swelling, followed by warm salt-water soaks or compresses, can assist your healing system in this work.

Lacerations are full, linear-shaped breaks in the skin where bleeding occurs. Stitches may be required if a laceration is extensive and the bleeding is profuse. Once the edges of the wound are brought together, your healing system takes over and heals the wound, in many cases with barely a scar. Even large lacerations that are not stitched will still heal with the help of your healing system, but they will generally take longer and may cause a scar.

Puncture wounds are stab-type wounds that pierce the skin. If they are not too deep, and with proper care, your healing system can usually mend puncture wounds quite easily.

Abscesses

Abscesses are swellings in the skin, most often caused by a bacterial infection. Many surgeons will lance an abscess with a scalpel, or drain an abscess with a needle. But if you begin treatment in the earlier stages and work with your healing system by applying warm salt soaks and pharmaceutical-grade clay (bentonite) packs, many abscesses will disappear on their own. Natural sunlight, aloe vera, salt-water compresses, and a non-oily diet can also be helpful to assist your healing system in healing abscesses.

Acne

Acne occurs in both males and females, most commonly during the onset of puberty, but it may linger for many years. Acne is caused by minute infections that occur in the oily buildup of the hair follicles. If scratched or picked, acne can cause permanent scarring and be disfiguring. Acne occurs most commonly on the face, which can have tragic consequences if scarring and disfigurement result.

The same natural treatments for abscesses can also be effective for acne. Drying agents, including alcohol, can also be helpful. Oily, fatty, rich diets, along with stress, can make acne worse. People with naturally oily skin need to pay particular attention to their diets. A *macrobiotic* diet (a very low-fat, plant-based diet that originated in Japan) can often clear up stubborn cases of acne in a short time. In many cases, conventional medicines may also be necessary. These medicines include topical drying agents, such as those that contain *benzoyl peroxide,* or internal preparations, such as *accutane,* a vitamin-A derivative, which, when prescribed under the care of a knowledgeable dermatologist, can be highly effective.

Boils, Carbuncles, Furuncles

These are infectious swellings in the skin similar to abscesses. Many start with just a simple ingrown hair, but they may become irritated, painful, and often quite large, especially if they are squeezed or picked. They can also become unsightly, especially if they are on the face or shoulder.

Natural treatments that work best with your healing system include soaking or compressing in warm, concentrated salt solutions, applying clay packs, exposing to sunlight, treating with alcohol and other drying agents, and keeping all dirt, oil, and bacteria away from the affected area. If boils, carbuncles, or furuncles are severe and are allowed to progress, antibiotics and/or lancing may be necessary to help your healing system repair these conditions.

Burns

Burns to the skin are relatively common, but if they are severe and extensive enough, they can cause much harm, even death. First-degree burns cause redness, pain, and swelling, but no blistering. When blistering occurs, second-degree burns have been sustained. Third-degree burns, the most serious type of burn, result when nerve endings are burned and the sensation of pain is lost. If you sustain a burn and it hurts, consider yourself lucky because it means that you don't have a third-degree burn.

Burns can be extremely painful, but, if they are not extensive, your healing system can handle them with little intervention. Burns should be kept clean, dry, and free from excessive moisture and dirt. Topical agents that are cooling, including ice in the initial stages, generally reduce swelling and pain. Antibiotic cremes, such as Silvadene cream, or a natural agent such as zinc oxide, can keep the skin from drying out and cracking and prevent infection. Aloe, vinegar, honey, and bee propolis may also be effective.

If the burn is extensive, covering it with light gauze dressings and nonstick bandages, and then leaving it undisturbed for at least 24 to 48 hours, possibly longer, might be necessary. Any dressing that gets wet, however, needs to be changed because wet dressings suffocate healing tissues and can promote infection. Pain medications may also be appropriate for one to two days or more. For second-degree burns with blisters, it is best not to pop the blisters because they serve as a natural protective barrier that your healing system employs to protect the new skin that is forming underneath.

In the later stages of healing burns, you can assist your healing system with natural topical applications such as aloe vera, comfrey root poultices, vitamin E cream, calendula, and turmeric cream.

Cysts

Cysts look very similar to abscesses, but they are often more chronic and have a tendency toward periodic swelling. Conservative treatment is similar to treatment for abscesses and boils, including soaking, sunlight, and using drying agents. Cysts may need to be lanced and drained if they become excessively large or intrusive. Once they have been lanced or drained, your healing system can take over and complete the healing process.

Folliculitis

This common condition represents inflammation and infection of the hair follicles, hence the name, *folliculitis*. Folliculitis looks like acne, but it may show up in areas of the skin away from the face, such as in the groin area or under the armpits. It can be very painful and itchy and is best treated with salt soaks, clay packs, and natural sunlight. If folliculitis is severe and is allowed to progress, antibiotics may also be required.

Impetigo

Impetigo, caused by bacteria and poor skin hygiene, is a rapidly spreading infection with a brownish-colored, crusty rash. Impetigo is common in children and may be spread at day-care centers. Bathing and good hygiene help to eliminate the organisms that cause this infection. Once impetigo has been contracted, antibiotics may be necessary to eliminate it. Salt soaks, clay packs, aloe vera, and sun baths can also be effective if it is caught early on. You can easily prevent impetigo by observing good skin hygiene.

Skin Rashes

In certain generalized infections, characteristic rashes appear on the skin as toxins make their way out of the body's deeper structures. We commonly see these rashes in childhood illnesses such as *measles, chicken pox, rubella (German measles),* and other viral diseases. If contracted at an early age, these conditions, although uncomfortable, are usually self-limiting and do little harm in Western populations. Certain food allergies, and immune-system disorders such as *lupus,* may also show up on the skin in the form of a rash. Even nutritional deficiencies, such as *pellagra,* can show up as a rash on the skin.

While you are treating any skin rash, it is important to work with your healing system by addressing the underlying causes of the rash. Drinking plenty of fluids will support your healing system in eliminating toxins if an underlying disease is present. There are many other methods to work with your healing system in these cases, such as getting plenty of rest, eating lightly, and taking certain herbs and plant remedies. Natural salves, ointments, and clay plasters applied topically to the skin may also be helpful. However, it is important to remember that a rash may have deeper origins than just the skin.

Because of its rich nerve supply, your skin is highly sensitive to pain and itching. When a rash itches, you will invariably scratch it, which will only make matters worse. An important part of the treatment of any rash is to stop the itch so the problem doesn't escalate while you are working to discover and treat the underlying causes. In addition to soothing topical creams, such as those that contain aloe, calendula, chamomile, or turmeric, conventional creams and ointments that contain *hydrocortisone,* and other over-the-counter conventional medicines, such as *antihistamines* or *analgesics,* can also effectively eliminate itching and prevent the rash from escalating.

Allergic Rashes

Rashes can appear in response to skin irritants and chemicals, such as those found in various sunscreen agents, soaps, and solvents. Rashes can even appear in response to naturally occurring substances found in plants, such as in mangoes, poison ivy, and poison oak. Skin allergies can also result as complications from insect bites, including bee stings, spider bites, and jellyfish stings.

Once again, while you are treating these rashes and controlling the itch and spread of the rash, the key to eliminating them permanently is to identify the offending agent and avoid all further contact with this agent. Many remedies, both conventional and natural, can be helpful in these cases. If you remove the offending agent, and control the itching and scratching, your healing system can usually heal the rash and restore your skin to its natural state of health.

Infectious Rashes

Many rashes are the result of skin infections, most commonly, fungal infections such as *athlete's foot* and *ringworm*. Bacterial infections, parasites (including *scabies*), and viruses such as *herpes simplex* (which causes cold sores) also can cause rashes. In each case, prevention is the key to avoiding infection in the first place. For example, fungi and most bacteria prefer wet, warm, dark places to breed and flourish. The feet, groin, buttocks, abdomen, and underarms are common sites of infection from these organisms. Environmental factors also play a role. For example, infectious rashes from fungi and bacteria are more common in the tropics, or during summer, when the weather is often more humid.

Once a skin infection is accurately diagnosed, natural remedies, including tea-tree oil, clay, and other drying agents, in addition to a wide range of medicated creams and ointments, are readily available to treat it. Of course, in difficult cases, additional conventional medicines may be required. This is particularly true for scabies. Keeping the skin clean and free from excess moisture, and allowing it to breathe and be exposed to fresh air and adequate sunlight are the best approaches for working with your healing system to prevent and eliminate skin infections.

Nerve-Related Rashes

Because the skin is intimately connected to the nervous system, many chronic rashes that don't easily go away have their origins in such conditions as chronic anxiety, stress, tension, or other emotional and nervous-system disorders. These are often classified as nerve-related rashes, and they include the following:

Eczema

Eczema is a chronic skin condition characterized by intense itching and a scaly, spreading rash that at times can be disfiguring. To aid your healing system, you can best treat this condition by applying topical soothing creams, taking pain medications if needed, using herbs or medicines that calm the nervous system, and eliminating caffeine and nicotine from your system. Emollient creams and various oily preparations applied continuously to the eczema can help prevent the constant drying out and loss of natural body oils that occur with eczema. Because this skin condition flares up during times of stress and anxiety, stress-management techniques can also be very effective in controlling it. Eating a wholesome diet and drinking lots of fluids can also be helpful with this condition.

Psoriasis

Psoriasis is a chronic skin condition that is common in the areas around the knees, elbows, scalp, feet, and back. Psoriasis flares up during times of anxiety and tension. Foods that stimulate the nervous system, such as caffeine and nicotine, can also aggravate this condition. Sunlight is often prescribed for psoriasis, as are suppressive medications and various corticosteroid creams. Addressing the underlying causes through such methods as diet and stress-management training, while gently relieving the symptoms of itching and scratching, can often reverse even long-standing cases of psoriasis.

Shingles

Shingles is caused by the *H. Zoster* virus, which stays in your body in a dormant stage but can flare up during times of stress and/or immune dysfunction. To aid your healing system, you can best treat this condition by applying topical soothing creams, taking pain medications if needed, using herbs or medicines that calm the nervous system, eliminating caffeine and nicotine from your system, drinking lots of fluids to flush toxins from your body, and practicing stress-management techniques.

Problems of the Head

Disorders and symptoms in the head are very common. Because the head contains the brain, which is sensitive to subtle changes in your body's internal environment, these problems may reflect imbalances in other parts of the body. For example, with *anemia*, not enough red blood cells and oxygen reach the brain, and headaches may occur. In addition, if you have anemia, you might be unable to think clearly. Weakness, along with dizziness and fainting, especially when you are standing up or making sudden movements with your head, may also occur.

Proper treatment of problems in the head requires understanding the underlying causes and working with your healing system to correct these problems.

Dizziness and Vertigo

Dizziness and vertigo are two common symptoms that, like headaches, may have simple causes or may represent more serious conditions, such as brain tumors, impending stroke, heart problems, dehydration, anemia, or infection. They may also signal a metabolic problem, such as low blood sugar, as in diabetes.

The most common underlying causes of dizziness and vertigo include dietary imbalance, including excess caffeine or nicotine; problems with sugar metabolism; stress; lack of sleep; muscle tension in the face, neck, and upper back; motion sickness; middle- and inner-ear problems (including a persistent viral infection); and dehydration. When symptoms are severe, nausea and vomiting can result.

Treatment should be directed toward the underlying causes. If a proper medical evaluation determines nothing serious, try working with your healing system by taking a week away from your hectic schedule and focusing on a healthy, wholesome diet with plenty of fiber, less caffeine, and plenty of water. In addition, receive a massage of the upper back, neck, and face, and make sure you get enough sleep. Acupuncture and other natural treatments can also be effective when no serious underlying problem exists.

Headaches

Headaches are one of the most common reasons people go to see a doctor. And even though most are easily corrected and have simple causes, headaches can be caused by more serious illnesses and problems. The head is a sensitive barometer for physiological imbalances that may be occurring in other parts of your body. For this reason, you should not ignore headaches, or merely suppress them with pain medication, particularly if they are persistent.

Headaches might occur as the result of fatigue, dehydration, anemia, indigestion, sinus infections, ear infections, having overdone certain foods or substances such as alcohol and caffeine, and as a result of other conditions, including stress. Headaches also commonly occur during regular monthly cycles of ovulation and menstruation. More serious causes of headaches include meningitis, encephalitis, stroke, and brain tumor. Headaches can also be the result of head trauma that causes increased pressure and swelling in the brain, caused by fluid.

Your healing system can heal most headaches once the underlying problems are corrected. However, if a headache is severe, persistent, keeps you awake at night, or interferes with your ability to work or function, it is time to go and see your doctor to be properly evaluated.

Cluster headaches appear predominantly in males and are similar to migraines in their cause and treatment. Cluster headaches commonly appear around the eye on one side of the face, and they come and go in waves of pain. They are also influenced by stress and dietary imbalances, and they often respond well to dietary moderation, including decreased caffeine and nicotine, and increased fluids. Massage, particularly of the upper back, neck, and facial muscles, along with acupuncture, chiropractic treatment, and gentle yoga stretching can often help your healing system eliminate cluster headaches.

Migraine headaches can be severe and disabling. Migraines were previously thought to be caused by swelling in the blood vessels of the head, but recent research has shown they are similar in origin to tension headaches, only more prolonged and severe. Diet and lifestyle, in addition to hormonal fluctuations, may also be contributing factors. In their worst presentation, migraines, with their symptoms of nausea, vomiting, visual disturbances, and loss of balance, might force you to be incapacitated for hours and sometimes days at a time. You might temporarily require strong pain medications. Natural migraine treatment methods that support your healing system include eating a wholesome diet, drinking plenty of fluids, and practicing stress-management techniques. Massage, particularly of the upper back, neck, and facial muscles, acupuncture, chiropractic treatment, and gentle yoga stretching are also often effective. Migraine headaches can often be relieved by getting rid of negative "emotional baggage," taking soothing herbs that calm the nerves and relax the muscles, and applying topical heat balms.

Tension headaches are caused by stress and tension; they also can be related to dietary imbalances, including excesses of caffeine or nicotine, and other factors. Conventional medicines may temporarily help relieve a tension headache, but most just suppress the pain. Implementing diet and lifestyle changes that reduce tension and stress, practicing daily stress-management techniques, and increasing fluids to eliminate toxins can all assist your healing system in relieving tension headaches. Massage, particularly of the upper back, neck, and facial muscles, in addition to acupuncture, chiropractic treatment, and gentle yoga stretching, can also be effective. Tension headaches are often relieved by soothing herbs such as feverfew and chamomile, which calm the nerves and relax the muscles, and by topically applied heat balms.

Head Injury

Because the brain is so important, head injuries can have serious consequences. With a severe head injury, prompt and responsible action can mean the difference between life and death. When a concussion occurs as a result of head trauma, and there is associated loss of consciousness, the possibility of damage to internal structures always exists, and immediate evaluation and medical attention are required. If no nausea, vomiting, lethargy, loss of memory, undue sleepiness, or other neurological symptoms develop during a 24- to 48-hour period following a head injury, then there is a high degree of probability that nothing serious has occurred internally. If no loss of consciousness occurred during head trauma, it is also highly unlikely that something serious has occurred. Anyone who has suffered a concussion, with reported loss of consciousness, should go immediately to the nearest emergency room to rule out the possibility of brain hemorrhage or other serious injury.

Amazingly, in spite of the potentially serious consequences, the majority of head injuries are not serious and respond favorably to your healing system's internal repair and restoration mechanisms. As with any other injury, however, your healing system works best when you cooperate with it by getting plenty of rest and making sure you are drinking enough fluids and eating wholesome, nutritious food.

Eye Disorders

Our eyes are the most dominant and important sense organs in our bodies. Additionally, because our eyes are so sensitive, problems in other parts of the body often affect them. In this regard, our eyes are a reflection of our overall general health. For instance, high blood pressure can erode and rupture the fragile blood vessels in the retina, a condition that a doctor can diagnose with a simple eye exam. Diabetes, which also causes changes in the appearance of the blood vessels in the back of the eye, can similarly be detected from a simple eye exam. Because our eyes are so important, a specialty in medicine, known as *ophthalmology*, exists just to tend to their needs.

Many chronic eye conditions are related to underlying problems elsewhere in the body, so these conditions are often preventable. Many of these disorders often reflect poor overall health, and so working with your healing system to improve your overall health can often improve such eye conditions. For example, when I was a flight surgeon in the U.S. Air Force, it was common knowledge that even among young, healthy fighter pilots, those who smoked had poorer night vision. They were considered a combat risk when they were flying night missions because the increased carbon monoxide and decreased oxygen in their blood as a result of smoking negatively affected their vision.

Good nutrition is very important to the health of your eyes. Vitamin A, which comes from beta carotene and is found in most yellow and orange fruits and vegetables, participates in the chemistry of vision. Eating a diet rich in beta carotene, and taking herbal medicines such as bilberry extract, help promote the health of your eyes. In addition, regular exercise, which improves blood flow and oxygenation of the eyes, and specific eye exercises also work with your healing system to promote eye health.

Conjunctivitis

Known as *pink eye, conjunctivitis* is a common condition in children that can sweep through schools in epidemic fashion. Conjunctivitis is often caused by viruses or bacterial agents, and it can occur when air quality is poor or adverse environmental conditions are present. It can also be associated with respiratory infections. Conjunctivitis appears as a reddish or pinkish color in the whites of the eyes. Usually only one eye is affected, but about 40 percent of the time it can occur in both eyes.

Conjunctivitis can be itchy and sometimes even painful. In the morning, the crusted secretions that have hardened during the night may cause the eyes to be glued shut. Warm compresses can be helpful to free the glued eyelids.

If you can avoid itching and scratching, your body's healing system can often eradicate this condition on its own in three to five days. Salt-water eye drops and natural sunlight can be very helpful. A gentle herbal eyewash such as *hyssop* or *chamomile* may also be helpful. Conventional treatments with anti-itch oral medications, including mild, over-the-counter anti-inflammatory medicines, analgesics, antihistamines, and antibiotic drops, can be helpful to prevent complications and control the itch as your healing system does its job.

Corneal Abrasions

Corneal abrasions occur when the surface of the eye has been scratched. This can be a very painful condition, as most contact-lens wearers know. However, because your eyes are so important, your healing system can initiate a rapid response to these injuries and usually repair them within 24 to 48 hours. If you have a corneal abrasion, an eye patch and antibiotic drops are customarily administered to rest and protect your eye, and to prevent it from becoming infected while your healing system does its important repair work.

Styes

Styes are small, inflamed swellings that occur as minute infections in the follicles of the hairs that line the edges of your eyelids, commonly known as your eyelashes. Styes are common when dust, oil, or foreign particles clog the pores of the skin near the eye. They are common with carpenters and construction laborers who are inclined to work around dusty construction sites. They may also occur when you inadvertently and repeatedly wipe your oily, dusty, or dirty hands in your eyes.

Warm salt-water compresses and natural sunlight usually cure styes in one to three days. Occasionally, in more difficult cases, topical antibiotic drops or ointments may be required. Natural eyewashes may also be helpful. Even though they are close to the eyes and can be unsettling, styes are more inconvenient than dangerous, and, thanks to your healing system, they usually heal on their own without any further complications.

Ear Problems

Your ear consists of three distinct parts: your external ear, your middle ear, and your inner ear. Each part carries with it its own special set of problems and, because those problems are treated differently, we will consider each ear part separately.

Impacted Ear Wax

Impacted ear wax is a common cause of hearing problems, discomfort, and outer-ear infections because the wax blocks the ear canal, can trap water, and can prevent sound waves from reaching your ear drum. Ear wax serves a beneficial function as both a lubricant to the ear canal and a natural antibiotic. However, to prevent excessive ear-wax buildup, you can help your healing system by gently flushing your ear canal with warm water and hydrogen peroxide in a 6:1 ratio, using a bulb syringe readily available from your nearest pharmacy. This flushing should take a maximum of 30 minutes. Ear candling is also becoming popular for this purpose. Most of us have been told never to stick anything in our ears smaller than our elbows, but I must confess that, after a hot shower, if the need presents itself, I will occasionally use a cotton-tipped swab to gently and carefully remove any excess wax that may have formed in my ear canal.

Meniere's Disease

Also known as *labyrinthitis*, this condition is marked by inflammation of the delicate inner-ear structures. Meniere's disease, which affects balance and hearing, is thought to be caused by a virus, which may follow on the heels of a respiratory infection. Meniere's disease often occurs only once, but it may recur from time to time. Natural approaches to inner-ear problems that support the work of your healing system include acupuncture, nutritional support, the use of specific herbs such as *gingko biloba*, cranial-sacral therapy, yoga, acupuncture, chiropractic care, and physical therapy.

Middle-Ear Infections

Middle-ear infections are quite common in infancy and early childhood, and they can be serious. They often cause fever and pain, and they can be accompanied by loss of hearing, loss of balance, vertigo, nausea, and vomiting. In children, under extreme conditions, a middle-ear infection runs the risk of spreading to the brain and causing *meningitis*. Because the passage that leads to the middle ear, the *eustachian tube*, is directly connected to the back of the nose, middle-ear infections occur as extensions of respiratory infections that may start as a cold, runny nose, sore throat, sinus infection, or chest congestion.

The key to treatment of middle-ear infections involves understanding the relationship between the middle ear and the respiratory system. You must cooperate with your healing system by focusing on prevention, and by treating respiratory infections in their early stages to preclude the possibility that they may spread to the middle ear. Diet also can play a role in preventing middle-ear infections. For example, by reducing intake of fats and oils and drinking plenty of fluids, you can help thin out the mucous, phlegm, and congestion in the respiratory system, which helps the body to eliminate toxins more readily. Good posture, gentle chiropractic adjustments, and deep breathing also appear to improve lymphatic drainage of the middle ear and can help prevent ear infections. Herbal remedies, such as *echinacea*, *astragalus*, and *wasabe* (Japanese horseradish) may also be helpful. When middle-ear infections are in their full-blown stages, antibiotics are usually required, especially to prevent the possibility of meningitis. But avoid the continuous use of antibiotics to treat this common problem.

Noise-Induced Hearing Loss

Hearing loss caused by noise damages the sensitive hair cells in the inner ear that conduct sound to the brain. Such loss is common in people who have worked around heavy equipment and loud machinery, and it is now showing up in ex-rock musicians, who have blasted their ears for years with screeching guitars and loud amplified music. Noise-induced hearing loss is particularly common in people who work around airplanes and man the flight lines at airports. These people are now required by law to wear ear protection to prevent this unnecessary condition.

Hearing aids are common in the elderly and can be effective to help people compensate for inner-ear hearing loss. Delicate surgical techniques involving the implantation of electronic sound-amplification devices are usually reserved for severe cases. Natural approaches to inner-ear problems that support the work of your healing system include acupuncture, nutritional support, the use of specific herbs such as *gingko biloba*, cranial-sacral therapy, yoga, acupuncture, chiropractic care, and physical therapy. Other methods may also prove helpful in certain cases of inner-ear problems, particularly if they are initiated in the early stages of these disorders. Because your ability to hear is a precious gift, and these conditions are often difficult to treat, prevention of noise-induced hearing loss is critical.

Outer-Ear Infections

Often known as *swimmer's ear* infections, outer-ear infections can be extremely painful and are common where people spend a lot of time in the water or where humidity is high. If you develop an outer-ear infection, antibiotic drops and keeping your ear dry to discourage bacterial growth allow your healing system to restore health to your ear, usually in less than seven days. Several natural eardrops, such as *gentian violet* and *mullein oil*, are also available and can be effective treatments. You can prevent or heal outer-ear infections by keeping your ears clean and dry. If you spend a lot of time in the water, you can help your healing system prevent outer-ear infections by applying alcohol and vinegar ear drops, or using a blow dryer after swimming. These can help keep your ears dry, which inhibits bacterial growth and minimizes the possibility of an outer-ear infection.

Perforated Ear Drum

This condition occurs as a result of increased pressure in the middle ear, which causes the eardrum to rupture. Perforated ear drum is common in divers, people who fly when they have respiratory infections, and people who are hit on the side of the head and the ear is traumatized. Symptoms may include pain, hearing loss, a bloody ear canal, and vertigo. Thanks to your body's healing system, if the tear is not too large, a ruptured eardrum will usually heal on its own in one month's time. During this healing period, it is important to support the work of your healing system by not getting water into your ears, which might cause a serious infection. If the rupture is very large, surgical grafting of a new eardrum may be required; but, thanks to your healing system, doing this is not common because your ear usually can heal on its own.

Surfer's Ear

Known as *exostosis,* surfer's ear occurs when the bones in the ear canal grow together, obstructing the ear canal and causing water to be trapped. This condition can lead to chronic outer-ear infections. Surfer's ear is common not only in surfers who frequent cold waters, but also in skiers, hunters, farmers, and other outdoor-oriented people who live in cold climates.

An operation to scrape away the extra bone growth is conventionally offered; however, if you return to the cold environment after surgery without sufficient ear protection, the bone growth will also return. The recurring bone growth is actually a compensatory protective mechanism of your healing system in its attempt to keep the sensitive and delicate ear drum warm enough to efficiently conduct sound waves so that hearing is not impaired. Ear plugs or other ear protection keeps the ears warm and helps your healing system to prevent this condition from developing.

Tinnitus

Also known as ringing in the ears, *tinnitus* is a problem of the inner ear, and may or may not accompany hearing loss. Tinnitus is a troubling condition not often responsive to conventional medical treatment.

Natural approaches to inner-ear problems such as tinnitus that support the work of your healing system include acupuncture, nutritional support, the use of specific herbs such as *gingko biloba*, cranial-sacral therapy, yoga, acupuncture, chiropractic care, and physical therapy. Other methods may also prove helpful in certain cases of inner-ear problems, particularly if they are initiated in the early stages of these disorders. Because your ability to hear is a precious gift, and these conditions are often difficult to treat, prevention is very important.

Respiratory System Disorders

Asthma

This chronic respiratory condition is characterized by congestion, coughing, wheezing, and constricted airways. During flare-ups, these symptoms can be severe and even life-threatening. Throughout the world, asthma appears to be on the rise, a fact that many experts attribute to increasing urbanization and air pollution. Other possible causes and triggers for asthma include respiratory infections, respiratory allergens, aerosol pollutants (including the inhalation of toxic fumes or vapors), climatic changes, dehydration, poor diets, and stress and emotional upheaval, among others. Conventional Western medicine has developed many effective medications for airway management to lessen the strain of breathing for persons who have asthma. Although many of these medications are invaluable, even life-saving, particularly in urgent and emergency situations, most do not address the underlying causes of asthma.

Treatment of asthma includes drinking plenty of fluids to help lubricate the lungs and decrease mucous and phlegm. You can also aid your healing system by breathing good, clean, wholesome air; avoiding dust, irritating aerosol chemicals, and other triggers; and keeping warm to avoid catching a cold. Also, stay away from fats and oils during flare-ups, practice stress-management and relaxation methods, release unhealthy emotions, and practice breathing exercises. All of these steps can be extremely effective in treating asthma. In addition to the medications your doctor may prescribe, natural, alternative medicines and treatments that work with your healing system also can successfully treat asthma.

Bronchitis

Bronchitis, one of the most common respiratory infections of the lungs, is most often caused by viruses or bacteria that have slipped past the body's primary defenses and entered into the airways. Bronchitis is characterized by inflammation and infection in the bronchi and bronchial tubes, which are the breathing passages in the lungs. Coughing and congestion are persistent, and fever may also be present. Conventional doctors usually prescribe antibiotics and cough medicines for this condition. (See the section on pneumonia for additional suggestions.)

Colds

Common colds are invariably associated with runny noses. When you catch a cold, usually the nose is the first organ affected because the thousands of bacteria, viruses, and other microorganisms in the air first come in contact with your body through the nose. Nasal congestion and inflammation can often be relieved by working with your healing system in several ways. These include breathing good air; avoiding dust, smoke, or polluted environments; keeping warm; eating lightly (focusing on soups and hot teas); and drinking plenty of fluids. Steam inhalation, saline nose drops, and other natural remedies, including horseradish, Chinese mustard, and wasabe (Japanese horseradish), can also be effective to help keep your nose and respiratory system healthy. Again, prevention is the key to avoiding the common cold; if this is not possible, your goal should be to initiate treatment in the earliest stages.

Emphysema and COPD
(Chronic Obstructive Pulmonary Disease)

These two respiratory-system disorders are usually related to long-term cigarette smoking, but they may also be linked to repeated exposure to asbestos or other chemicals that are harmful to the lungs, especially over a substantial time period. The best way to assist your healing system in the treatment of these conditions includes breathing good air, doing breathing exercises, and drinking plenty of fluids. Certain natural remedies, including vitamin C and herbs that stimulate repair of damaged tissues, such as comfrey and aloe, may also be helpful. Again, prevention is much more effective and easier than attempting to cure either of these conditions once the disease has established itself. Because of the body's healing system, however, even people with long-term smoking habits can improve their breathing and the health of their lungs if they quit smoking before irreparable damage has occurred.

Pharyngitis

Pharyngitis is an inflammation of the pharynx that frequently results in a sore throat. Pharyngitis often begins when the body is chilled, and bacteria have entered past your body's primary defenses. Often, you will need a prescription for an antibiotic. Other, more natural methods that support your healing system to overcome pharyngitis include eating fewer fats and oils, drinking plenty of fluids, keeping warm, managing stress, and getting adequate sleep and rest. Ginger-root tea can also be very effective in treating pharyngitis. To make ginger-root tea, grate fresh ginger root, put it in boiling water, and steep for 5 to10 minutes; then add lemon and honey before you drink the tea.

Pneumonia

Pneumonia is an extension of bronchitis and an invasion of the infection into the air sacs and deeper recesses of the lungs. Fever and night sweats are often present with pneumonia, and because oxygen is unable to enter the bloodstream as a result of the infection, over-all weakness is common. Before the advent of antibiotics, pneumonia was one of the leading causes of death. As with all respiratory infections, pneumonia is usually a reflection of decreased immune function as the result of certain stresses on the body, such as an unhealthy diet and lifestyle. In addition to whatever medications you might require, including antibiotics, and the use of other natural remedies, such as plant- and mineral-based medicines, it is important to assist your healing system by following these recommendations:

1. Drink plenty of fluids.

   Your body is 70 percent fluid, and so the more fluid you bring into your system, the faster your body can eliminate the toxins from the infection. Additionally, it is important to avoid fats and oils until you are better because they tend to create more phlegm and mucous, which increase congestion and clog your airways.

2. Keep warm.

   Your body likes to stay warm, around 98.6 degrees. When you become chilled, your immune system is impaired as a result of the stress of your body attempting to restore proper temperature. You can keep warm by wearing a sweater or windbreaker, drinking plenty of warm liquids such as soups and herbal teas, and avoiding air conditioning, fans, or exposure to cold weather.

3. Rest.

   When you are sleep deprived or chronically fatigued, your immune system and healing system bog down and you become more susceptible to illness. It is difficult to get better and heal if you are not getting adequate rest because your healing system does most of its best work when you are resting or sleeping.

Respiratory Allergies

Respiratory allergies come in various forms and commonly afflict the nose and sinuses. A few of the more common varieties include *rhinitis, hay fever,* and *allergic sinusitis.* Many people report the source of their allergy to be specific plant materials, such as pollens, grasses, or fungal spores, but many others tend to have worse symptoms while they are indoors. This suggests that chemicals, dust, dust mites, mold, and other potentially allergic material in the ventilation systems at work or in the home may be responsible for most allergies. Additionally, the way people breathe can affect their susceptibility to a respiratory allergy. For example, people who breathe exclusively through their mouths have higher rates of respiratory allergies. This is probably because the air they are breathing does not have the opportunity for the nose to filter and clean it.

Following are six simple tips for helping your healing system eliminate a respiratory allergy:

1. Pay attention to the quality of the air you breathe.

2. Learn to switch to nasal breathing.

3. Eliminate or minimize fats and oils in your diet, including heavy, rich, fried foods, which tend to increase mucous and phlegm in the respiratory system.

4. Try natural plant medicines, such as echinacea, wasabe, Chinese mustard, horseradish, astragalus, ginger, and stinging nettles.

5. Reserve suppressive medications, including steroids, antihistamines, and decongestants, for urgent situations only, and don't rely on them for long-term treatment.

6. Try sunbaths, exercise, yoga, acupuncture, chiropractic care, and other natural methods that work with your healing system and that can play a supporting role in managing and overcoming respiratory allergies.

Sinus Infections

Sinus infections are some of the most common of all respiratory infections and one of the most common reasons people visit the doctor's office. Sinus infections occur when respiratory infections, which begin in the nose and throat area, spread to the sinuses. The sinuses are small, cavernous air pockets that play an important role in defense, balance, and buoyancy of the head.

Antibiotics are often prescribed and effective in acute cases of sinus infection, but chronic conditions respond better to more natural methods that support your healing system. These methods include drinking more fluids; breathing steam; applying salt-water cleanses, sprays, or irrigation; and breathing good air. Natural sunbaths, acupuncture, yoga, gentle massage, and cranial-sacral bodywork may also be helpful to your healing system. In addition, reducing fats and oils in your diet can help. Natural plant remedies such as wasabe, horseradish, Chinese mustard, echinacea, and astragalus may also be helpful. (An excellent book about sinus infections is *Sinus Survival*, by Dr. Rob Ivker, past president of the American Holistic Medical Association and former chronic sinusitis sufferer.)

Strep Throat

Strep throat is caused by various types of *streptococcal* bacteria and is more common when the weather turns colder, often coinciding with the beginning of flu season. We used to consider strep throat highly contagious, but recent evidence points more toward changes in weather, stress, and compromised host-resistance factors, which lowers immune function.

Under most conditions, strep throat does not affect other organs and systems of the body; however, because of the rare complicating factors that can affect the kidneys and heart, doctors routinely treat it with antibiotic therapy. The key to treating this condition, again, lies in prevention. You can also assist your healing system by keeping your body warm, drinking plenty of fluids, avoiding stress, and getting sufficient rest, sleep, and adequate exercise. Ginger, in addition to other herbs, and salt-water gargles, can also be helpful.

Tonsillitis

Until recently, the tonsils were routinely removed if they were continually swollen. We now know, however, that the tonsils perform an important immune function and, if possible, are better left in.

Although antibiotics may be required to effectively treat tonsillitis, dietary management involving decreased dairy, fats, and oils, and drinking plenty of fluids, helps thin the mucous and aids your healing system in eliminating toxins. Keeping warm, getting plenty of sleep and rest, and managing stress all appear to be helpful in aiding your healing system in the treatment and prevention of tonsillitis. Ginger-root tea can also be very effective in treating tonsillitis. To make ginger-root tea, grate fresh ginger root, place it in boiling water, and steep for 5 to 10 minutes; then add lemon and honey before you drink the tea.

Tuberculosis

Tuberculosis (TB) is common where adverse environmental conditions such as poor air quality, lack of sunlight, and inadequate ventilation exist in conjunction with inadequate nutrition, poor sanitation, and lowered immunity. This illness more commonly occurs in developing countries or in populations that are destitute and despairing, such as alcoholics and people who are chronically malnourished.

Treatments exist to cure this illness, but if the underlying causes are not addressed, curative medications may last only temporarily. The problem may come right back after treatment has been completed because re-infection is likely. Conversely, once you cooperate with your healing system by addressing the underlying causes, symptoms of TB will often improve on their own. TB sanitariums, which still exist in many parts of the world, emphasize the importance of daily sunbathing and proper diets, factors that support the body's healing system.

Digestive System Disorders

Problems in the digestive system are common and are often the result of a faulty diet, in combination with stress. These problems can range from such common conditions as heartburn, acid indigestion, *esophageal reflux*, minor upset stomach, and *gastritis*, to more serious conditions.

You can often prevent and treat these conditions by working with your healing system. This means paying closer attention to the foods you eat, drinking more water, practicing stress-management techniques, and avoiding irritating or harmful substances such as coffee and alcohol. The digestive system is very susceptible to stress because of the sensitive lining of the intestines, and the rich nerve supply that connects these structures to the brain and nervous system. Increasing water intake; decreasing irritating and toxic substances such as coffee and alcohol; avoiding or minimizing acidic foods, such as vinegar, orange juice, and citrus juices; avoiding too many fried foods, fats, and oils; and going long periods without any food or liquid intake whatsoever are a few of the specific ways that you can work with your healing system to overcome most digestive-system problems. Natural remedies such as peppermint and chamomile tea, *slippery elm, deglycyrrhizinated licorice*, and aloe vera, can also be helpful. Maintaining adequate fluid and fiber intake is important to ensure timely elimination of toxins and waste products while preserving the health of your intestinal tract.

Appendicitis

In this country, *appendicitis* has traditionally been regarded as a surgical emergency because people who fail to receive timely treatment can rupture their appendix and suffer serious and sometimes fatal consequences. In fact, during abdominal surgery for other reasons, a surgeon will often remove the appendix as a preventative measure at no extra charge. Low-residue foods and foods that are highly processed, along with excess fat in the diet, can be contributing factors to appendicitis.

Appendicitis, strangely enough, is not routinely operated on in China, as it is here; rather, if the inflammation is caught in its earlier stages, it is often successfully treated with fluids and certain herbs. Even in this country, if caught early, many cases of appendicitis will respond well to clear-liquid diets. Diets high in fiber and low in fat can often help prevent this problem. Because little research has been done on the dietary influences on appendicitis, however, there is still a tendency to regard surgery as the only solution to the condition. Prevention, including the regular ingestion of adequate fiber and fluids, will help your healing system maintain the health of your appendix.

Colon Cancer

A leading cause of death in the U.S., *colon cancer* is remarkably absent in most developing countries where little meat and refined food products are consumed. The now-famous study by Dennis Burkitt, M.D., reported that there were no cases of colon cancer in African villages where people subsisted largely on vegetarian diets. Similarly, in Seventh Day Adventists, who are known vegetarians, colon-cancer rates are very low compared to the mainstream U.S. population.

In addition to diet, apparent contributors to colon cancer are dehydration, chronic constipation, stress, and emotional factors. Learning how to relax, practicing stress management, following the dietary suggestions given earlier, and instituting measures aimed at good bowel hygiene will aid your healing system and prevent colon cancer from occurring, even if it has a high rate of occurrence in your family.

Constipation

Constipation is the most common condition of the colon, or large intestines, and is most often caused by poor diet, lack of fiber, not enough fluids, stress and anxiety, and a sedentary lifestyle. The problem with constipation is that it causes toxins to back up in your system, which can contribute to other disease processes. If it is allowed to progress, constipation can result in *bowel obstruction*, which is a surgical emergency.

Increased fluid and fiber, relaxation and stress management, and increased exercise, which increases blood flow to the colon, are usually quite helpful to your healing system in preventing constipation. You can also occasionally use gentle conventional and natural laxatives for acute episodes of constipation.

Gastritis

Gastritis results most commonly from a combination of faulty diet and stress. Causes include improper food combinations, eating in a hurry, ingesting certain toxic substances such as strong coffee and alcohol, and certain carbonated sodas, acidic foods, or excessive fried or fatty substances. These substances serve to increase acid production in the stomach, which irritates the lining.

Removing these factors while drinking plenty of water and nonacidic, soothing liquids will aid your healing system in eliminating this condition. Eating more bland and soothing foods, especially during flare-ups; managing stress; and using natural soothing compounds such as aloe vera juice, deglycyrrhizinated licorice, peppermint, chamomile, and slippery-elm teas can also be quite helpful.

Gastroenteritis

Gastroenteritis is a general term that refers to irritation and inflammation of the entire gastrointestinal tract, which includes the stomach and the small and large intestines. Mild cases of food poisoning represent the ingestion of contaminated foods and are among the more common causes of gastroenteritis. Some of these cases can be severe, but most last no more than a few days. Symptoms often include nausea and vomiting, abdominal pain with cramping, and diarrhea. Fever may or may not be present.

Treatment is directed toward supporting the body's healing system, which can flush out the intestinal contaminants with the vomiting and diarrhea, especially if no solid foods are eaten. Take clear liquids in abundance for the first 48 hours, without any solid foods. It is important not to introduce solid food that can feed the offending organisms and slow down your body's healing processes. If fever is present, antibiotics may be necessary for a few days, particularly if you are traveling overseas or are in an exotic tropical locale where your body may not be used to the local flora and contaminants in that part of the world.

Hepatitis

Inflammation of the liver is called *hepatitis*, and there are many causes for the different types of hepatitis. Cases of hepatitis can be acute and isolated, or chronic and debilitating. *Viral hepatitis* is contracted through various infectious sources. Viral hepatitis now appears in multiple forms, including hepatitis A, B, C, non-A, non-B, and many more. Hepatitis A is usually contracted by eating or drinking contaminated food or water, or through sharing contaminated eating utensils. Most other forms of hepatitis, such as B, C, and others, are most commonly contracted through unsafe sexual practices, contaminated needles, or blood transfusions. *Alcoholic hepatitis* is due to the chronic irritation and consumption of alcohol and can lead to *cirrhosis* of the liver, which causes scarring, abnormal growth, and other complications, including *liver cancer*.

Conventional Western medicine has little to offer in the way of medications to improve the health of the liver. Most treatments for hepatitis, as in chemotherapy for cancer, are aimed at attacking the supposed agents of disease, and they may be even more damaging to the liver than the agents themselves.

Diet is extremely important in supporting your healing system when you have hepatitis. Nutritional elements that help support the health of your liver include foods high in beta carotene, including turmeric and all yellow and orange vegetables and fruit. Consuming plenty of fiber and fluids is also important. High-fat diets and low-residue foods seem to aggravate liver conditions. The herb milk thistle and its extracted alkaloid, *silymarin*, can be helpful for certain liver conditions. Traditional medicines from India and China also appear to be promising. Stress management, visualization and guided imagery, and emotional release of anger can also be very helpful for liver conditions. Because the liver is so important and so difficult to treat, practicing preventive medicine is essential to avoid these liver conditions.

Inflammatory Bowel Disease

Inflammatory bowel disease includes a large category of intestinal conditions such as *colitis, irritable bowel syndrome, spastic colon, Crohn's disease,* and *ulcerative colitis.* Diarrhea, abdominal pain, and cramping are common during flare-ups in patients with inflammatory bowel disorders, which behave similarly to autoimmune diseases. Like other chronic intestinal diseases, these conditions are influenced by dietary factors and stress. During times of stress, the nerves in the intestines can become hyperstimulated and irritate the delicate intestinal lining. For these reasons, these conditions have a higher occurrence in people who are under long-term stress, those who are high achievers, and those with perfectionist tendencies.

Conventional treatments, including drugs and surgery; a combination of stress-management techniques, including guided imagery and visualization; and special dietary practices are most helpful to the healing system in managing these conditions. An effective diet for these disorders is one that is bland, gentle, and soothing, and that consists of adequate fiber. Okra is ideal for people with inflammatory bowel problems because it contains adequate fiber and is also gentle and soothing, a rare dietary combination. Other natural substances that can assist your healing system in helping to soothe and heal inflamed intestinal surfaces are water, slippery elm and chamomile teas, aloe vera, and deglycyrrhizinated licorice.

Alternative approaches, including Ayurvedic medicine, Chinese herbal medicines, acupuncture, and yoga, can also assist your healing system to help reverse these conditions. Addressing problems related to these disorders early on is important because these conditions can contribute to problems elsewhere in the body. Those problems include anemia, vitamin deficiencies, and syndromes related to poor absorption of essential nutrients; if not brought under control, those conditions can worsen.

Stomach Ulcers and Duodenal Ulcers

Commonly referred to as *peptic ulcers, stomach ulcers* and *duodenal ulcers* are areas of the stomach that become deteriorated by stomach acid. Indigestion and abdominal pain in the upper abdomen and lower chest often accompany stomach ulcers, and, sometimes, the ulcers can bleed. Stomach ulcers often have similar causes to inflammatory bowel disease, but they represent a more persistent and chronic imbalance in the digestive system. In recent years, a bacterium known as *H. pylori* has been implicated in the cause of certain ulcers, but stress also is known to be a big factor in these conditions.

In the acute stages of an ulcer, treatment depends on stopping the bleeding if it has already begun. A more long-term approach includes learning how to manage stress and changing your eating habits to support your healing system. Drinking more water and eating a blander, more neutral, gentle, soothing, less acidic, less flesh-oriented diet that consists of non-irritating foods are most helpful. Eliminate caffeine, nicotine, and alcohol from your diet if you have ulcers. Acting early to institute these measures will help prevent ulcers from developing in the first place. Stress-management techniques and learning how to relax are extremely helpful for the treatment and prevention of ulcers. Many gentle, soothing natural supplements, such as peppermint and chamomile tea, deglycyrrhizinated licorice, slippery elm, in addition to the more traditional antacids and acid-blocking drugs, are often effective to help your healing system in the short- and long-term management of ulcers.

Urinary System Disorders

The kidneys are the main filters and organs of your body that eliminate liquid waste products. Your kidneys require adequate fluid intake and regular flushing, and they can become unhealthy if you don't drink enough fluids. Other factors that can be harmful to your kidneys include the regular ingestion of certain toxic substances, and long-standing high blood pressure and diabetes, conditions that, if treated early or prevented, will most often not harm your kidneys.

Kidney Stones

Kidney stones are another fairly common and very painful problem. Kidney stones are made of stone-like material that forms in the kidneys and then attempts to pass down from the ureters into the bladder, and from the bladder through the urethra. Kidney stones can be extremely painful, and they almost always cause a small amount of blood in the urine. If kidney stones are large, they can block the ureters and may require surgical removal.

Some stones can be blasted out by sound waves, a technique known as *lithotripsy*. Stress, dehydration, hormonal imbalance, faulty diet, and excess caffeine and nicotine can all contribute to the formation of kidney stones. Stress management, drinking plenty of fluids, and avoiding alcohol and caffeine all help to support your healing system to prevent and eliminate kidney stones.

Urinary-Tract Infections

Urinary-tract infections include *bladder infections*, which are more common in women than in men and can lead to serious kidney infections. Urinary-tract infections can easily be prevented if good bladder and bowel hygiene are maintained. Once you have contracted a urinary-tract infection, however, antibiotic therapy is mandatory to prevent further spread and damage to the kidneys. In adult women, the most common activity associated with urinary-tract infections is sexual intercourse, and most women instinctively know to urinate after sex to prevent this from happening. Another more prudent preventive measure is to take a bath or shower in the morning after you have moved your bowels. Doing this will eliminate the bacteria that are associated with these infections. Along with lots of fluids, certain herbs, such as *uva ursi*, juniper berries, and other natural substances such as cranberry, can help your healing system maintain the health of your kidneys, bladder, and urinary tract.

Female Reproductive System Disorders

The female reproductive system is extremely sensitive and complex. It operates on a cycle, responding to nerve transmissions from the brain and hormonal messages from the pituitary gland. At the same time, it is producing its own hormones in the form of estrogen and progesterone that feed back to these other organs.

Problems in the reproductive system may reflect hormonal imbalances that originate in other parts of the body, and such problems often flare up during times of mental and emotional stress. An unhealthy diet, including excess caffeine, nicotine, and alcohol, and other harmful lifestyle factors may also contribute to problems of the female reproductive system. Sexually transmitted diseases can also damage the reproductive system. To help your healing system maintain the health of your reproductive system, follow the recommendations for overall health given in previous chapters, try appropriate natural herbs, and eat a wholesome, healthy diet. An excellent resource on how you can improve the health of your reproductive system is Dr. Christiane Northrup's best-selling book, *Women's Bodies, Women's Wisdom.*

Cancer of the Female Reproductive System

The female reproductive system is one of the most common sites for cancer to appear. There are two reasons for this. First, the female reproductive system is extremely sensitive and vulnerable, and it intimately interacts with other systems in your body. Second, the cells of this system are some of the most rapidly dividing, active, and volatile cell populations of any tissue in the body. *Cervical cancer, ovarian cancer, uterine cancer,* and *breast cancer* are the predominant types of cancer, male or female, on this entire earth. I address the subject of cancer and how to deal with it in more detail later in this chapter.

Menopause

It is during this time in a woman's life that ovulation and menstruation gradually end, resulting in diminishing levels of estrogen in the blood. The question of estrogen (hormonal) replacement therapy to prevent osteoporosis and heart disease that can occur following menopause is an ongoing area of debate among experts. Although estrogen replacement may be appropriate in certain cases, it also has an associated risk of increased reproductive-system cancer. Because of this risk, the use of natural, plant-derived estrogens and substances that work with the healing system are becoming more popular. These options are generally safer, gentler, and often just as effective as more conventional forms of estrogen. Also, new evidence with NASA astronauts who experienced osteoporosis while they were in prolonged zero-gravity conditions showed that their osteoporosis could be reversed by their resuming normal weight-bearing activities once they were back on earth. The late actor, Christopher Reeve, a quadriplegic, who also developed osteoporosis due to inactivity, was able to reverse this condition as well by resuming weight-bearing exercises. Clearly, there is more to osteoporosis than merely menopause and estrogen.

In generations past, menopause was accepted as a natural condition of life, with little evidence that it caused increased risk of heart disease or osteoporosis. While the lack of estrogen may play a role in these conditions, certainly, other more important risk factors also need to be considered.

Premenstrual Syndrome (PMS)

Premenstrual syndrome, or *PMS*, is a common, painful disorder that occurs around the time of menstruation and involves cramping of the uterine muscles. It may also include headaches and other associated symptoms, sometimes so severe that they can be disabling.

Stress, tension, emotional upheaval, lack of exercise, poor diet, dehydration, and excessive caffeine and alcohol can make PMS symptoms worse. For women who are always on the go, it is important to ease back a little on normal activities and listen to their bodies during menstruation, a time of blood loss and sloughing of reproductive tissues. Drink plenty of fluids, decrease caffeine and alcohol intake, practice stress-management and visualization techniques, and rest to support your healing system at these times. Natural herbs, such as *cramp bark*, raspberry tea, and *dong quai*, can help alleviate PMS symptoms. Acupuncture, gentle yoga stretching, breathing, and massage may also be helpful. Other disorders of the female reproductive system, such as *endometriosis, uterine fibroids, ovarian cysts,* and *fibrocystic breast disease* often reflect hormonal imbalances, which, if caught early, can successfully respond to methods that work with your healing system. Some of these methods are proper diet, stress management, increased fluid intake, and natural medications and treatments.

Male Reproductive System Disorders

Male Menopause

Recent research shows that men may go through a male equivalent to female menopause, when, around the ages of approximately 45 to 65, their testosterone levels become diminished, and they can suffer from mood swings and depression. Standardized doses of testosterone are currently available to supplement low testosterone levels, and natural sources of testosterone that work more harmoniously with your healing system are also currently being researched.

Prostate Cancer

Prostate cancer has now become one of the most common types of cancer in men. New research on prostate health and prostate cancer, being conducted by Dr. Dean Ornish, Dr. Ruth Marlin, and others at the University of California, San Francisco, and at Sloan Kettering Cancer Institute in New York, is showing that diet and emotional factors, including stress, play a significant role in prostate cancer and other disorders of the prostate. In addition to these studies, many case reports and books are beginning to demonstrate successful treatments for overcoming prostate cancer using methods that naturally work with your body's healing system. *Prostate Health in 90 Days* is an excellent book by Larry Clapp, a lawyer who had prostate cancer and successfully overcame it with methods that work with the body's healing system.

Prostate Enlargement

Also known as *benign prostatic hypertrophy*, or *BPH*, this condition compresses and encroaches upon the urethra, which is the tube leading from the bladder through the penis. Prostate enlargement makes passing urine difficult. In advanced cases, a man may have to wake up 6 to10 times or more a night to urinate because with BPH, the bladder never fully empties.

In addition to conventional medicines, *saw palmetto*, a natural herb that works with your healing system by shrinking and reducing swelling in the prostate, can often be very helpful for BPH. A low-fat diet, increased fluids and fiber, and reducing overall body tension by learning how to relax can also support your healing system in preventing and minimizing symptoms of BPH. BPH is not related to prostate cancer.

Testicular Cancer

This form of cancer frequently afflicts younger males. If testicular cancer is caught in its early stages and given appropriate medical treatment, accompanied by lifestyle changes that help support the body's healing system, it is often curable. The subject of cancer is discussed more thoroughly later in this chapter.

Lymphatic System Disorders

Your lymphatic vessels, channels, and lymph nodes make up your lymph system, which shares an important relationship with your body's immune and healing systems. The white blood cells of your immune system, which help fight infection and keep your blood clean, circulate in the lymph fluid. Lymph-node enlargement, which represents white-blood-cell proliferation and activation, occurs in response to infections.

Serious disorders of the lymphatic system include *Hodgkin's disease, lymphoma,* and other *lymphatic cancers*, which represent generalized, weakened conditions of the body. Conventional treatments such as radiation can often be helpful for these conditions, but it is also important to use natural methods that work with your healing system, such as stress management, eating a healthy, wholesome diet, increasing fluid intake, and using other natural medicines and herbs. If caught early, these conditions of the lymphatic system are easier to eradicate. A famous success story of a person who overcame lymphatic cancer is Lance Armstrong, legendary *Tour de France* champion and author of *It's Not About the Bike.*

Nervous System Disorders

Disorders of the nerves are some of the more complex and difficult of all conditions to treat. These challenges are because of the intricate interactions between your brain, your nervous system, your mind, and your emotions.

Central Nervous System Disorders

Central nervous system disorders often involve the brain and are usually serious. They include such conditions as the following:

- *Alzheimer's disease*, characterized by a loss of short-term memory.

- *Cerebral palsy*, which appears early in life and is a debilitating condition related to birth trauma or other congenital problems; cerebral palsy results in speech and movement disturbances.

- *Epilepsy*, which includes a wide range of conditions that cause seizures.

- *Multiple sclerosis*, thought to be an autoimmune disease, with symptoms including progressive weakness, loss of balance, lack of coordination, and speech and visual disturbances.

- *Parkinson's disease*, characterized by tremors, a shuffling walk, and rigidity.

- *Spinal-cord disorders*, which are usually trauma related and result in life-altering paralysis of one degree or another.

Because of the seriousness of central nervous system disorders and the difficulties in treating them once they are established, the focus should be on working with your healing system to prevent them. Conventional medicines may be necessary to help manage these problems once they are established, supported by good nutrition and natural medicines. *Gingko biloba*, which has been shown to increase blood flow to the brain, may be helpful in selected cases of Alzheimer's and Parkinson's diseases. Stress management, including relaxation training and breathing techniques, have a natural calming effect on the mind and brain, and they help manage these conditions by stabilizing the electrical activity of the nervous system. Stress-management techniques are also effective in relieving pain and tension resulting from these conditions. Gentle yoga techniques can also support the healing system by improving balance and coordination. Acupuncture, music therapy, and massage can also be helpful.

The most important thing you can do is pay attention to the underlying causes of these conditions and start treatment in the earliest stages when symptoms are less severe. Exciting new research in the field of nerve regeneration is investigating procedures that support the healing system's ability to mend damaged nerves and create new pathways for victims of spinal cord injury and other diseases of the central nervous system.

Peripheral Neuropathies

Peripheral neuropathies are nerve disorders that usually involve the extremities. These disorders include *diabetic neuropathy, sciatica* and *"pinched nerves,"* and *nutritional neuropathies,* such as those caused by vitamin B_{12} deficiency, (*pernicious anemia),* or thiamin deficiency, (*beriberi).* Because these conditions are often associated with other health problems that are both correctable and preventable, addressing those underlying factors is the key to working with your healing system to improve and reverse the nerve disorders. Paying attention to good nutrition and incorporating stress management and other natural methods that work with your healing system can go a long way toward improving these conditions.

Musculoskeletal Disorders

Problems in the muscles and bones are common and range from bruises and contusions to fractures and other conditions.

Fractures

Fractures heal best with adequate calcium and vitamin D, rest, immobilization, plenty of fluids, natural sunlight, proper nutrition, and natural medicines that support your healing system. Because of your healing system's amazing ability to mend and remodel bone, most fractures heal uneventfully once the bones are held in place by either a cast or splint. The largest bone in the body, the femur, takes just six weeks to heal from a simple fracture.

Some complex fractures might require assistance with methods such as bone setting and open surgical reduction using plates, rods, screws, and pins, as well as electrical bone stimulation, but most fractures may not even require casting. This was demonstrated in a well-known study involving Nigerian bone doctors, who never went to medical school, yet they showed that the fractures they treated using only sticks healed in the same amount of time as those treated with modern methods in a large hospital in America.

Muscular Injuries

Injuries of the muscles are common. If muscles are strong and overdeveloped, but not flexible or relaxed, the likelihood of injuries increases because of their stiffness and rigidity. Additionally, because your muscles are connected to your nerves, mental tension and stress can also cause muscular tension and stiffness. These conditions contribute to muscle pain, and they are often contributing factors to many muscular and neuromuscular disorders, including back pain and *fibromyalgia*. Dietary factors and other lifestyle and personal health habits also play a major role in these conditions.

A healthy muscle is one that is strong, flexible, and relaxed; so regularly stretching and relaxing all the muscles in your body, in addition to exercising, are important. Yoga is a gentle, systematic approach to ensuring proper health of your muscles through exercises that lengthen, stretch, and relax the muscles while building tone and strength. Anyone with a muscular condition would do well to investigate the possibility of adding yoga to his or her overall healing program.

Osteoporosis

Common in post-menopausal women, *osteoporosis* represents a loss of bone density and strength. Many experts believe this condition is caused by a lack of estrogen; however, newer research on astronauts shows that a lack of weight-bearing exercise may play a larger role. There is evidence that stress, which affects the endocrine system and influences calcium metabolism, and high-protein diets, which can leech calcium from bone, may also contribute to the condition.

Osteoporosis can be prevented and often reversed by regular weight-bearing exercise and stretching, adequate vitamin D and calcium, stress management, and a healthy, wholesome diet that supports your healing system.

Joint Disorders

Because you are constantly moving, your joints are subject to wear and tear, and they are a common site for painful problems and disturbances. Joint diseases are particularly common in the Western developed world. Ironically, these conditions are relatively rare in most developing countries where activities and lifestyles are less sedentary.

Gout

Known as the "rich man's disease," *gout* is caused by excess uric acid production, often the result of rich foods such as meat and flesh products. Gout is virtually absent among poor populations, which subsist predominantly on vegetables and grains. Gout is entirely curable and preventable, and it responds well to reducing or abstaining from all meats, fowl, and seafood. In addition, increasing fluid intake and avoiding coffee and alcohol can prevent flare-ups of this condition.

Osteoarthritis

Most doctors believe that *osteoarthritis* is caused by the steady wear and tear of joints. This condition can be prevented and reversed by following methods that work with your healing system. These include gentle stretching of the muscles that surround the affected joints, and increased consumption of fluids, including fruit and vegetable juices. Movement therapies such as yoga, tai chi, and swimming; acupuncture; and visualization and guided imagery can also be very helpful for this condition. Certain foods and natural supplements such as *glucosamine* may also be helpful.

Rheumatoid Arthritis

Now considered an autoimmune problem, *rheumatoid arthritis* is caused by dysfunction in the lines of communication among the immune system, the endocrine system, and your brain. Emotional upheaval often precedes painful flare-ups of rheumatoid arthritis. Dr. George Freeman Solomon, at UCLA, who is one of the world's foremost authorities on rheumatoid arthritis, has identified several psychological factors, such as repressed anger, that can alter the chemistry of your internal environment and trigger destructive autoimmune responses that affect joint surfaces. Other factors may also be present in this condition. If caught in its early stages, rheumatoid arthritis often responds well to physical therapy, stretching, diet, and stress-management practices, including breathing and imagery, all strategies that help support your healing system.

Disorders of the Hands, Feet, and Extremities

Hand Problems

The hands are subject to overuse and abuse, and consequently they are a common site for the occurrence of arthritis, particularly in later years. This arthritis is often due to chronic tension in the fingers, which eventually causes the muscles to fix the joints in a particular position, which subsequently leads to irritation, swelling, inflammation, and joint pain.

Working with your healing system by addressing the underlying causes of these problems, along with regular gentle extension of the muscles and tendons that control the movement of the fingers, can help reverse and prevent this problem. Arthritis of the hands is easier to manage or cure if you catch it early and if you incorporate methods that work with your healing system into your daily life.

Carpal Tunnel Syndrome

Carpal tunnel syndrome is a chronic condition of the wrists related to overuse of the wrist joints. Surgery is often performed in more severe cases. However, this condition responds well to methods that work with your healing system, such as physical therapy and gentle, persistent stretching like that found in yoga therapy. In fact, the effectiveness of yoga therapy for carpal tunnel syndrome was documented in a study that appeared in the *Journal of the American Medical Association.*

Foot Problems

Your feet bear the entire weight of your body, and if you do not properly care for them, they can cause endless misery—so much so, that an entire specialty, known as *podiatry*, exists just to tend to the feet alone.

Corns, Heel Spurs, Plantar Fasciitis, and Plantar Warts

Corns, heel spurs, plantar fasciitis, and plantar warts are all common conditions of the feet. They are often caused by improperly fitted shoes, or imbalances created by improper movement while walking, standing, jogging, or participating in sports and other strenuous activities. Although these conditions are so painful at times that they can be incapacitating, they can usually be reversed quite readily once the underlying causes are addressed. Stretching the muscles of the feet, toes, and legs; taking warm foot baths; going barefoot whenever possible; and applying gentle, soothing natural creams such as turmeric or calendula that soften the skin and support healing processes all serve as valuable aids to your healing system as it works to alleviate these conditions. Additionally, wearing roomy, comfortable shoes and getting regular foot massages can often help your healing system correct these problems. *Reflexology* is a type of massage that involves nerve meridians that connect areas of the feet to other parts of the body; it can be very effective for problems involving the nerves and muscles of the feet.

Disorders of the Spine

Spine disorders represent a special and more complex aspect of musculoskeletal joint diseases. There are 24 joints in the human spine, and each one is subject to a potential problem if it is not properly cared for.

Back Pain

Back pain is the single most common cause of work disability in the United States. Approximately 100 billion dollars is spent annually on this problem. Back pain comes in various forms and severity and is associated with common diagnostic names such as *spinal arthritis, spondylosis, spondylolisthesis, degenerative disc disease, ankylosis spondylitis, scoliosis, herniated* and *ruptured discs, spinal stenosis,* and *sciatica.* Long-standing histories of poor posture, stress, physical abuse, repetitive injuries, and inadequate diet often contribute to these conditions.

Even long-standing, stubborn cases of back pain can be reversed if you address the underlying causes and use methods that work with your healing system, such as developing proper spine mechanics, gentle stretching, eating a healthy, wholesome diet, and managing stress. In my previous book, *Healing Back Pain Naturally*, I address the underlying causes, treatment, and ways to prevent this common, debilitating group of maladies in a simple, organized manner that will allow you to work with your healing system to overcome these problems.

Circulatory System Disorders

Heart Disease

Heart disease is the number-one killer in the Western world, and it comes in several forms. The most common type of heart disease, known as *coronary artery disease*, is caused by *atherosclerosis*, or clogging of the arteries of the heart. Coronary artery disease can lead to sudden death from heart attack and claims more lives than all other diseases combined, including cancer, diabetes, accidents, or infections.

High-fat diets, stress, lack of exercise, repression of anger and inhibition of emotions, social isolation, and a lack of intimacy all have been shown to be significant contributing factors to heart disease. Dr. Dean Ornish's groundbreaking work on the reversal of heart disease without drugs or surgery is based on a program that incorporates simple, yet powerful, natural methods that work with your healing system. These include eating a low-fat diet, performing moderate but regular exercise, practicing stress management and relaxation, and learning how to express emotions and share feelings in a supportive group environment. When you learn to work with your healing system, even the worst and most dangerous disease in the world can be healed naturally.

High Blood Pressure

Also known as *hypertension*, *high blood pressure* is referred to as "the silent killer." It is a serious circulatory disease that, if not treated properly, can cause heart disease and stroke. This common disease is caused by constriction and narrowing of the arteries and smaller blood vessels, which increases the pressure of the blood flow inside them. The effect is similar to what happens when you place your thumb or finger over the end of a garden hose to spray the water out further and faster.

Because the smooth muscles that control the diameter of your blood vessels are, in turn, controlled by nerves that are connected to your brain, your blood pressure can become elevated when you are under stress. This can occur when you are upset, excited, frightened, or worried. Conversely, when you are calm and relaxed, your blood pressure tends to automatically become lower.

Medicines are available to artificially control high blood pressure, but many of them have side effects that can interfere with the quality of your life. Whether or not you are currently taking medications, it is critical for you to work with your healing system by learning how to relax and manage your stress to help bring your blood pressure down. Lowering your blood pressure this way will lower your risk of stroke and heart disease and reduce your dependence on medications. Losing weight has also been shown to reduce blood pressure, as has exercise. In addition to cutting out caffeine and nicotine, which are both known to elevate blood pressure, some natural medicines can aid your healing system by supporting circulation and keeping your blood vessels calm and relaxed.

Stroke

Stroke is a well-known circulatory disorder most often caused by underlying complications of long-standing high blood pressure. The prolonged, increased pressure in the blood vessels that go to the brain eventually causes the vessels to burst, rupture, and bleed. A second mechanism that causes stroke occurs when small blood clots, usually generated from an irregularly beating heart, become lodged in the brain's circulatory paths and clog the blood vessels that nourish the brain.

Stroke, which can be severely incapacitating and even fatal, most commonly results in paralysis of one side of the body, typically an arm and a leg. Other structures on the face may also be affected, such as the tongue, mouth, lips, and cheeks. Speech and swallowing are often affected. Memory loss and loss of other mental faculties can also occur.

For those who can keep their spirits up during the hard work of the stroke rehabilitation phase, the body's healing system can often restore the body to practically normal functioning, although this process might take months or even years. The body can do this by accessing duplicate information on the undamaged side of the brain and transferring it to the affected side, and connecting new nerve pathways to compensate for the damaged portion that previously controlled these functions. Once the brain learns to make the necessary new connections, seemingly dead, paralyzed limbs and muscles miraculously can come back to life. Because of the body's healing system, even under circumstances where all hope appears lost, many people have been able to resume normal lives once again after they have suffered a stroke.

Endocrine System Disorders

The endocrine system consists of important organs and glands that produce powerful hormones that are involved in a wide range of functions. Because of its extensive connections, the endocrine system may become imbalanced and dysfunctional as the result of underlying problems elsewhere in the body. For example, nutritional and metabolic problems can affect the endocrine system, and vice versa. The most common endocrine disorder is *diabetes*, which is a derangement of sugar or glucose metabolism, usually caused by insulin deficiency.

Chronic Fatigue Syndrome

Chronic fatigue syndrome is a relatively new disorder that is more common in women and also is somewhat baffling to treat by conventional medical practices. Experts who specialize in the treatment of the disorder believe exhaustion of the adrenal glands may be an important factor. Prolonged stress and a lack of rest appear to be major factors in chronic fatigue syndrome. Many patients with this syndrome report extreme fatigue after living hectic, fast-paced lives, in which the pressures that surround them are enormous and they haven't rested or relaxed for many years. When the body is under considerable stress and lacks quality sleep and rest, it is only natural that it will suffer from a lack of energy and eventually become fatigued.

With chronic fatigue syndrome, there may other concomitant problems, such as yeast infections and fibromyalgia, in addition to accompanying depression and other psychological factors that further deplete physical energy and prevent the condition from healing sooner. Psychological factors might include the fear of getting well and becoming overwhelmed again by the demands of work and other responsibilities. These factors may serve as impediments to the healing system's ability to do its job in a timely and efficient manner. To prevent this from happening, and to work with your healing system to restore natural health and energy, it is imperative to incorporate adequate sleep and rest into your lifestyle; focus on a healthy, wholesome diet; drink plenty of fluids; practice stress management; and participate in a regular physical exercise and movement program.

Diabetes

There are several ways to classify *diabetes* and the stages of this illness. The two main types of diabetes have traditionally been broken down into *Type I, juvenile onset, insulin-dependent diabetes* and *Type II, maturity onset,* or *adult diabetes*, which often starts out as non-insulin dependent, but may become insulin dependent over time. *Insulin dependent* refers to the need to inject insulin from a syringe into your body to help bring your blood sugar under control.

The danger of high blood sugar, which is the common denominator of all types of diabetes, is that it can damage blood vessels in the eyes, causing blindness. It can also damage the kidneys, causing kidney failure, and contribute to other problems, such as nerve damage, and chronic skin ulcers on the feet and ankles, as well. There also is a strong associated risk of heart disease in people who suffer from diabetes.

Adult, or maturity onset, Type II diabetes has been traditionally linked to obesity, a diet high in sugar, and a lack of exercise. It also appears to be related to stress, depression, emotional upheaval, and unresolved grief, conditions that influence personal health habits and diet, which in turn significantly influence the course of this disease. Although some researchers have tried to link this form of diabetes to genetic causes, the evidence clearly points more toward lifestyle factors, including stress and diet, since this type of diabetes is rare in developing countries, but on the rise in Western countries. The good news is that this type of diabetes can be reversed when you catch it early and apply methods that work with your healing system.

The juvenile form of diabetes, Type I, occurs at a much younger age and can often be severe. In the past, many experts believed that juvenile diabetes was an autoimmune illness triggered by a virus or another infection, but newer research points toward stress and deranged mind-body interactions that occur during periods of intense emotional upheaval in the individual or family, or during gestation. This changed perspective is due in part to the discovery that insulin communicates directly with the brain and is now classified as a *neuropeptide* or *neurotransmitter*, rather than as a pure hormone. The current view is further based on the scientific observation that more insulin can be found at any one time in the brain than in any other organ or structure in the body.

Newer treatments for diabetes that address the underlying causes, rather than merely manage the symptoms, involve methods that work with your healing system. These treatments include eating a proper diet, getting adequate exercise, practicing stress-management techniques, drinking plenty of water, taking natural medications, and addressing the deeper emotional, mental, and spiritual factors that may be driving this unhealthy condition. These strategies are obviously more effective if they are instituted in the early stages of the illness. Insulin may be required until these other methods are well established, but a large number of patients have successfully weaned themselves from insulin dependence in a relatively short period of time. During my tenure as a medical student more than 20 years ago, getting patients off insulin was considered an impossibility. If diabetes happens to run in your family, focus on incorporating preventive strategies before the illness has a chance to surface in your body.

Thyroid Dysfunction

Thyroid dysfunction is more common in women than in men, and it occurs fairly frequently. It occurs in several forms, most commonly *hypothyroidism,* or low production of the thyroid hormone, which usually requires supplementation. When low thyroid function is corrected with thyroid hormone replacement, there is an increase in metabolism, greater energy, improved mood, and loss of weight. These are desirable qualities for an overweight person who may suffer from fatigue and depression, but the long-term effects of supplementing with thyroid hormone when it may not be absolutely necessary are unknown.

Additionally, because the thyroid gland is under the domain of the pituitary gland, which is under the domain of the hypothalamus and the brain, thyroid dysfunction usually indicates problems higher up the chain of command, which need to be addressed if one is to get to the root of the problem. Unfortunately, Western medicine usually ignores these underlying causes in the treatment of thyroid conditions.

In many cases, you can support your healing system by addressing the underlying factors that may be responsible for thyroid dysfunction, such as stress, dietary imbalances, lack of exercise, and an unhealthy lifestyle. Implementing the methods that strengthen and fortify your healing system, as shared in previous chapters, can be most helpful.

Immune-System Disorders

Very little was known about the powerful and sophisticated intricacies of the immune system before the onset of the devastating AIDS epidemic. We still have a long way to go, but, because of AIDS and the HIV virus, today we know much more than ever before.

Allergies

Every person is created as a unique individual and as a result may have specific sensitivities to certain substances or environmental conditions. These sensitivities, if prolonged or pronounced, can develop into an allergy. The most common types of allergies affect the skin and respiratory system, and we have already discussed those under these separate headings.

Allergies are often system specific. This means that only one system at a time may be sensitive to a particular substance. For example, if dust is breathed into the lungs, the dust may cause coughing, wheezing, and a runny nose, but if it is placed on the skin, dust may not cause any reaction at all. A substance that causes an allergic rash may not cause any reaction whatsoever when it is placed on the skin, chewed, swallowed, and eaten.

To overcome allergies in general, focus on building up the health of the specific system that is affected by the allergy. Employ the methods discussed in previous chapters that strengthen and fortify your healing system as it relates to the affected system.

Chemical and Drug Allergies

Chemical and drug allergies are common with medications and in medical settings. These include allergies to medicines such as penicillin and other antibiotics; mineral dyes, such as iodine; and other drugs or chemicals. These allergies may show up in the form of a skin rash, or they may even result in a serious, life-threatening situation.

Effective conventional medications are currently available to help manage and suppress the acute symptoms of allergy from whatever cause. For long-term treatment, however, it is better not to suppress your symptoms, but instead to work with your healing system to overcome the allergy. You can do this by carefully observing how your body interacts with each and every suspected allergen in your environment. Even though discovering the true source of any allergy may require a bit of tedious detective work, if you cooperate with your healing system in this manner, sooner or later you will be able to identify the offending agent, take precautions to avoid further exposure or contact with it, and eliminate its unhealthy influence on your body.

Food Allergies

Food allergies are less common than those of the skin and respiratory system. Food allergies include conditions that may not be true allergies, such as *lactose intolerance,* one of the most common of all suspected food allergies. With lactose intolerance, the body lacks a specific enzyme and is simply unable to digest foods that contain lactose, which is a simple sugar found in dairy products. This enzyme is lacking in the majority of people from the Orient and many other parts of the world. In fact, lactose intolerance is not a true allergy but merely a normal variant found in certain ethnic groups. Many other suspected allergies have similar stories.

Many synthetic chemicals used in industry are harmful and irritating to the human body. Because new synthetic chemicals are continuously being introduced into our food supply, it is not surprising to find that food-related allergies are becoming more common. To minimize the risk of exposure to such allergens, it is important to know exactly what you are introducing into your body when you eat. Variety is the spice of life, but to avoid food allergies, avoid foods with chemical additives whenever possible.

Cooperate with your healing system by eating foods from organic and natural sources that are free from chemical pesticides, pollutants, and additives. You can also work with your healing system to keep your digestive system free from irritating and toxic substances by consuming plenty of fluids and fiber, and practicing good intestinal hygiene.

Acquired Immune Deficiency Syndrome (AIDS)

AIDS is an example of what can happen to your body when the immune system is impaired. When the immune system is compromised, your body can become afflicted by organisms that cause infections and disorders that, under normal circumstances, would not occur.

Where the HIV virus initially came from is still controversial, but it is clear that those whose immune systems are already impaired and worn down are at higher risk. This virus can be found among people with multiple sexual partners, repeated intravenous drug use, or poor personal health habits.

AIDS is entirely preventable by practicing safe sex, abstaining from illegal intravenous drug use, and avoiding blood transfusions from unknown sources. The additional good news is that many people currently afflicted with HIV are learning to work with their healing systems to improve their health. This approach includes concentrating on healthy diets, drinking plenty of fluids, exercising, practicing stress management, including visualization/imagery techniques, and relying on natural medicines and modalities that support the rebuilding and restoration of the immune system. Many people with HIV are now symptom free, and, in selected cases, a complete conversion from HIV positive back to HIV negative has been reported.

In the beginning much shame was associated with HIV infection, but those with this condition who are able to love and accept themselves, and to open up to the loving support that is available from their families, friends, and communities, seem to have the greatest success in dealing with this difficult problem. As infected individuals learn to strengthen, fortify, and cooperate with their bodies' healing systems, it is highly likely that this disease will one day be declared completely curable, as has happened with other dreadful diseases from the past.

Anaphylaxis

Anaphylaxis is a less common but more serious form of an allergic reaction that can occur with bee, wasp, and other insect stings; jellyfish stings; and bites by other venomous animals. Anaphylaxis also can occur as a reaction to other substances, including pharmaceuticals.

Keeping your mind calm and relaxed is critical in the early stages of severe allergic reactions that might possibly become anaphylactic reactions. Remaining calm is essential because psychological factors such as stress, anxiety, and tension can increase the symptoms. Stress management and breathing techniques can be helpful for anaphylaxis, but, as explained in an earlier chapter, it is best to learn these techniques before any medical emergency occurs. To prevent anaphylaxis, be careful with new foods, especially when you are traveling, and exercise caution when you introduce new drugs or substances into your body.

Autoimmune Diseases

This rapidly growing category of illnesses describes conditions that occur as a result of a derangement in the immune system that causes it to attack normal body tissues. Illnesses in the autoimmune disease category include *rheumatoid arthritis, ankylosing spondylitis, lupus, Sjogren's syndrome, scleroderma,* and *multiple sclerosis,* among many others. Some researchers feel that viruses and certain bacteria can trigger the immune system to attack normal body tissues, but new research suggests that these conditions represent complex mind-body interactions because they almost always worsen during times of stress. Behavioral scientists also believe that autoimmune dysfunction may be a reflection of deep-seated hostility, self-hatred, or resentment that causes elements of the immune system, acting under orders from the brain, to inadvertently attack the body. These scientists believe that self-destructive thoughts, if persistent and prolonged, can lead to physical self-destruction through powerful neurochemicals released from the brain. As the eminent cardiologist Dr. Robert Eliot said, "The brain writes prescriptions for the body." It is becoming increasingly clearer over time that this is indeed true, so this current perspective is not an unreasonable explanation for the origin of many difficult-to-treat autoimmune illnesses.

Ankylosing Spondylitis

Ankylosing spondylitis is a severe form of arthritis of the spine. Stress and emotional trauma appear to worsen this condition. Conventional treatment is largely focused on suppressing the symptoms, and it is not very effective. Working with methods that support your healing system, such as stress management, gentle yoga stretching, and a wholesome, natural diet, can be extremely helpful for this condition. In his best-selling book *Anatomy of An Illness*, Norman Cousins described his journey of complete recovery from an advanced case of ankylosing spondylitis. He attributed his success to learning to use the powers of his mind and body while he incorporated other, simple, natural methods, including large doses of vitamin C and laughter, which activated his healing system to overcome this autoimmune disorder.

Multiple Sclerosis

In her groundbreaking book *Who Said So? A Woman's Fascinating Journey of Self Discovery and Triumph over Multiple Sclerosis*, Rachelle Breslow documented the mind-body factors that contributed to her own case of multiple sclerosis. She was told by her conventional doctors that her condition was incurable, but she proved them wrong. By learning to work with her healing system, eating a healthy, wholesome diet, incorporating stress-management strategies and positive mental programming, and initiating other beneficial lifestyle changes, she was eventually able to overcome this so-called incurable disease.

These strategies are entirely consistent with a comprehensive program based on the principles of working with the body's healing system, and they demonstrate what is also possible for you.

Autoimmune Disorders and Your Healing System

In addition to the experiences of Rachelle Breslow and Norman Cousins, there is now growing evidence, from both clinical case reports and laboratory data collected from various research programs around the country, that immune function, operating under the direction of the brain and nervous system, is strongly influenced by your thoughts, attitudes, beliefs, and emotions. By learning to harness these forces in a constructive way, you may be able to activate your healing system and overcome any one of a number of diseases with suspected autoimmune origins.

Strategies that may be effective for autoimmune disorders include the following:

- Mind-body strategies, including visualization and guided imagery

- Stress-management techniques

- A wholesome, healthy diet

- Release of unhealthy emotional baggage

- Exercise

- Group support

- Strengthened social intimacy

- Love

By incorporating these strategies into your life, you can work with your healing system to significantly increase your chances of overcoming autoimmune disorders.

Cancer

Before I discuss the strategies for healing cancer, I need to address four common myths about cancer. First, cancer does not come out of the blue to attack people randomly. It also is not caused by the demons of fate. As with any illness, there are definite causes, events, and circumstances that allow cancer to take root in the body, even though these factors may seem hidden, obscure, or elusive. Second, cancer is not just one disease, but rather an entire category of illnesses, each with its own specific contributing causes. Third, even though cancer may congregate in families, the overwhelming majority of cancer cases do not have a genetic basis. Fourth, and perhaps most important, by all measurements, standards, and definitions, cancer is an unnatural illness and disease that can be prevented, and in many cases overcome, particularly if it is caught early.

Cancer appears more commonly where nature's laws of health have been violated. As such, it is not surprising to see the highest cancer rates among the more modern, industrialized nations of the world, where synthetic, artificial chemicals and substances are used in abundance, and where lifestyles are becoming increasingly hectic, stressful, and unhealthy. This scenario represents a distinct departure from the simpler, more wholesome ways of life that our forefathers and ancestors enjoyed, when cancer was almost nonexistent. In developing nations, where these simpler, healthier lifestyles are still somewhat more preserved today, cancer rates are, not surprisingly, significantly lower than those in modern industrialized nations.

To understand the origins of cancer a little better, it will be helpful to remember the following important universal scientific principle that operates in nature and the world of living organisms: "Any stimulus or force, when applied to a system, will generate a specific response in return." For example, when the wind blows against a tree, it causes the tree to bend. When the sun shines, a plant or flower will grow toward the direction of the sunlight. When the sex hormones emitted by females of most species are released in the air, they create a powerful stimulus that attracts male animals to their source.

Problems in nature develop when artificial or unnatural stimuli are superimposed on systems that have been programmed to react to specific, natural stimuli in predictable ways. For example, deer and frogs, two nocturnal animals that become more active at night, become mesmerized and freeze in their tracks in response to automobile headlights. They do this because the headlights are artificial stimuli not part of their normal nighttime environment. This abnormal response to an unnatural stimulus is hazardous to the health of both deer and frogs, and it often causes them to be hit and run over by passing cars. Moths get into similar trouble because their nighttime navigational systems are naturally programmed for starlight and moonlight, but not for artificial lights or flames, which are nearer and of much brighter intensity. To the unsuspecting observer, a moth's propensity to fly straight into a bright light or flame appears to be nothing short of a suicide mission. In reality, the movement is caused by an unnatural response to an artificial, unnatural stimulus.

What occurs in the cells of normal tissues in humans and how these cells turn cancerous is not unlike the plight of deer, frogs, and moths when they are confronted with unnatural stimuli. The story of cancer begins here, for it is here, on the cellular level, that cancer first starts to grow, undetected and invisible, until many years later when it may first be discovered as a blip on an X-ray or a lump underneath the skin.

Before we can continue our story, it is important for you to know more about normal cells, how they grow, and how they evolve. This information will help explain how your body naturally works, so you will understand the underlying causes of cancer more clearly.

Normal Cellular Evolution

From the moment of conception, your body's original two cells multiply, divide, grow, and evolve into three distinct, primitive germ-cell tissues known as *ectoderm, mesoderm,* and *endoderm.* This stage is completed after just three weeks of gestation. From this stage, according to precise division-of-labor requirements, your cells embark upon an orderly, supervised journey of further multiplication, differentiation, segregation, and migration. They are eventually assigned to a particular organ or tissue, where they are programmed to carry out a specific function. For example, a neuron in the brain is programmed to conduct electrical impulses and discharge information to nerve tracts located throughout your body. A cell in your skin is programmed to help grow hair, absorb sunlight, and regulate sweating and body temperature. Although these cells look completely different and participate in completely different tasks, in reality, they have come from the same identical, primitive germ-cell lines, which, in this particular example, is ectoderm tissue. As different as they appear and behave when they have reached full maturity, these cells continue to communicate with each other and remain functionally connected throughout your life, through the same organizing intelligence that created them.

Evolution of a Cancer Cell

Cancer represents a departure from the highly ordered, natural state of health that exists within the cells of all living systems. When any cell or tissue is subjected to repeated irritation and disturbance from an unnatural stimulus, the cell begins to respond to this stimulus by defending itself against further irritation and injury. In so doing, it changes its appearance and function. In contrast to the high degree of differentiation all normal cells exhibited, cancer cells, irrespective of the organ or tissue from which they may have originated, represent a reversion to a more primitive state. In this regressed state, a cancer cell no longer functions in its previous, highly developed capacity.

As cancer cells regress from their highly differentiated structure and function, and take on more primitive roles, they relinquish their connection to the natural, orderly form and function they exhibited previously. It is as if these cells rebel against the cooperative organization and orderliness of the body that characterizes its natural state of health and instead break away to form their own aberrant colony.

These changes do not occur overnight, but slowly, sometimes over many years. These new, more primitive cells now react directly with the stimulus that caused them to change and adapt, and they become their own independent, self-assertive, abnormal mass of cells.

These abnormal cells multiply and reproduce at an accelerated speed to improve their chances of survival. At the cellular level, cancer is nothing more than a maladaptive response to an abnormal, unnatural, persistent, irritating, injurious stimulus.

Let's look at a common example of how the evolution of cancer might come about from smoking, where, in the lungs, cancer has been clearly linked to repeated exposure to cigarette smoke.

- Cigarette smoke, which is unnatural and unhealthy, introduces harsh particles and noxious chemical compounds into the lungs, where they cause irritation and injury to the cells of the lungs.

- The cells in the lungs attempt to mend the damage from the irritation and injury the smoke has caused. At the same time, the cells also attempt to defend themselves from further damage as more smoke continues to enter into the lungs.

- As the cells work without any rest to try to repair the damage to the lungs and to prevent further damage, the continued input of smoke disrupts normal mechanisms of healing and repair.

- Over the days, weeks, months, and years that a person continues to smoke, damage to the cells in the lungs is never allowed to heal. On top of this, more damage is created as more smoke enters into the lungs.

- The continuous and persistent damage from the smoke causes the delicate cells that are in the lungs to react in a defensive, protective manner. Because the cells are now in "survival mode," the smoke begins to change their basic characteristics. This process is called mutation. Mutation is an adaptation response of the cell to changes in the external environment. In this case, mutation is a way that the lung cells can adapt and survive in the face of the continuous irritation from the cigarette smoke.

- A mushrooming growth, characteristic of a cancerous tumor, eventually appears after many years in response to the repeated unnatural, injurious stimulus of the smoke.

- In many cases, if smoking ceases and continuous damage to the cells of the lungs stops, healing processes in the lungs can resume and continue undisturbed. Cessation of the unhealthy stimulus allows the healing system to repair and regenerate new, healthy tissues, replacing the mutating cells with normal, healthy, lung cells.

From this example, it is obvious that a cancer cell is nothing more than a good cell turned bad in an effort to heal from repeated abuse, irritation, and injury. This cell eventually turns the region into the monster called cancer that we all so dreadfully fear. Cancer can occur anywhere in your body that an irritating, disruptive, unnatural stimulus is repeatedly applied to the cells of otherwise normal, healthy tissues. Once the injurious stimulus is removed, however, your healing system always has the ability to repair damages and restore normal health and functioning to any organ or tissue in your body.

Unnatural stimuli that cause cancer can come in many forms. For example, excessive exposure to the sun's powerful ultraviolet rays can cause skin cancer. Excessive radiation exposure from atomic-bomb or nuclear-energy leakage, as witnessed at both Hiroshima and Chernobyl, causes cancers of the skin, immune system, and other internal organs. In most cases, however, cancer is a gradual process, requiring many years of repeated unnatural irritation and injury to tissues at the cellular level.

Cancer is also linked to toxic drugs or chemicals. Intestinal cancers can often occur with the repeated ingestion of certain foods, substances, or chemicals that continually irritate the lining of the stomach or intestines. This commonly occurs in Japan, where high rates of stomach cancer have been linked to excessive amounts of smoked fish, which contain toxic, irritating substances. Too much alcohol can cause liver cancer. Certain medicines and drugs can also cause cancer, as occurred with the drug DES, which caused thyroid cancer in the children of mothers who took this medication.

Additionally, the irritating stimulus that precipitates cancer may be a natural substance produced by your own body, but in excess. An example of this might be hydrochloric acid, secreted in normal amounts by your stomach during digestion. During times of increased stress and mental agitation, however, hydrochloric acid can be produced in excess. Excess hydrochloric acid can cause irritation, inflammation, and ulcers in your stomach and intestines, which can evolve into cancer.

Neurotransmitters, chemical messengers, and other powerful hormones produced by your brain and endocrine system can also exert an irritating, injurious effect on specific organ tissues. When stress or unhealthy moods or emotions repeatedly generate excessive amounts of these chemicals over an extended period of time, they can become powerfully unhealthy, irritating, and abnormal stimuli to the cells of specific organs. This constant stimulation results in the disruption of normal tissue structure and function, and can eventually lead to cancer. The largest number of cancers now occurring fall into this category.

Cancer Prevention

The promise of finding a cure for cancer lies in understanding its origins and focusing more on prevention than on treatment. Many experts advocate early screening measures to detect cancer; but, in many cases, by the time the cancer is detected, it may already be well established and difficult to eradicate. Although cancer is certainly easier to treat if it's caught in its early stages, it is still far better to prevent it before it has a chance to take hold in the body.

Studies conducted in places around the world where cancer is noticeably absent can provide important clues to the direction we need to take with cancer research and prevention. Some of the critical factors to consider include lifestyles, health habits, foods, medicines, beliefs, and mental attitudes of the populations being studied. We can be hopeful about the possibility of a cancer-free future if we begin to learn from these cancer-free societies, and institute changes in our own lives that support and strengthen our healing systems, incorporate ideas and methods from those cultures that place a strong emphasis on prevention, and continue cancer research and our quest for a cure.

Working with Your Healing System to Heal Cancer

As our knowledge and understanding increase, more people today than ever before have gone into complete remission and have overcome cancer. Currently, 8 million Americans who have gone into remission after their medical treatments are now cancer free. Many of these cures have come about using conventional treatments, such as surgery, drugs, and radiation, while others represent a combination of conventional and alternative therapies. These methods include the use of natural medicines, exercise, diet and lifestyle changes, and specific mind-body techniques that work to activate and stimulate the body's healing system. Guided-imagery and visualization techniques successfully employed by cancer specialists Dr. O. Carl Simonton and Dr. Bernie Siegel, as well as others, have been extremely effective in helping motivated people overcome their cancers. Learning to express emotions in a healthy way and reaching out for loving support are also highly effective in helping the healing system overcome cancer. And although there are times when surgery, radiation, and chemotherapy may be necessary to shrink tumors and remove cancerous lesions from your body to aid the work of your healing system, it is important to remember that ultimately you must not view cancer as something that has invaded your body from the outside, but rather, as a disease primarily of internal origins and causes. External agents of healing may be helpful, but your internal resources for healing are far more vast and powerful, and you should not ignore or neglect them.

Remember that cancer represents a regression of form and function by a specific group of your body's cells as the result of an unhealthy stimulus that has caused them to lose their unique identity, design, and purpose. In addition, this unhealthy stimulus has broken the connection these cells have to the rest of your body. If you can discover the unhealthy stimulus in your life and remove it, you will be well on your way to healing. Additionally, if you can bring your mental energies, awareness, and desire to cooperate with your healing system to deep inside your body, you will be in a much better position to overcome your illness and reclaim your natural state of health.

Here are a number of effective measures you can take to heal cancer:

- Remove all toxic, offending stimuli and substances from your body, such as cigarette smoke, alcohol, and junk food, as well as all toxic environmental stimuli.
- Eat a wholesome diet, with lots of fresh fruits, vegetables, and natural fiber.
- Drink plenty of fluids.
- Exercise regularly but not strenuously for at least 30 minutes each day.
- Focus on your healing system and internal resources for healing.
- Remember that your thoughts and attitudes affect your physiology. Use the power of your mind to create healthier internal chemistry for your body.
- Release all tension, anger, hostility, resentment, and grudges from your mind and body.
- Release all self-destructive thoughts, all thoughts of worthlessness and self-condemnation, and all negative beliefs about yourself.

- Learn to relax your body and mind completely. Practice stress management and meditation to the point that you can access your natural state of peace and inner tranquility regularly.

- Practice forgiveness of yourself and others.

- Use guided-imagery and visualization techniques that are appropriate for your condition. Make them deeply personal and detailed, according to your own specific needs. Use these techniques to dialogue with your body and establish a line of communication with your cancer cells. To boost your confidence in healing, focus on the elements of your body that are healthy and functioning well. Talk to your healing system. Enlist its help. In your internal imaging dialogue, remind the cancer cells that, based on the precise division of labor for which they were originally created, you value and appreciate their role, and that, in the spirit of cooperation for the greater health of your body, you sincerely request their assistance in healing.

- Use discretion and common sense in choosing your treatments, but be open-minded. Consider all available means at your disposal, including all conventional and natural methods that have proven track records. Continue to focus all your energies and intentions on reversing the disease process until your natural state of health has been restored.

- Understand that reversing cancer may be a gradual process. For the cancer to develop, evolve, and grow in your body was a gradual process, and you must allow at least an equal amount of time for the cancer to disappear back into the matrix of your body's naturally healthy cells, organs, and tissues. Just as Rome was not built in one day, so, too, restoration of health may take time. Never act out of a sense of desperation or hurry, because true healing cannot take place under these circumstances. Remember that your healing system works best in a quiet, calm, relaxed internal and external environment.

- Make healing your number-one priority in life. Remember that by bringing your awareness deep inside of your body, you have the power to activate your healing system and positively influence the health of every single organ, tissue, and cell. Remember that your natural state is health.

Closing Thoughts on
Conquering Health Conditions

Your healing system has been designed and built to keep you healthy through every conceivable challenge life could possibly throw your way. Even illnesses believed to be incurable can be overcome when you set into motion the chain of events necessary to stimulate the activity of your healing system. Naturally, the longer you have had a particular disease, the longer the period of time required for healing. In this respect, it is important to cultivate the fine art of patience as you set about the diligent work of incorporating all of the ideas and methods outlined in this and previous chapters. Patience and perseverance are required to support the work of your healing system so it can restore your body to its natural state of health in the shortest time period.

As long as you are alive, you have healing power. Even as you age, there are ways to stay healthy and overcome illness by keeping your healing system in tip-top shape. Because you have a healing system, if your commitment and resolve are sufficient, there isn't a disease on the face of this earth that can stand in the way of reclaiming your natural state of health.

Additional Relaxation Methods, Breathing Techniques, and Guided-Imagery Techniques to Strengthen Your Healing System

In this section of the book, you'll learn additional techniques and methods for tapping into the extraordinary power of your healing system.

Relaxation Methods to Strengthen and Fortify Your Healing System

Like any artist who requires a quiet, peaceful, uplifting environment to concentrate and perform his or her best work, your healing system does its best work when you are relaxed. When you are relaxed, your mind, your nervous system, and your body's internal environment provide the ideal backdrop in which your healing system can optimally perform its reparation and restorative work for your body.

Nature, in her infinite wisdom, has created the natural sleep cycle because the relaxation you get from sleep is essential to your health and well-being. When you are sleeping, your body's physiological processes are minimized, your internal environment quiets down, and your healing system can work optimally to restore your health. After a good night's sleep, you should feel refreshed, renewed, and invigorated to begin the new day. When responding to their patients' health problems, many doctors will tell them,

"Take two aspirins and call me in the morning." They know that most problems are not as serious the next day, thanks to the magical, healing, and restorative powers of sleep.

When we have trouble getting to sleep, and when we fail to take advantage of the natural, restorative powers of sleep, insomnia can set in. Health suffers and illness can easily take hold when we don't get enough sleep.

During our waking hours, however, it is also important to be relaxed. In fact, one of the major causes of insomnia is the inability to relax during waking hours. Relaxation used to be a natural aspect built into our lifestyles, but today our lifestyles have become so fast-paced that we don't have time to relax. Further, even if we had the time, we wouldn't know how to do it.

When we are not relaxed, but are instead tense or excited, the fight-or-flight response can become activated. As you may recall from our earlier discussions (see Chapter 6), the fight-or-flight response occurs whenever we are frightened, tense, or feeling threatened in any way. This response results in the release of adrenaline, which causes the speeding up of our heartbeat and breathing, among other things. The fight-or-flight response is definitely helpful when our life is actually being threatened; however, when the response is elicited frequently and sustained over time, it drains vital energies, weakens host-resistance factors, lowers our bodies' defenses, and interferes with the work of our healing systems. For these reasons, when tension becomes chronic and long lasting, it is easy for illness to step in and invade our bodies. In fact, long-standing tension is one of the key underlying factors in the development and progression of many chronic degenerative diseases.

To neutralize the harmful effects of tension and reverse the damaging effects of the fight-or-flight response, it is important to learn how to relax. In so doing, you will be strengthening and fortifying your healing system in a most fundamental way.

I am continually amazed at how many people don't know or never learned how to relax. When I inquire, most people report to me that they need some kind of external prop or activity, such as reading or watching TV, a mind-altering substance such as alcohol or a tranquilizer, or a combination of these, to wind down from their busy days and help relieve their tensions. These methods and activities often feel relaxing, but, in most instances, the mind is still actively engaged. Or, at the cost of achieving mental relaxation, consciousness, proper judgment, and the body's health (most commonly the liver's) are sacrificed. At best, these methods and devices are only temporary and achieve only a small fraction of the relaxation that the healing system requires to function optimally. Additionally, they usually have harmful side effects that neutralize whatever benefits they might contribute.

In our high-speed modern lifestyles, learning how to relax is, unfortunately, a lost art, and one reason why many stress- and tension-related disorders are on the increase in North America and Europe. These diseases are not in the minor leagues, either; rather, recent research has determined that they include some of the heaviest hitters in the annals of international public health. As mentioned earlier, among these diseases are heart disease (the world's number-one killer), high blood pressure, diabetes, asthma, and cancer. To overcome these diseases and improve our health, it is imperative that we relearn what once was a natural process, built into our simpler, more organic lifestyles: how to relax.

True relaxation involves the natural quieting down and calming of your mind to a point at which a feeling of deep peace and comfort permeates every part of your body. True relaxation improves your overall health by calming and soothing your body's internal environment so your healing system can function and perform at its best.

As we learn, practice, and experience regular relaxation, many illnesses and diseases can be totally eradicated, never to return again—including the heavy hitters previously mentioned. Many scientific studies can attest to the power and efficacy of relaxation, which is an essential ingredient for lifelong, natural health. I might add that beyond the immediate benefits of the actual relaxation practices and techniques, a spillover effect occurs in the rest of your waking hours. These benefits accrue over time to produce greater health, much like a high-interest-bearing account grows larger and stronger over time.

In preparation for practicing the relaxation techniques, it is important to secure a 20- to 30-minute time slot for yourself during which you can be quiet and alone. Make sure you won't be disturbed during this period, and that you have no responsibilities to attend to—no phone or pager to answer, no diapers to change, no stove or oven to turn off, and so on. Find a room where you can close the door and be free from all distractions. (You may need to wear earplugs or headphones if it is noisy.) Make sure you are not cold. Whatever your position, you may need to place blankets or pillows under your knees, head, or back to ensure your comfort.

Normally, when you are performing relaxation techniques or breathing exercises, it is preferable to breathe through your nose. Before you proceed with any of the following techniques, you might find it helpful to get a small tape recorder and record your voice as you read the instructions out loud, slowly and calmly. After you have recorded your words, you will have your own voice recorded, to guide you any time you wish. Or, if you wish, you can just read through each technique once or twice before you attempt to practice it.

Progressive Relaxation for Your Healing System

This is a wonderful relaxation technique for people who are chronically tense or "high strung." It is especially useful for people who have never experienced what it feels like to be relaxed. For people who have trouble with the Deep Relaxation technique described earlier in Chapter 6, Progressive Relaxation offers another simple yet powerful way to learn how to relax.

The Technique

- Lie down in a comfortable position with your feet about shoulder width apart. Keep your hands along the side of your body, with your palms facing up. Adjust any part of your body to make sure you are comfortable before you proceed.

- Gently close your eyes, and bring your awareness inside of your body.

- Now, shift your awareness to your feet and toes. Take a long, deep breath as you tighten and tense all the muscles in your feet and toes. Squeeze as hard as you can, and hold all the muscles in your feet and toes in a tight, contracted state. Count to eight in your mind as you squeeze the muscles tight. Do not force or strain, but hold your breath as you are squeezing.

- After a good, long, strong squeeze, let go of your squeezing as you slowly let your breath out. Allow these muscles to let go of their tension and relax as you slow and deepen your breathing, gently, without forcing or straining. Continue to relax your muscles, and gently slow your breathing. With each exhalation of your breath, allow whatever tension exists in these muscles to leave your body.

- Next, bring your awareness to your ankles, lower legs, knees, and thighs. Take a long, deep breath as you tighten and tense all the muscles in your ankles, lower legs, knees, and thighs. Squeeze as hard as you can, and hold these muscles in a tight, contracted state while you slowly count to eight in your mind. Hold your breath as you are squeezing. After a good, long, strong squeeze, let go of your squeezing and at the same time slowly let your breath out, allowing these muscles to relax on their own. Allow these muscles to relax as you slow and deepen your breathing, gently, without forcing or straining. Continue to let go of all muscular efforts of squeezing these muscles. Continue to relax your muscles while you gently slow your breathing. With each exhalation of your breath, allow whatever tension exists in these muscles to leave your body.

- Now, bring your awareness to your hips, pelvic area, buttocks, and lower spine. Take a long, deep breath as you tighten and tense all the muscles in your hips, pelvic area, buttocks, and lower spine. Squeeze as hard as you can, and hold these muscles in a tight, contracted state while you slowly count to eight in your mind. Hold your breath as you are squeezing. After a good, long, strong squeeze, let go of your squeezing while you slowly let your breath out, allowing these muscles to relax on their own. Allow these muscles to relax as you gently slow and deepen your breathing, without forcing or straining. Continue to let go of all efforts to squeeze these muscles. Continue to relax your muscles and your breathing. With each exhalation of your breath, allow whatever tension exists in these muscles to leave your body.

- Next, bring your awareness to your stomach, abdomen, and chest. Take a long, slow, deep breath as you tighten and tense all the muscles in your stomach, abdomen, and chest. Squeeze these muscles as hard as you can, and hold them in a tight, contracted state while you slowly count to eight in your mind. Hold your breath as you are squeezing. After a good, long, strong squeeze, let go of your squeezing, and at the same time let your breath out, allowing these muscles to relax on their own. Allow these muscles to relax as you gently slow and deepen your breathing, without forcing or straining. Let go of all efforts to squeeze these muscles. Continue to relax your muscles and your breathing. With each exhalation of your breath, allow whatever tension exists in these muscles to leave your body.

- Now, bring your awareness to the muscles in your middle and upper back, including the area between your shoulder blades. Take a long, slow, deep breath as you squeeze these muscles as hard as you can, drawing your shoulders back slightly while you gently arch your spine. Hold these muscles in a tight, contracted state while you slowly count to eight in your mind. Hold your breath as you are squeezing. After a good, long, strong squeeze, let go of your squeezing, and at the same time let your breath out, allowing these muscles to relax on their own. Allow these muscles to relax as you slow and deepen your breathing, without forcing or straining. Let go of all efforts to squeeze these muscles. Continue to relax your muscles and your breathing. With each exhalation, allow whatever tension exists in these muscles to leave your body.

- Next, bring your awareness to your shoulders, arms, forearms, wrists, hands, and fingers. As you draw in a long, deep breath, squeeze the muscles in your shoulders, arms, forearms, and wrists as hard as you can, and hold them in a tight, contracted state. Make tight, clenched fists with both of your hands while you slowly count to eight in your mind. Hold your breath as you are squeezing. After a good, long, strong squeeze, let go of your squeezing, and at the same time let your breath out, allowing these muscles to relax on their own. Let go of all efforts to squeeze these muscles. Allow these muscles to relax as you slow and deepen your breathing, without forcing or straining. Continue to relax your muscles and your breathing. With each exhalation of your breath, allow whatever tension that exists in these muscles to leave your body.

- In a similar manner, systematically tense, squeeze, and then relax all the muscles in the back of your neck and head, as well as those on the top of your head.

- In a similar way, systematically tense, squeeze, and then relax your forehead, and all the muscles around your eyes, ears, and jaws, and all the muscles on your face.

- In a similar manner, systematically tense, squeeze, and then relax all the muscles in your body, until all your muscles have been tensed and relaxed in this fashion.

- Next, allow your entire body to lie limp and relaxed, with the only movement being the automatic, involuntary movement of your stomach and abdomen as they rise and fall rhythmically, in conjunction with the movement of your breath as it flows in and out of your body. Every time the breath leaves your body, feel all the muscles in your body releasing tension and becoming more relaxed.

- Now slowly bring your awareness to the tip of your nose, where your breath is flowing in and out of your body through your nostrils.

- Notice the gentle, flowing movement of your breath as it comes in and out of your body at this point, without trying to control the rate or depth of the movement.

- Observe your breath as if it were something different from yourself.

- As you continue to observe your breathing for at least 5 to 10 minutes, or longer if you desire, let your mind and body relax completely.

After you complete this exercise, gently open your eyes and stretch your entire body. Don't rush to your next activity. Take the time to savor the calm and relaxed state you have just experienced. Know that this is not an artificial or contrived state, but rather your natural state of being. Focus on remaining in this calm and relaxed, natural state throughout the day, until the next time you are able to do this exercise.

Regularly practicing Progressive Relaxation helps to strengthen and fortify your healing system in a powerful way. If you are currently battling a health disorder, practice twice a day for a minimum of six weeks, and you should see significant gains in your health. If you are currently healthy, practice Progressive Relaxation once a day for 20 to 30 minutes to prevent illness from invading your body.

Blue Sky Floating on Your Back Relaxation

This relaxation technique begins like the Deep Relaxation technique (see Chapter 6), but this method also incorporates the soothing natural imagery of water and sky. If you have an affinity for these elements, this technique can be extremely effective and powerful.

The Technique

- Make sure you are in a comfortable position on your back.

- Keep your hands along the side of your body, with your palms facing up, or fold your hands on top of your stomach and abdomen. Gently close your eyes, and bring your awareness inside of your body.

- Notice in the area of your stomach and abdomen the slight up and down movement that occurs in conjunction with the movement of your breath as it flows in and out of your body.

- Notice that when the breath flows into your body, your stomach and abdomen gently rise, gently expand.

- Notice that when the breath flows out of your body, your stomach and abdomen gently fall, gently contract.

- Without trying to control the rate or depth of this movement, allow your mind to be a passive observer to the rhythmical flow of your breath as it moves in and out of your body, causing your stomach and abdomen to rise and fall.

- Every time the breath leaves your body, feel all the muscles in your body releasing tension and becoming more relaxed. (Note: There is a natural relaxation phase in your body that occurs during each exhalation of the breath. When you pay close attention to your body and its breathing processes, you can feel this relaxation phase quite distinctly.)

- Now, bring your awareness down to your feet and toes. Use your breath and the natural relaxation phase that occurs during each exhalation to gently relax all the muscles in your feet and toes.

- Relax all the muscles in your ankles, lower legs, knees, thighs, hips, pelvic area, buttocks, and lower spine.

- Relax all the muscles in your stomach, abdomen, and chest, as well as the muscles in your middle and upper back, including the area between your shoulder blades.

- Relax all the muscles in your shoulders, arms, forearms, wrists, hands, fingers, and fingertips.

- Relax all the muscles in the back of your neck and head, and the top of your head.

- Relax your forehead, and all the muscles around your eyes, ears, and jaws, and on your face.

- Relax all the muscles in your body.

- Continue to observe your breathing, noticing the gentle up and down movement in your stomach and abdomen. Continue to feel more relaxed with each exhalation.

- Now, keeping your eyes closed, imagine that you are floating on the surface of a quiet, serene lake, and there is blue sky above and all around you. (If you are not comfortable being directly in the water, you can imagine yourself floating on a strong and secure rubber inner tube in the water. Above all else, it is important to feel completely safe and secure with this imagery and this technique.)

- As you continue to breathe in and out in a gentle and relaxed manner, notice how the water beneath you is soothing and refreshing to your body. Notice how the vast blue sky above you is peaceful and refreshing to gaze upon, as if your entire being is embracing infinity and merging into the heavens.

- Notice a feeling of lightness and peace in your mind that extends into every part of your body as you continue to float on the surface of the water, gazing up into the blue sky. Allow yourself to feel this peaceful sensation of lightness and relaxation from the top of your head to the tips of your fingers and toes.

- As you continue to float on the surface of the water, look up at the blue sky above you, and allow yourself to feel as if you are melting into the expansiveness of the sky and all of creation.

- Continue to breathe and relax, drinking in the peace and serenity of this experience.

After you complete this exercise, gently open your eyes, and stretch your entire body. Make sure you don't rush to your next activity. Take the time to savor the calm and relaxed state you have just experienced. Know that this is not an artificial or contrived state, but rather your natural state of being. Focus on remaining in this calm and relaxed natural state throughout the day, until the next time you are able to do this exercise. Practicing this exercise regularly brings the most effective benefits.

Breathing Techniques That Strengthen and Fortify Your Healing System

Breathing is an activity that you probably take for granted because your body can breathe on its own, automatically. It usually does so 24 hours a day, seven days a week, without your even being aware of it. But breathing is a powerful physiological activity that can be modified, either to your benefit or detriment, and it can aid or hinder the functioning of your healing system.

As we discussed in Chapter 6, breathing works on many different levels to influence your body's health and the performance of your healing system. And although there is no right or wrong way to breathe, many people have developed habits of breathing that do not optimize the performance of their healing systems.

On a mechanical level, breathing affects your posture. Because the muscles of respiration move your rib cage and chest, which connect to the vertebrae in your spine, every breath you take influences the alignment of your spinal column. For example, people with asthma and other chronic breathing problems are typically shallow breathers, and they tend to develop restrictive, hunched-forward positions in their spine, known as *kyphosis*. Kyphosis further restricts deep breathing and deprives the body of adequate oxygenation. An extreme example of kyphosis could be seen in the Hunchback of Notre Dame.

Breath is also the link between your body and mind, and it exerts a powerful influence on your nervous system. For example, when you are agitated or upset, your breathing becomes shallow and rapid. Conversely, when you are relaxed and peaceful, your breathing becomes slower and deeper. The processes are interrelated. In fact, by practicing slow, relaxed, deep breathing, you can calm and relax your mind and nervous system, while you improve the oxygenation of your body's tissues.

By learning to practice these simple, easy breathing techniques, which are based on ancient yoga techniques from India, you can bring more *prana*, or energy, into your body, and strengthen and fortify your healing system.

Because breathing, for the most part, is such a natural, unconscious activity, many people have a strong aversion to learning how to breathe in a way that may initially feel different or unnatural. However, based on my 25 years of experience as a doctor who has studied breathing, and on new scientific studies of breathing, I can assure you that taking a closer look at your breathing, and committing yourself to just one or two of the following simple breathing techniques, will enable you to notice a tremendous improvement in your overall state of health.

Of all the physical activities you can do to improve your health and influence your healing system, breathing is one of the most powerful of all.

Breathing Techniques

Breathing techniques are traditionally done in a sitting position, but you can also do them while you're lying down. The important thing is to make sure you are in a comfortable position. If you are doing breathing techniques while you are sitting, keep your spine straight and your shoulders relaxed. If you are doing these while you are lying down, you can assume a similar position to that of the Deep Relaxation (see Chapter 6) or Progressive Relaxation (see the section in this chapter on relaxation methods) techniques. Whatever your position, you may need to place blankets or pillows under your knees, head, and back to ensure your comfort. Make sure you are not cold.

Normally, when you are performing breathing exercises, as with other relaxation techniques, breathing through your nose whenever possible is preferable.

The beauty of breathing exercises is that you can do them at numerous intervals throughout the day, from one minute's duration, up to 30 to 60 minutes, depending on your schedule. Obviously, the longer you can do them, the more powerful their effect. But even if you have only a few brief moments at selected times throughout the day, breathing exercises can make a tremendous difference in your overall health because of their cumulative effects. Breathing exercises are ideally practiced with your eyes closed, but you also can practice them with your eyes open. Breathing exercises are quiet and gentle, and they require no external props. So you can perform them effortlessly without anyone else knowing what you are doing when you're on long airplane flights, a bus or train, stuck in rush hour commuter traffic, or in the midst of boring meetings. Again, although they are simple and easy, and they feel good, breathing exercises are powerful in their ability to strengthen and fortify your healing system.

Breathing practices have a relaxing effect, so, in the beginning, you should not perform them while you are driving or operating mechanical devices or equipment. In time, as you become more accomplished, you may find that you can do them while you are carrying on your normal activities. Even though breathing practices are initially calming and relaxing, they can be extremely energizing in the long run.

Before you proceed with any of the following techniques, you might find it helpful to get a small tape recorder and record your voice as you read the instructions out loud, slowly and calmly. After you have recorded your words, you will have your own voice recorded to guide you any time you wish. Or you might wish to just read through each technique once or twice before you attempt to practice it.

In and Out Breath

This is a very simple yet powerful breathing technique that helps to quiet down your mind, calm and purify your nervous system, and strengthen and fortify your healing system. You can do the In and Out Breath technique either lying down or in a seated position. It is preferable to do it while you're seated, so you can do it in your spare moments in the midst of your busy days; but, in the beginning, it may be more convenient to learn this technique while you're lying down.

The Technique

- Make sure you are in a comfortable position, lying down or seated. Use blankets, pillows, cushions, pads, or other necessary support to help you get comfortable.

- Once you are comfortable, close your eyes, and bring your awareness inside of your body.

- Relax all the muscles in your body as you focus on the gentle movement of your breath flowing in and out of your body.

- Notice the slight movement in your stomach and abdomen every time your breath flows in and out of your body.

- Notice that when your breath flows into your body, your stomach and abdomen gently rise and expand. Notice that when your breath flows out of your body, your stomach and abdomen gently fall and contract. Without trying to control the rate or depth of this movement, just allow your mind to be a passive observer of this automatic movement of your breath as it flows in and out of your body.

- Continue to watch your stomach and abdomen move up and down every time your breath flows in and out of your body.

- Every time the breath leaves your body, feel all the muscles in your body releasing tension and becoming more relaxed.

- After you feel somewhat relaxed, gently shift your awareness to the tip of your nose, where your breath is flowing in and out of your body through your nostrils.

- Visualize your breath as if it were something different from yourself.

- Continue to observe the rhythmical flow of your breath as it flows in and out of your body through your nose.

- As you continue to observe your breathing, allow your mind and body to relax more deeply.

- After you have observed your breathing for several minutes, notice that the air flowing out of your nose is slightly warmer than the air flowing into your nose. Or you can notice that the air flowing into your nose is slightly cooler than the air flowing out of your nose. At first, focus your awareness on whichever sensation is easier for you to feel. Notice this temperature difference between the air moving into your nose and the air moving out of your nose as you continue to breathe with this increased awareness. Continue to breathe this way for one or two minutes.

- After one or two minutes, on your next exhalation, as you breathe out, follow the breath as it leaves your nose, and see how far you can feel it moving away from your body.

- In the beginning, you can place a hand in front of your nose to help you feel the movement of your breath. As your breath strikes your hand, keep moving your hand further away from your nose. As you continue to breathe, keep moving your hand further and further away until you can no longer feel your breath striking your hand. (After you get good at this, you will no longer need to use your hand.) Now bring your hand back slightly until you can still just barely feel your breath. As you continue to breathe this way, be aware of how far your breath flows out of your body.

- Continue to hold your awareness at the point at which you can just barely feel your breath. Continue to hold your awareness at this point, only now, see whether you can do it without using your hand. (Adjusting your awareness may take a few moments.)

- At the furthest point away from your body at which you are still able to just barely detect your outgoing breath, start to focus your awareness on the incoming breath. See whether you can begin to feel the slightly cooler air coming into your body from this same point. Continue to focus at the point of origin of the cooler air as it begins to enter into your body.

- As you breathe in, follow the cooler air entering into your body and notice the place at which it comes in contact with your nose. Feel the cooler air gently striking your nose as it enters into your body, and then continue to follow this air as it moves into your throat and lungs. Follow your breath further into your body as it causes your stomach and abdomen to rise and expand. Feel your breath spreading throughout your entire body with each inhalation that you take.

- With each breath you take, continue to follow your incoming breath as it flows into your body, watching it cause your stomach and abdomen to rise and expand.

- Continue to observe the gentle movement of your stomach and abdomen as your breath flows in and out of your body.

- Now, gently shift your awareness back to the most distant point at which you could detect the movement of your breath.

- Simultaneously feel both of these points: 1) the point that is furthest away from your body at which you can detect your breath, and 2) the most interior point within your body at which you can still feel the presence of your breath.

- Hold your awareness between these two extreme points as you continue to observe the automatic, flowing movement of your breath as it flows in and out of your body.

- After 5 to 10 minutes, slowly open your eyes, stretch your body, and release yourself from your seated or lying-down position.

"The Pause That Refreshes" Breathing Exercise

This is a simple and easy breathing exercise that you can do anytime, anywhere, while you are sitting or lying down. The more you do it, the easier it gets, and the more natural it feels. When you perform this exercise correctly, it is extremely pleasurable. Even though it is simple and easy, and feels so good, don't underestimate its power and effectiveness in strengthening and fortifying your healing system.

The Technique

- Although it is preferable to sit, you may also lie down in a comfortable position for this breathing technique. Close your eyes, bringing your awareness into your body. Relax your shoulders and all the muscles in your body.

- Bring your attention to the area of your stomach and abdomen. Notice in the area of your stomach and abdomen the slight up and down movement that occurs in conjunction with the movement of your breath as it flows in and out of your body.

- Notice that when the breath flows into your body, your stomach and abdomen gently rise, and when it flows out of your body, your stomach and abdomen gently fall.

- Without trying to control the rate or depth of this movement, just allow yourself to be a passive observer to the natural flow of your breath as it moves in and out of your body. Breathe like this for several minutes, until you begin to feel a sensation of relaxation sweeping over your entire body.

■ Next, as you notice yourself becoming relaxed, gently slow and deepen your breathing, so that the time of your inhalation and exhalation are slightly prolonged. Note, however, that it is extremely important to do this gradually, without forcing or straining. Above all else, make sure you are comfortable with your breathing.

■ Now, as you continue to gently lengthen, deepen, and slow your breathing, notice that right before your breath flows into your body, and right before it begins to flow out again, there is a slight pause between these separate phases of your breathing. These phases are known as inspiration and expiration, respectively. Notice that there are a total of two pauses built into your body's natural breathing cycle.

■ As you continue to breathe in and out slowly, notice these two distinct pauses between inspiration and expiration.

■ Now, during the next pause after inspiration, right before you exhale, gently lengthen the time of the natural pause before you commence exhaling. Do this in a gentle and soothing way, without forcing or straining. If you do it right, you should feel a slightly pleasurable sensation, especially when you exhale. As you hold this pause, you may want to gently press your tongue against the back of your teeth or the top of your palate to make sure no air escapes during this period.

■ Now, after a brief and slight breath pause of one or two seconds, when you have temporarily suspended movement in your normal breathing rhythms, gently release the pause and let your breath out slowly and smoothly, as you would during normal breathing.

■ When you are ready, after the next full inspiration, and right before expiration, at the time of the next natural pause or break in your breathing, once again gently prolong and lengthen this pause for one or two seconds before you let your breath out naturally, as you would during your normal breathing cycle.

■ Continue to breathe this way, gently prolonging the natural pause that occurs with each cycle of breathing between inspiratory and expiratory phases.

■ During this pause, take a brief inventory of how you feel in your body and mind. Make sure you are not forcing or straining, and that you are comfortable with your breathing.

■ Make sure you are comfortable at all times while you are performing this powerful breathing exercise. If you try to prolong the pause longer than you can handle, you will experience breath deprivation, discomfort, and a sensation of forcing or straining. Additionally, the rhythm of your breathing will not be smooth and flowing, but rather jerky and interrupted. As you breathe out, and then again as you breathe in, and even during the pause, your breath should be smooth and flowing, and you should feel comfortable and pleasurable sensations.

■ In the beginning, do this breathing exercise for no more than 3 to 5 minutes at a time, and not more than four times a day, no matter how pleasurable and relaxing you may find it. Even though it is gentle and soothing, this technique is also extremely powerful and subtle, and you can overdo it, especially in the beginning. In time, you can build up to 20 to 30 minutes at a time.

■ Also, over time, you can gently prolong the pause between each inspiration and expiration for up to one minute, or even longer. Remember to focus your awareness within, and take a brief inventory of your body and mind during this pause. During the pause, which is a time of complete cessation of respiration, an accompanying slowing down of physiological processes and mental activities occurs. This slowing down can be calming and peaceful, and it is extremely beneficial to your healing system, which, as you'll recall, does its best work when your body's internal environment is quiet and calm.

Breathing exercises calm the mind and body, and they are extremely beneficial to your healing system. Incorporate these exercises into your daily routine, and before long you'll begin to see their remarkable effects.

Guided Imagery to Strengthen and Fortify Your Healing System

Your brain translates mental images into electrical and chemical signals that are transmitted to your body. Because of this deep connection between your brain and your body, the techniques of visualization or guided imagery can be a powerful way to activate, strengthen, and fortify your healing system. Many studies have shown the health-enhancing benefits of guided imagery and visualization techniques in helping motivated patients overcome serious illnesses, including cancer and heart disease. (For more information on guided imagery and visualization, see Chapter 6.)

"Meeting Your Healing System" Guided-Visualization Technique

Begin this technique as you would the relaxation techniques described earlier in the book, such as Deep Relaxation, Progressive Relaxation, or Blue Sky Floating on Your Back Relaxation. Read through the directions completely once or twice before you attempt to practice it. You may also want to get a tape recorder and record your own voice as you read through this exercise. Then you will be able to close your eyes and listen to your own voice guide you through the imagery.

Follow these simple steps to do this technique:

- Make sure you are in a comfortable position, lying on your back with your eyes closed.

- Focus on your breathing as you allow your mind and body to relax completely.

- As you begin to feel yourself becoming relaxed, take a deep, sighing breath. As you breathe out, let all the tension leave your body.

- Take a second, deep, sighing breath, and, as you breathe out, allow your mind and body to be completely relaxed. Make sure you feel completely relaxed before you proceed further with this exercise. It is important not to hurry or rush through this step.

- After you are somewhat relaxed, keep your eyes closed, and allow an image to form in your mind of any quiet, serene, uplifting place. Your image could be a beautiful outdoor setting or inside in a favorite, cozy room of a house. It could be a place you have actually been to in real life, a place you saw in a picture, or a totally fresh image that you have never seen before. Whatever image begins to appear, do not force or strain with the imagery, and do not judge it in any way.

- As you continue to breathe and relax, be patient with the imagery. Allow it to keep forming in your mind until you have a fairly clear picture of the place.

- Once your special place begins to come into focus, and you have a fairly clear idea of where you are, continue to breathe deeply and relax.

- Allow the image to become clearer and more well defined.

- Notice all the senses, and answer these questions in your mind:♦

  ♦ What are the sights? What are the sounds? What are the smells?

  ♦ What kind of day is it? What does the sky look like? Where is the sun?

  ♦ What does the countryside or surrounding environment look like?

  ♦ What sensations are you feeling on your skin?

  ♦ What is the air quality? Is it cool or warm? Is there humidity, or is it dry? Are there any breezes?

  ♦ What are you wearing?

- Breathe deeply and relax as you allow your mind to absorb the images.

- Find a place to sit down (or, if you feel more comfortable, to lie down, or even stand) in your quiet, special place. In your image, make sure you are in a comfortable position.

- Once you are comfortable in your special place, allow your awareness and imagination to go inside your body.

- See yourself examining the inner workings of your body as you gently survey the landscape.

- As you move around within the various structures and tissues of your body, imagine yourself going on a journey of discovery.

- Find a quiet place, deep within the recesses of your body's internal environment, where you feel safe and protected.

- Stop and relax once you've found a place where you feel comfortable. Let your intuition guide you.

- Breathe deeply, and allow yourself to relax in this quiet place within your body.

- See yourself waiting with anticipation, as you prepare to meet your healing system.

- Wait for the first image to form as your healing system begins to come into view.

- As you begin to get the first glimpses of your healing system, allow whatever image is developing to form on its own. There is no right or wrong here, so there is no need to judge anything about the image. If an image forms that is totally unexpected, which is often the case, welcome it. Do your best not to reject or be afraid of the image of your healing system that your imagination presents to you.

- Allow the image of your healing system to come into clearer focus. Notice all you can about its shape, dimensions, color, texture, and whether it is moving or still.

- Your healing system may even appear in the form of a person, animal, or some other creature. It might even have a face or a name.

- When you have a fairly clear picture of your healing system in your mind, allow yourself to come close enough to it so you can have a conversation with it. Or it may be so powerful that you are more comfortable stepping back and creating distance. Find the distance that feels best for you, and adjust your position to the image so that you are comfortable.

- Just as you would upon meeting a new friend for the first time, introduce yourself to your healing system. Or you may feel as if you are meeting an old friend after a long time, and you are reintroducing yourself.

- You may want to tell your healing system how you feel. If you are in pain, you may want to share this, or you may be angry with it because you think it's not been doing such a good job of protecting your health. Tell it this. Or you may feel more comfortable asking your healing system more questions and getting to know it first, before you tell it how you feel.

- If you are in pain, you may ask your healing system how it can heal your pain. If you are sick or have an illness, you may want to ask it how to heal and get better.

- Ask your healing system whether you might be doing something that is interfering with its work. Ask whether there is something you are neglecting to do to keep your healing system strong and vibrant. Ask how you can improve your lifestyle and your daily personal health habits in support of its work.

- Ask your healing system how you can get to know it better, and what it needs to be healthy and strong.

- Continue to ask as many questions as you like.

- Remember to listen attentively to the answers that will be forthcoming. There may be a slight delay in receiving the information, so don't rush the responses, or be in a hurry.

- When you are done, remember to say "Thank you" to your healing system.

- Find out when you can meet again.

- Schedule an appointment for the next time you will meet. Doing this is very important to help you stay accountable for your role in this ongoing internal dialogue with your healing system. Because your healing system is punctual and always available to you, it will definitely show up at whatever time and date you specify, but you must be specific.

- When you are finished, say "Goodbye" to your healing system.

After you have completed this guided imagery/visualization exercise, take a few moments to reflect on the experience. Take a pen and notebook and write down as much information about the experience as you can remember. What new insights did you gain? Make an action plan based on new ideas or information that your healing system has shared with you in your imagery dialogue.

Now it is up to you to implement these ideas in your daily life. So, what are you waiting for? Do it today! If you stay in touch with your healing system, you'll see that it will function better and work harder to keep you healthy and strong.

RESOURCES

Recommended Reading

General Healing

Batmanghelidj, F., M.D. *Your Body's Many Cries for Water*. Falls Church, VA: Global Health Solutions, Inc., 1998.

Bennet, Hal Zina. *The Doctor Within*. New York: Clarkson N. Potter, 1981.

Bennett, Cleaves, M.D. *Control Your High Blood Pressure Without Drugs*. Garden City, NY: Doubleday, 1986.

Benson, Herbert, M.D. *The Wellness Book*. New York: Birch Lane Press, 1992.

Borysenko, Joan. *Minding the Body, Mending the Mind*. New York: Bantam Books, 1988.

Breslow, Rachelle. *Who Said So?: A Women's Fascinating Journey of Self Discovery and Triumph over Multiple Sclerosis*. Berkeley: Celestial Arts, 1991.

Brownstein, Arthur, M.D. *Healing Back Pain Naturally*. Gig Harbor, WA: Harbor Press, 1999.

Cawood, Frank W. *High Blood Pressure Lowered Naturally*. Peachtree City, GA: FC, & A Publishing, 1996.

Chopra, Deepak, M.D. *Ageless Body, Timeless Mind*. New York: Bantam Books, 1993.

Chopra, Deepak, M.D. *Quantum Healing*. New York: Bantam Books, 1990.

Cortis, Bruno, M.D. *Heart and Soul*. New York: Villard Books, 1995.

Cousins, Norman. *Anatomy of an Illness*. New York: Bantam Books, 1985.

Cousins, Norman. *Head First: The Biology of Hope*. New York: E.P. Dutton, 1989.

Dossey, Larry, M.D. *Healing Words*. San Francisco: Harper Collins, 1993.

Eliot, Robert, M.D. *Is It Worth Dying For?* New York: Bantam Books, 1989.

Golan, Ralph, M.D. *Optimal Wellness*. New York: Ballantine Books, 1995.

Goleman, Daniel and Joel Gurin. *Mind Body Medicine: How to Use Your Mind for Better Health*. Yonkers, NY: Consumer Reports Books, 1993.

Hay, Louise. *You Can Heal Your Life*. Carlsbad, CA: Hay House, 1997.

Hirshberg, Caryle and Marc Ian Barasch. *Remarkable Recovery*. New York: Riverhead Books, 1995.

Hirshberg, Caryle, et. al. *The Art of Healing*. Atlanta: Turner Publishing, 1993.

Ivker, Rob. *Thriving*. New York: Crown Publishers, 1997.

Jampolsky, Gerald, M.D. *Forgiveness*. Hillsboro, OR: Beyond Words Publishing, 1999.

Jampolsky, Gerald, M.D. *Love Is Letting Go of Fear*. Berkeley: Celestial Arts, 1988.

Laskow, Leonard, M.D. *Healing with Love*. San Francisco: Harper Collins, 1992.

Locke, Steven, M.D. *The Healer Within: The New Medicine of Mind and Body*. New York: E.P. Dutton, 1986.

Myss, Caroline. *Why People Don't Heal and How They Can*. New York: Three Rivers Press, 1997.

Northrup, Christiane, M.D. *Women's Bodies, Women's Wisdom*. New York: Bantam Books, 1998.

O'Regan, Brendan and Caryle Hirshberg. *Spontaneous Remissions*. Sausalito, CA: Institute of Noetic Sciences, 1993.

Ornish, Dean, M.D. *Dr. Dean Ornish's Program for Reversing Heart Disease*. New York: Random House, 1990.

Pagano, Jon. *Healing Psoriasis*. Englewood Cliffs, NJ: The Pagano Organization, 1991.

Pinckney, Neal. *Healthy Heart Handbook*. Deerfield Beach, CA: Health Communications, 1996.

Pleas, John. *Walking*. New York: Norton Books, 1987.

Roizen, Michael, M.D. *RealAge*. New York: Cliff Street Books, 1999.

Schatz Pullig, Mary, M.D. *Back Care Basics*. Berkeley: Rodmell Press, 1992.

Siegel, Bernie, M.D. *How to Live Between Office Visits*. New York: Harper Collins, 1995.

Siegel, Bernie, M.D. *Love, Medicine & Miracles*. New York: Harper and Row, 1986.

Siegel, Bernie, M.D. *Peace, Love & Healing*. New York: Harper and Row, 1989.

Siegel, Bernie, M.D. *Prescriptions for Living*. New York: Harper Collins, 1998.

Simon, David, M.D. *Vital Energy*. New York: John Wiley and Sons, 2000.

Simonton, O. Carl, M.D. *Getting Well Again*. New York: Bantam Books, 1988.

Simonton, O. Carl, M.D. *Healing Journey*. New York: Bantam Books, 1992.

Sinatra, Stephen, M.D. *Optimum Health*. New York: Lincoln-Bradley Publishing Group, 1996.

Teitelbaum, M.D. *From Fatigued to Fantastic*. New York: Avery Publishing Group, 1996.

Weil, Andrew, M.D. *Spontaneous Healing*. New York: Knopf, 1995.

Whitaker, Julian, M.D. *Reversing Diabetes*. New York: Warner Books, 1990.

Whitaker, Julian, M.D. *Reversing Heart Disease*. New York: Warner Books, 1988.

Yanker, Gary and Kathy Burton. *Walking Medicine*. New York: McGraw-Hill, 1990.

Stress Management, Relaxation, Meditation, Breathing, and Imagery

Benson, Herbert, M.D. *The Relaxation Response*. New York: Avon Books, 1976.

Carrington, Patricia. *Freedom in Meditation*. Garden City, NY: Anchor Books, 1978.

Monroe, Robin, R. Nagararhna, M.D., and H. R. Nagendra. *Yoga for Common Ailments*. New York: Fireside Books, 1990.

Nagendra, H.R., *Pranayama*. Bangalore, India: Vivekananda Yoga Institute Publications, 1999.

Payne, Larry and Georg Feurstein. *Yoga for Dummies*. Foster City, CA: IDG Books, 1999.

Payne, Larry. *Yoga Rx.* New York: Broadway Books, 2002.

Rossman, Marty, M.D. *Healing Yourself: A Step-by-Step Program for Better Health Through Imagery.* New York: Pocket Books, 1989.

Sedlacek, Keith, M.D. *Finding the Calm Within You.* New York: Signet Books, 1990.

Srikrishna, M.B.B.S. *Essence of Pranayama.* Bombay, India: Kaivalyadhama Press, 1996.

Zinn, Jon-Kabat. *Full Catastrophe Living.* New York: Delta Books, 1990.

Nutrition

Agatston, Arthur, M.D. *South Beach Diet.* Emmaus, PA: Rodale Press, 2003.

Balch, James F., M.D. and Phyllis A. Balch. *Prescription for Nutritional Healing.* Garden City Park, NY: Avery Publishing Group, 1990.

Ballantine, Rudolph, M.D. *Diet and Nutrition.* Honesdale, PA: Himalayan International Institute, 1978.

Barnard, Neal, M.D. *Food for Life.* New York: Crown Publishers, 1993.

Griffith, H. Winter, M.D. *Vitamins.* Tucson, AZ: Fisher Books, 1988.

Haas, Elson, M.D. *Staying Healthy with the Seasons.* Berkeley: Celestial Arts, 1981.

Lane, Theresa (Ed.). *Foods That Harm, Foods That Heal.* Pleasantville, NY: Reader's Digest Books, 1997.

Lappe, Francis Moore. *Diet for a Small Planet.* New York: Ballantine Books, 1982.

Melina, Vesanto, Brenda Davis, and Victoria Harrison. *Becoming Vegetarian.* Summertown, TN: Book Publishing Company, 1995.

Nedley, Neil, M.D. *Proof Positive: How to Reliably Combat Disease and Achieve Optimal Health Through Nutrition and Lifestyle.* Ardmore, OK: Nedley Publishing, 1998.

Null, Gary. *Complete Guide to Health and Healing.* New York: Delta Books,1984.

Ornish, Dean, M.D. *Eat More, Weigh Less.* New York: Harper Collins, 1993.

Robbins, John. *Diet For a New America.* Walpole, NH: Stillpoint Publishing, 1987.

Rubin, Jordan. *Patient Heal Thyself.* Topanga, CA: Freedom Press, 2003.

Sears, Barry. *The Zone.* New York: Harper Collins, 1995.

Shintani, Terri, M.D. *Eat More, Weigh Less Diet.* Honolulu, HI: Halpax Publishing, 1993.

U.S. Dept. of Agriculture. *Handbook of the Nutritional Contents of Foods.* New York: Dover Publications, 1975.

Weil, Andrew, M.D. *Eating Well for Optimum Health.* New York: Knopf, 2000.

Natural Healing

Chan, Luke. *101 Miracles of Natural Healing.* Cincinnati, OH: Benefactor Press, 1997.

Guinness, Alma E. (Ed.). *Family Guide to Natural Medicine.* Pleasantville, NY: Reader's Digest Books, 1993.

Page, Linda. *Healthy Healing.* Carmel Valley, CA: Traditional Wisdom, 2000.

Weil, Andrew, M.D. *Natural Health, Natural Medicine.* Boston: Houghton Mifflin, 1990.

Organizations for Healing

Academy For Guided Imagery
30765 Pacific Coast Highway #369

Malibu, CA 90265
800-726-2070
www.interactiveimagery.com

American Holistic Health Association
P.O. Box 17400
Anaheim, CA 92817-7400
714-779-6152
www.ahha.org

American Holistic Medical Association
12101 Menaul Blvd. NE, Suite C
Albuquerque, NM 87112
505-292-7788
www.holisticmedicine.org

Association for Applied Psychophysiology and Biofeedback
10200 West 44th Avenue, Suite 304
Wheat Ridge, CO 80033
www.aapb.org

Center for Attitudinal Healing
33 Buchanan Drive
Sausalito, CA 94965
415-331-6161
www.attitudinalhealing.org

Center for Mind-Body Medicine
5225 Connecticut Ave. NW, Suite 414
Washington, DC 20015
202-966-7338
www.cmbm.org

Commonweal Cancer Help Program
P.O. Box 316
451 Mesa Road
Bolinas, CA 94924
415-868-0970
www.commonweal.org

Hawaii State Consortium of Integrative Medicine
932 Ward Ave. Suite 600
Honolulu, HI 96814
808-535-5559
www.blendedmed.net

Institute of Noetic Sciences
101 San Antonio Road
Petaluma, CA 94952
707-775-3500
www.noetic.org

Integrative Medicine Alliance
180 Massachusetts Ave.
Arlington, MA 02474
617-648-9866
www.integrativemedalliance.org

Mind/Body Medical Institute
824 Boylston St.
Chestnut Hill, MA 02467
617-991-0102
Toll free: 866-509-0732
www.mbmi.org

National Center For Complementary and Alternative Medicine
National Institutes of Health
Bethesda, MD 20892
www.nccam.nih.gov
info@nccam.nih.gov

Preventive Medicine Research Institute
900 Bridgeway
Sausalito, CA 94965
415-332-2525
www.pmri.org

Program in Integrative Medicine
Dr. Andrew Weil
University of Arizona
www.drweil.com
www.integrativemedicine.arizona.edu

Scripps Center for Integrative Medicine
10820 North Torrey Pines Road
La Jolla, CA 92037
858-554-3971
www.scrippsfoundation.org

Simonton Cancer Center
P.O. Box 6607
Malibu, CA 90264
818-879-7904
Toll free: 800-459-3424
www.simontoncenter.com
simontoncancercenter@msn.com

Cousins Center for Psychoneuroimmunology
UCLA Neuropsychiatric Institute
300 UCLA Medical Plaza, Suite 3109
Box 957076
Los Angeles, CA 90095-7076
310-825-8281
www.npi.ucla.edu/center/cousins

About the Author

ART BROWNSTEIN, M.D. has been talking with his patients about the body's extraordinary ability to heal itself for almost as long as he's been a doctor. In his long and distinguished career as an award-winning physician, educator, and speaker he has witnessed thousand of cases of extraordinary healing achieved by patients who were able to tap into their own healing powers. His own remarkable recovery from debilitating back pain, without the use of drugs or surgery, inspired his first, highly successful book, *Healing Back Pain Naturally.*

Dr. Brownstein is a Diplomate of the American Board of Preventive Medicine and a Founding Diplomate of the American Board of Holistic Medicine. He is also Assistant Clinical Professor of Medicine at the University of Hawaii, and for many years he was Director of the Princeville Medical Clinic in Princeville, Hawaii. Dr. Brownstein has worked with Dr. Dean Ornish in Dr. Ornish's very successful program for reversing heart disease, which relies heavily on the body's ability to heal itself.

Dr. Brownstein lives with his wife and son in Hawaii.

Also by Dr. Brownstein

In his first book, *Healing Back Pain Naturally: The Mind-Body Program Proven to Work,* Dr. Art Brownstein tells how he learned to permanently cure himself after enduring 20 years of crippling back pain.

Dr. Brownstein incorporated the lessons of his own extraordinary healing into the revolutionary and world-famous Back to Life program, which has since cured thousands of other patients without drugs or surgery. In *Healing Back Pain Naturally,* Dr. Brownstein leads you through the program step-by-step, showing how you, too, can triumph over pain and rediscover the joy of living.

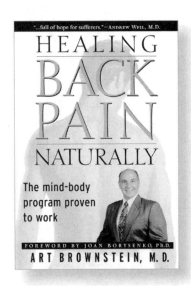

"...full of hope for sufferers."—ANDREW WEIL, M.D.

HEALING BACK PAIN NATURALLY

The mind-body program proven to work

FOREWORD BY JOAN BORYSENKO, Ph.D.

ART BROWNSTEIN, M.D.

"*Dr. Brownstein has written a personal, practical, and informative book to help people prevent and treat back pain. Its approach is consistent with the philosophy of integrative medicine that I teach, and its content is both scientifically accurate and full of hope for sufferers.*"

—Andrew Weil, M.D.
Founder, The Center for Integrative Medicine
Author of *Natural Health, Natural Medicine;
Spontaneous Healing;* and *8 Weeks to Optimum Health*

Order *Healing Back Pain Naturally* online at
www.harborpress.com.
Or to order by phone, call toll-free 888-851-9090.